Exploring the World of Parasites

Edited by Salvatore G. De-Simone and Guilherme C. Lechuga

Published in London, United Kingdom

Exploring the World of Parasites
http://dx.doi.org/10.5772/intechopen.1004958
Edited by Salvatore G. De-Simone and Guilherme C. Lechuga

Contributors
Ahmed Amin Ahmed Saleh, Ahmed Shamkhi Jabbar, Ali Idan Al-Musaedi, Anita Yadav, Cheryl Cooper, Cátia Lourenço-Marques, Diana María Barrero-Torres, Eliézer Kouakou N'Goran, Fidèle Kouakou Bassa, Florbela Soares, Francisco Javier Martínez-Moreno, Gaoussou Coulibaly, Guillem Herrera-Torres, José Pérez, Leandro Buffoni, Luis Miguel Flores-Velázquez, Mamadou Ouattara, María Teresa Ruiz-Campillo, Monica E.T. Alcón-Chino, Márcio Moreira, Nana Rose Diakité, Pablo José Rufino-Moya, Prashant K. Mallick, Priya Agrohi, Raja Babu Kushwah, Rebecca Swindall, Rui Sousa, Salvatore G. De-Simone, Sandeep K. Malhotra, Valerie Smith, Verónica Molina-Hernández, William Sorensen, Álvaro Martínez-Moreno

First published in London, United Kingdom, 2025 by IntechOpen
IntechOpen is the global imprint of INTECHOPEN LIMITED, registered in England and Wales, registration number: 11086078, 167-169 Great Portland Street, London, W1W 5PF, United Kingdom

For EU product safety concerns: IN TECH d.o.o., Prolaz Marije Krucifikse Kozulić 3, 51000 Rijeka, Croatia, info@intechopen.com or visit our website at intechopen.com.

British Library Cataloguing-in-Publication Data
A catalogue record for this book is available from the British Library

Exploring the World of Parasites
Edited by Salvatore G. De-Simone and Guilherme C. Lechuga
p. cm.
Print ISBN 978-1-83634-356-1
Online ISBN 978-1-83634-355-4
eBook (PDF) ISBN 978-1-83634-357-8

Meet the editors

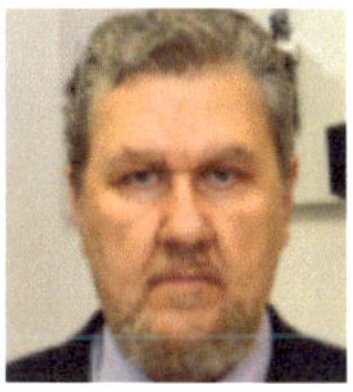

Salvatore G. De-Simone holds a BSc in Biomedical Sciences and an MSc/DSc in Biochemistry. He was a visiting researcher in France, the USA, and Germany and served as a Full Professor of Biochemistry at the Federal Fluminense University in Brazil. At the Oswaldo Cruz Foundation (FIOCRUZ), he led the Biochemistry of Protein and Peptides Laboratory and Peptide Synthesis Platform and led the Protein and Peptides Biochemistry group (CNPq). A key contributor to postgraduate programs, he has mentored over 90 postgraduate and postdoc candidates and coordinated numerous symposiums and research projects. Dr. De-Simone is an advisor for Brazilian universities and agencies, a reviewer for 100+ journals, a guest editor, a book editor, and an expert in health innovation, including diseases of neglected populations. He is affiliated with CDTS-FIOCRUZ, IDPN-CNPq, FAPERJ, and CNPq, advancing science and biotechnology globally.

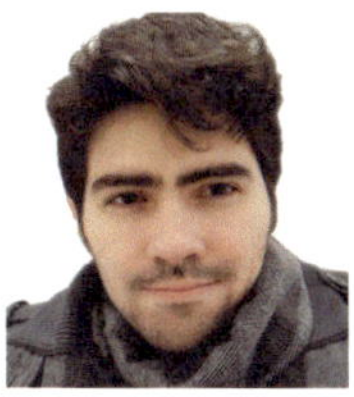

Dr. Guilherme Curty Lechuga is a postdoctoral fellow at the Center for Technological Development in Health (CDTS) at the Oswaldo Cruz Foundation (FIOCRUZ). He holds a BS in Biomedicine and an MS and Ph.D. in Science and Biotechnology from Fluminense Federal University (UFF; Brazil). His expertise spans cell biology, biochemistry, peptide synthesis, epitope mapping, and protein-protein interactions, focusing on preclinical drug development and diagnostics. His research includes investigating drug candidates for Chagas disease, heme, and iron dysmetabolism in COVID-19, studying humoral immunity in infectious diseases, and developing rapid diagnostic tests. Dr. Lechuga's contributions aim to advance understanding and innovation in biomedical sciences, particularly in infectious disease diagnostics and therapeutic development.

Contents

Preface

The field of parasitology has long captivated scientists and researchers, offering a window into the complex relationships between parasites and their hosts. This edited volume, *Exploring the World of Parasites*, brings together an array of studies highlighting the intricate dynamics and groundbreaking findings in this vital area of science. Parasitic diseases impose a significant economic burden and are often classified as neglected diseases. This book discusses some examples of parasites that affect health, economic production, and biological control. By providing insights into the biology, ecology, and impacts of parasitic organisms, this book not only seeks to enhance understanding but also to spark further inquiry among its readers.

The chapters within this volume present a comprehensive exploration of parasitology, covering a wide range of topics from fundamental biology to applied research. The opening chapter, "Host Manipulation by Parasites" by Ali Idan Al-Musaedi, explores the fascinating strategies parasites use to influence host behavior to their advantage. Following this, "Epidemiology of Urinary Bilharziasis in Taabo, South-Central Côte d'Ivoire" by Gaoussou Coulibaly, Nana Rose Diakité, Fidèle Kouakou Bassa, Mamadou Ouattara, and Eliézer Kouakou N'Goran, provides critical insights into the epidemiological aspects of schistosomiasis in a specific region.

In "An Update on the Control of Fasciolosis: Traditional and Alternative Treatments and Possible Future Approaches", Guillem Herrera-Torres and colleagues discuss current and emerging strategies to manage fasciolosis. The subsequent chapter, "Evolutionary Lineage of Invasive Anisakidae of Zoonotic Significance under Environmental Influence" by Sandeep K. Malhotra and Anita Yadav, delves into the evolutionary dynamics of marine zoonotic nematodes affected by environmental factors. Aquaculture health is addressed in "Amyloodiniosis in Semi-Intensive Aquaculture" by Florbela Soares, Márcio Moreira, Rui Sousa, and Cátia Lourenço Marques, which examines the challenges posed by parasitic infections in aquaculture systems. "Mass Production and Field Application of Some Parasitoids in Egypt" by Ahmed Saleh and Ahmed Shamkhi Jabbar explores innovative biological control methods using parasitoids, highlighting their role in integrated pest management.

Further broadening the parasitological scope, "From Helminths to *Blastocystis*: Intestinal Parasite Prevalence among Children of Northeast Texas" by William Sorensen, Rebecca Swindall, Valerie Smith, and Cheryl Cooper investigates the prevalence of soil-transmitted intestinal helminths in a vulnerable population. In "Understanding the Diagnosing of Canine Ehrlichiosis: A Comprehensive Review", Monica E.T. Alcón-Chino and Salvatore G. De-Simone provide an in-depth overview of the diagnostic methods and challenges associated with canine ehrlichiosis, a tick-borne disease of growing veterinary importance. Concluding the volume, "Aqueous Affairs of Red Blood Cell: Variations That Alter Parasite Growth" by Priya Agrohi, Raja Babu Kushwah and Prashant K. Mallick explores the volume regulation of erythrocytes and how these influence the development and survival of malaria parasites.

Breakthroughs in genomics and molecular biology have uncovered mechanisms of parasitic infection and resistance, paving the way for novel treatments and vaccines. For instance, efforts to combat diseases have led to the development of drugs targeting specific stages of the parasite's life cycle and innovative vector control strategies, such as genetically modified mosquitoes. Despite these advancements, challenges remain. Many parasites have resisted existing treatments, and the socio-economic factors associated with parasitic diseases often hinder eradication efforts. Climate change further complicates the picture, altering parasites' and their vectors' distribution, potentially exposing new populations to risk. Beyond their scientific and medical implications, parasites also serve as a lens to explore broader biological and philosophical questions. Their ability to manipulate hosts and their intricate life cycles challenge traditional notions of autonomy and interdependence in nature. They underscore the interconnectedness of life, where even the smallest organisms can exert profound influences on others. Exploring the world of parasites is a journey into the depths of nature's ingenuity. It reveals the challenges these remarkable organisms pose and the opportunities they offer for understanding life's complexity and developing innovative solutions to global health problems. In studying parasites, we uncover a delicate balance between harm and harmony, survival and symbiosis, ultimately enriching our understanding of the natural world.

This book is a testament to the collaborative efforts of researchers and practitioners dedicated to advancing parasitology. As editors, we are grateful for the invaluable contributions of the authors, whose expertise and insights have shaped the content of this volume. We extend our heartfelt thanks to the reviewers and co-editor, Dr. Lechuga, whose critical evaluations ensured the quality and rigor of the chapters. Special acknowledgment is due to the editorial and production teams at IntechOpen for their support and professionalism throughout the publication process. We invite you, the reader, to join us in this journey of exploration and discovery. We hope that *Exploring the World of Parasites* will catalyze further research and understanding in the field of parasitology. This book, a valuable resource for students, researchers, and professionals, contributes to a deeper understanding of parasitic organisms and their implications. We aspire to contribute to the global effort to mitigate the burden of parasitic diseases and improve economy and health outcomes worldwide. Let this book inspire you to delve deeper into the world of parasites and contribute to advancing science and global health.

Salvatore G. De-Simone and Guilherme C. Lechuga
Center for Technological Development in Healthy,
Oswaldo Cruz Foundation,
Rio de Janeiro, Brazil

Chapter 1

Host Manipulation by Parasites

Ali Idan Al-Musaedi

Abstract

When considering parasitic infections, our first thoughts often concern symptoms, prevention, and treatment. However, understanding how parasites spread from one host to another is a central topic in parasitology. Grasping these categories is crucial for applied fields like epidemiology and medicine and addressing fundamental biological questions. One key concept in this area is the host manipulation hypothesis. In this research, I explain what parasitic manipulation entails and highlight the key aspects of the hypothesis: first, the distinction between adaptive and nonadaptive manipulation; second, the dimensions of phenotypic alterations in the host and the mechanisms behind these alterations; and finally, the evolutionary and ecological implications of parasitic manipulation.

Keywords: manipulation, adaptive host, behavior, phenotype, mechanisms

1. Introduction

The world of parasitism is vast, encompassing a wide range of taxa, from unicellular organisms like bacteria, yeast, and protozoa to multicellular entities like worms and insects. These parasites have evolved various strategies, known as parasitism, to thrive. They often infect vertebrate hosts, significantly impacting their survival and reproductive success [1]. A key topic in parasitology is how parasites transfer from one host to another. Understanding these strategies is crucial for applied fields like epidemiology and medicine and addressing fundamental biological questions [2].

The host-parasite interaction is frequently depicted as a struggle over resources that the host perceives as its own. However, this struggle operates on multiple levels; for instance, the host's behavior affects itself and its parasites [3]. In this coevolutionary race, parasites employ various strategies to maximize their transmission and enhance their fitness. One such strategy is described by the host manipulation hypothesis, which posits that parasites can induce changes in the host's phenotypic traits to improve their survival and transmission success [4, 5]. Despite significant advancements in recent years, important knowledge gaps and new challenges remain to be addressed [6].

In this chapter, I present the results of a review of host-parasite manipulation and discuss the following topics: (1) the manipulation hypothesis, (2) adaptive and nonadaptive manipulation, (3) the mechanisms underlying these manipulations, and (4) the evolutionary and ecological aspects of manipulation.

2. Manipulation of host phenotypes

Parasitic organisms have evolved manipulation strategies to enhance their fitness. Evidence suggests that at least some species capable of host manipulation belong to the animal phyla Platyhelminthes (classes Trematoda and Cestoda), Acanthocephala, Nematoda, Nematomorpha, and Arthropoda, as well as various viruses, bacteria, fungi, and single-celled eukaryotes [7–9].

Early in the twentieth century, scientists recognized parasites could manipulate their hosts' phenotypes. A notable report [10] indicated that fish retrieved from cormorants, the definitive hosts, were significantly more likely to be intermediate hosts for the cestode *Ligula intestinalis* than fish caught by fishermen. Numerous studies have demonstrated that a wide range of host phenotypic traits—such as behavior, morphology, and physiology—can be altered by parasites, with changes varying from subtle shifts in activity levels to the emergence of complex and remarkable behaviors [9, 11]. Parasites can modify host traits to increase their chances of transmission; however, not all phenotypic changes following infection result from adaptive manipulation, as some are mere side effects of the infection [12, 13]. Such manipulative parasites can have harmful, even lethal, effects on their hosts. The debate over whether these alterations result from adaptive manipulation or by-products of infection has persisted for decades [12–14].

Host manipulation can lead to striking changes, such as limb malformations in amphibians infected with the trematode *Ribeiroia ondatrae*, or notable behavioral changes like the "death grip" observed in ants infected with the fungus *Ophiocordyceps unilateralis* [15, 16].

There are many examples of host manipulation. One of the earliest demonstrations involved amphipods infected with larval acanthocephalan parasites, which exhibited aberrant behavior and abnormal coloration, making them more susceptible to predation by the parasite's next host [17, 18]. This phenomenon has been documented across nearly all major groups of living organisms [7–9]. For instance, the tropical arboreal ant *Cephalotes atratus* displays a bright red abdomen after being infected by the nematode *Myrmeconema neotropicum*. These examples highlight the parasites' diverse strategies to manipulate their hosts, ultimately enhancing their survival and successful transmission.

Parasites may alter two or more phenotypic traits to enhance their transmission and, consequently, their fitness. While behavioral changes often reduce the host's fitness by compromising survival, parasites transmitted through trophic chains by ingestion typically manipulate their intermediate hosts to increase their exposure to predators (the definitive hosts) [12, 19]. For example, the manipulation caused by *Toxoplasma* emerged in the 1960s and 1970s, with reports indicating that congenital, acute, and chronic toxoplasmosis significantly affects the behavior of infected mice [20]. Regarding its impact on humans, studies have shown that about one-third of people worldwide with latent toxoplasmosis exhibit personality profiles that differ markedly from those of uninfected individuals [21]. *T. gondii* has been suggested to suppress the aversion of its primary host, the brown rat, to cat odor, facilitating the parasite's transmission to its definitive host, cats [22].

In addition to behavioral changes, parasites can induce morphological modifications in their hosts, such as color changes or the development of new structures, to enhance transmission [4, 23]. For instance, the tropical arboreal ant *Cephalotes atratus* displays a bright red abdomen after infection with the nematode *Myrmeconema neotropicum* [24].

3. Mode of manipulation

3.1 Adaptive manipulation

As we know, while parasites influence their hosts, hosts also influence parasites, prompting the latter to adapt to these pressures. There are various definitions of adaptation. For a specific trait to be considered an adaptation, it must be a response to a particular selective agent, requiring an inference about its evolutionary history [25]. Reeve and Sherman [26] defined adaptation as a phenotypic variant that maximizes fitness among a specific set of variants in each environment, focusing on the trait's current effects on reproductive success. They also noted that the adaptations leading to manipulation emerged under certain ecological conditions.

Certain parasites, known as manipulative parasites, induce changes in host phenotypes that enhance their own fitness while diminishing that of the host [18, 27, 28]. Over the past three decades, research has proposed three explanations for animal behavioral changes resulting from parasitic infection. First, the parasite may directly induce changes in the host's behavior that benefit the parasite. This classic explanation posits the existence of "manipulative" genes in the parasite's genome (**Figure 1**). Second, the changes represent an adaptive response by the host to combat the infection or mitigate its negative effects. Third, altered host behavior may be a by-product of pathology or other aspects of infection that fortuitously aid in parasite transmission [4].

Poulin [27] argued that alterations in host behavior following infection can only be considered adaptive if they meet certain criteria: (1) they should be complex, (2) they should show signs of purposeful design, (3) they are more likely to be adaptations if they arise independently in multiple host or parasite lineages, and (4) they must ultimately enhance the fitness of either the host or the parasite (**Figure 1**).

Thus, the altered phenotype of the host is expected to be under the genetic control of the parasite, representing its "extended phenotype" [29, 30]. Natural selection should favor parasite phenotypes that manipulate hosts in ways that enhance the parasite's fitness [31]. However, not all effects of infection are adaptive. Not every action the parasite takes qualifies as adaptive, as some may be by-products of infection. Determining whether a change is adaptive for the parasite, the host, or merely a by-product can be challenging. Decades of research have been required to explore the adaptive consequences of host manipulation for both hosts and parasites [32]. This complexity is part of the difficulty

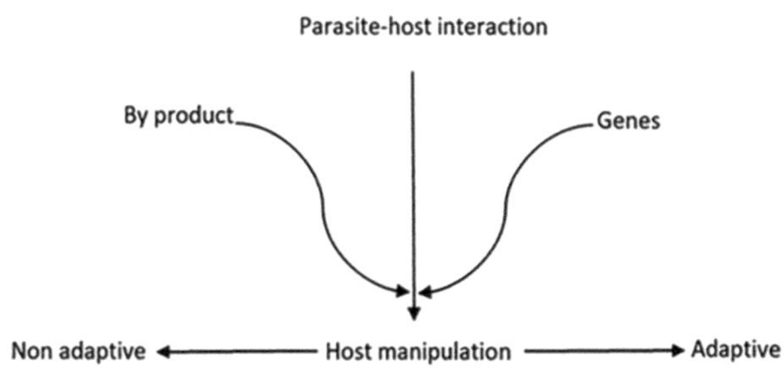

Figure 1.
The schematics illustrate the modes of manipulation. Parasitic manipulation is categorized into adaptive and nonadaptive types. Distinguishing which phenotypes are adaptive versus by-products can be challenging. The classic explanation for adaptive manipulation posits that "manipulative" genes exist in the parasite's genome [4]. According to the concept of the "extended phenotype," the host's altered phenotype is expected to be under the genetic control of the parasite [29, 30].

in identifying the mechanisms behind changed phenotypes [33]. Understanding these mechanisms will enhance our comprehension of the selection pressures on parasites that lead to host-mediated changes in behavior, the dynamics of host-parasite interactions, coevolution, and how parasites influence their hosts' evolution [34, 35].

So, what is a by-product? According to established definitions, "a by-product is a trait that evolved not because it was selectively beneficial, but because it was closely linked to another reproductively beneficial trait" [36].

The effects of parasitic infection are often complex and challenging to track. For instance, snails of *Potamopyrgus antipodarum* collected from the field and infected by the trematode *Coitocaecum parvum* were found to have smaller shell volumes than uninfected snails. Additionally, the internal shell volume available for parasite reproduction represented a larger proportion of the total internal shell volume. These findings led researchers to suggest that the parasite may manipulate infected snails to increase the relative shell volume despite a reduction in overall shell size, likely due to the energetic demands of infection. This suggests that adaptive parasitic manipulation could occur within the constraints imposed by infection [37].

However, a study on *P. antipodarum* snails infected with *Atriophallophorus winterbourne* trematode eggs showed that the altered shell growth observed in field snails was not a result of adaptive parasitic manipulation. Some researchers argue that it is difficult to distinguish between adaptive manipulation by the parasite and side effects of infection, as these could also represent host responses aimed at eliminating the parasites or compensating for the damage caused by infection [4, 27, 28].

4. Dimensions of a parasite affecting host phenotypes

Parasites can induce various host phenotypic changes, including morphological, behavioral, and physiological alterations, to enhance their transmission [9, 23, 38]. Parasites with complex life cycles often depend on their intermediate hosts being consumed by a definitive host, where the parasites reach sexual maturity and reproduce [23, 39]. Various forms of morphological manipulation support this trophic transmission. For example, the sporocysts of the digenean parasite *Leucochloridium macrostomum* transform the antennae of the snail *Succinea putris* into colorful, pulsating structures resembling blinking lights [40]. These altered snails are colloquially known as "lighthouse snails" and represent several examples of manipulated phenotypes alongside the well-known "zombie ants," both caused by trematodes. *Leucochloridium* species change the color and shape of their snail hosts' tentacles, causing them to pulsate in response to light, thereby attracting predatory birds, which act as the parasite's definitive host [41].

Another example involves the fish *Chaetodon multicinctus* from Hawaiian reefs, which prefers feeding on polyps infested by the trematode *Podocotyloides stenometra*. Infected polyps become swollen and pink, making them more visible and easier to capture [42]. Parasites can also negatively impact their hosts' physiology [43]. Some insect parasites secrete chemicals that manipulate the host's biology [44]. For instance, *Toxoplasma gondii* secretes proteins that interact in complex ways with the host's immune system [45], though these chemicals' exact nature and action remain unclear. The parasitic hairworm *Spinochordodes tellinii* produces chemicals that influence the development of its host's central nervous system, causing grasshoppers (*Meconema thalassinum*) to exhibit abnormal behaviors, such as jumping into the water, where the parasite reproduces [46].

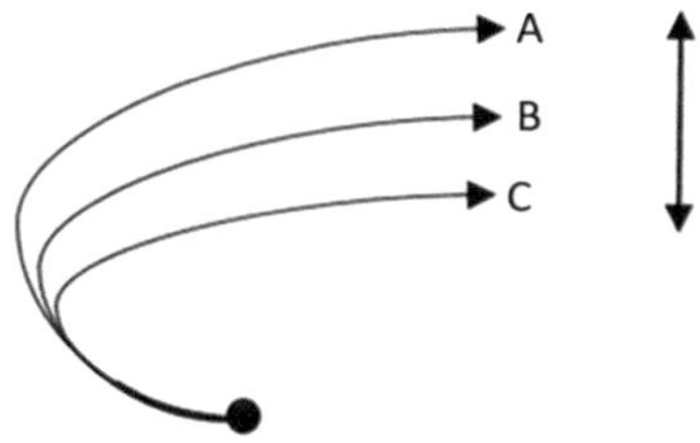

Figure 2.
The schematic illustrates multidimensional manipulation, with the black circle signifying its origin, leading to diverse phenotypic traits (A, B, C) through simultaneous or sequential changes. For instance, orthopterans parasitized by subadult hairworms exhibit erratic, photophilic behaviors, while adults trigger water-seeking behavior [55, 56].

Recent studies have begun to uncover mechanisms behind some host phenotypic changes parasites induce. For instance, *T. gondii* has been shown to alter levels of neurotransmitters like dopamine and hormones such as testosterone in mammals [47, 48]. These changes in behavior often benefit the parasite or its offspring by increasing transmission. Despite the commonality of such behavioral alterations, understanding the neural mechanisms involved is still in its early stages [44]. For example, the acanthocephalan parasite *Pomphorhynchus laevis* infects the gammarid *Gammarus pulex*, leading to significant behavioral changes such as reversed phototaxis and abnormal behaviors. These alterations make infected gammarids more susceptible to predation by fish, definitive host [49].

A well-known case of behavioral manipulation is the "fatal attraction" caused by the protozoan *T. gondii*, which makes rodents, such as brown rats, lose their natural aversion to cat odors, thereby increasing the likelihood of predation by cats, *T. gondii*'s definitive host. Infected rats lose their fear of cat odors and exhibit heightened general activity and slower reaction times, increasing their vulnerability to predation [4, 19, 22, 50–54].

Multidimensional manipulation involves at least two simultaneous changes across different phenotypes, such as behavior, morphology, or physiology (**Figure 2**) [57]. For example, a tropically transmitted parasite can significantly increase the detectability and susceptibility of its intermediate host to predation by its definitive host if it alters both the host's behavior and coloration [58, 59]. However, the mechanisms of this multidimensional manipulation remain poorly understood [60].

5. Mechanisms of host manipulation

The mechanisms by which parasites modify host behavior are complex and not yet fully understood, although certain components of these changes have been identified. Unraveling all the potential mechanisms remains a key area of collaborative research across parasitology, physiology, and neurobiology [61]. Current efforts are focused on understanding how parasites exert control over animal behavior. Given the broad taxonomic diversity of parasites—ranging from viruses and fungi to apicomplexans, worms, and parasitic insects—it is likely that the mechanisms of manipulation are equally diverse [62].

Parasites appear to employ at least three broadly defined mechanisms to alter host behavior: psychoneuroimmunological mechanisms, neuropharmacological mechanisms, and genomic or proteomic-based mechanisms. Additionally, symbiont-mediated behavioral manipulation has been proposed as another potential pathway, though research in this area is still in its early stages [63–65].

5.1 Neuroimmunological mechanisms

When a parasite infects a host, the immune system releases cytokines as part of the neuroinflammatory defense response, typically leading to "sickness behavior." These behaviors shift energy away from nonessential activities, such as reproduction or social interaction, to enhance the host's chances of recovery from infection [66, 67]. Cytokines can induce these behavioral changes because neurons have receptors in specific brain regions [68]. Parasites can manipulate host behavior by influencing the type, amount, or balance of cytokines released [69]. For instance, during the active phase of *Toxoplasma gondii* infection, a cascade of cytokines is released, including gamma interferons and pro-inflammatory mediators that are toxic to neurons [70]. *T. gondii* also triggers microglia activation by releasing nitric oxide, which impacts neurite outgrowth and acts as a neuromodulator [71].

Both vertebrates and invertebrates have bidirectional communication between the immune and nervous systems [68, 72, 73]. Some of these immune-neural interactions are thought to be evolutionarily ancient. In invertebrate hosts, behavioral changes resulting from cytokine manipulation tend to align more closely with the parasite's objectives, suggesting a more direct link between immune mechanisms and behavioral outcomes [74, 75]. This may be due to differences in complexity and phylogenetic factors between invertebrate and vertebrate hosts.

5.2 Neuropharmacological mechanism

Neuropharmacology studies how medications affect the nervous system [65]. Increasing evidence suggests parasites can release neuromodulators, hormones, or neurotransmitters that influence the host's central nervous system (CNS) [61, 63, 69, 76]. In some cases, these behavioral changes appear novel for the host [11], suggesting that certain parasites secrete substances that act directly on the host's nervous system. The secretion of such substances is not unusual, as many organisms produce compounds capable of altering neuronal activity [63]. However, the complex immune-neural interactions involved make it difficult to determine whether a behavioral change benefits the parasite or is simply a by-product of the host's immune response.

Additionally, some parasites mimic host immune system compounds. For example, the fluke *S. mansoni* releases endorphins and other opioid peptides [27, 77, 78], influencing immune and neural functions [77, 79].

5.3 Genomic-/proteomic-based mechanisms and symbiont mechanisms

Most reports of parasite-induced behavioral changes in hosts are based on observational data, while experimentally confirmed examples of specific parasite genes driving these changes remain limited [44, 80–83]. Neuroscientists have employed genomic and proteomic techniques to selectively manipulate gene expression and protein production, particularly those involved in neural function [84]. In the case of manipulated ants, changes in gene expression related to neuronal function may be due to compounds secreted by *Ophiocordyceps*. One hypothesis suggests that neurotransmitter receptors could be targets for the fungus's ADP-ribosylation toxins. In contrast, a potential aflutter alkaloid toxin may disrupt the host's nervous system, causing disease-like symptoms. Additionally, various uncharacterized secreted proteins provide candidate genes that could affect the nervous system or other host biology [85].

In some cases, the genetic basis of behavioral manipulation is being investigated in more detail. A striking example is a virus that manipulates caterpillars to remain exposed on leaf surfaces, where they are killed and their bodies are liquefied to spread viral particles. It was discovered that a single gene encoding the enzyme ecdysteroid UDP-glycosyltransferase (EGT) is responsible for this manipulation. EGT inactivates the host insect's ecdysteroid hormones, preventing insect moulting on the tree Furthermore, it keeps the insect feeding out on the leaves where it will die [62, 82, 86]. Identifying the genes critical to manipulation is more challenging for parasites with larger and more complex genomes and requires multiple independent lines of evidence [62, 82, 86].

As manipulators of host phenotypes, parasites typically target four key physiological systems: neural, endocrine, neuromodulator, and immunomodulator. Various neurotransmitters, neuromodulator chemicals, hormones, proteins, enzymes, and other molecules influence these systems. Parasites can manipulate these systems via genetic or epigenetic mechanisms, with epigenetic changes altering gene expression without changing the underlying DNA sequence [87–89].

Symbiont-mediated behavioral manipulation is another potential mechanism, although research in this area is still in its early stages [64, 65]. This form of manipulation involves a close relationship between two parasitic species, which may result in the behavioral manipulation of a shared host. For example, research suggests that behavioral changes in ladybeetles may be due to the parasitic wasp *Dinocampus coccinellae*'s symbiotic virus, *Dinocampus coccinellae paralysis virus* (DcPV), rather than direct manipulation by the wasp itself. DcPV, a neurotropic virus, is transmitted to the host during the wasp's larval development and replicates in the host's cerebral ganglia, leading to changes in behavior [64]. The presence of DcPV particles in the wasp's oviduct cells suggests that the virus could be transmitted to the wasp's eggs, further supporting the role of DcPV in host behavioral manipulation (**Figure 3**). Thus, the behavioral changes in ladybeetles likely arise from DcPV replication rather than direct parasitic manipulation by the wasp [64].

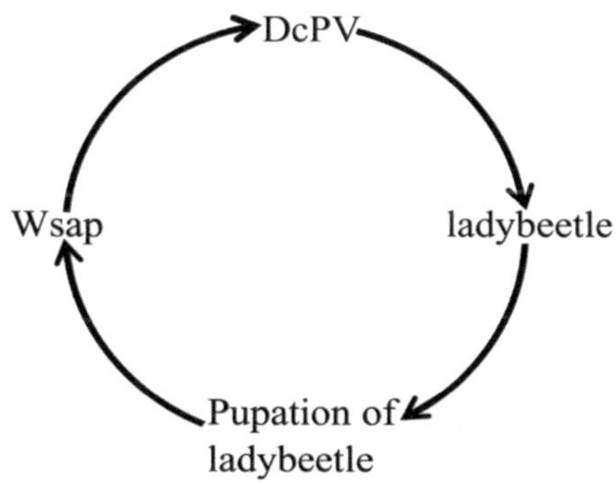

Figure 3.
The schematic illustrates symbiont mechanism. DcPV, a neurotropic virus, is transmitted to the host during the wasp's larval development and replicates in the ladybeetle's cerebral ganglia, leading to changes in behavior [64].

6. Host-parasite interaction: The evolutionary and ecological aspects in manipulation

Highlighting the evolutionary and ecological aspects of parasitic manipulation is essential, as they, alongside other factors, form the foundation for understanding the host-parasite relationship. Many studies on manipulation have overlooked these environmental and evolutionary dimensions, leading to gaps in our understanding of the phenomenon [28].

Behavioral changes in hosts may result from natural selection acting on the host-parasite interaction, but they can also be inherited traits from ancestors, which may or may not continue to provide a selective advantage to the parasite in the present system [2]. These host behavioral changes are often considered under the genetic control of the parasite, representing its "extended phenotype" [29]. However, from an evolutionary perspective, even when these changes benefit the parasite, they are not solely the result of its extended phenotype. Instead, they arise from natural selection acting on the parasite and the host genome [90]. This shared phenotype results from an evolutionary arms race shaped by the parasite's manipulative adaptations and the host's defensive countermeasures [90–92]. Natural selection favors parasites that can manipulate host behavior to enhance their transmission success [2, 91], as manipulation aims to increase the parasite's chances of transmission and complete its life cycle [11, 23, 28, 93].

The ability to manipulate host behavior has evolved independently multiple times across and within various parasite species [11, 93]. Interestingly, not all parasites exhibit manipulative traits, but in species like acanthocephalans, the entire group is manipulative, suggesting that this ability was inherited from a common ancestor and subsequently diversified into different behavioral modifications.

To better understand the manipulation hypothesis, it is helpful to consider three main evolutionary pathways: manipulation *sensu stricto*, the "mafia-like" strategy, and the exploitation of compensatory responses [81]. The mafia-like strategy is the most compelling example of the host-parasite interaction influencing host behavior [94, 95]. This hypothesis proposes that parasites impose additional fitness costs on noncompliant hosts, thereby selecting for cooperative behavior. The cuckoo's relationship with its host bird exemplifies this strategy: cuckoos force their hosts to tolerate non-self-eggs by making the consequences of rejecting them more costly than accepting them [94–96].

Understanding the manipulation process within an ecological context is crucial for studying manipulated hosts [96]. Parasites profoundly impact communities and ecosystems, often through density-dependent pathogenic effects on their hosts [97]. Ecological factors can influence the manipulation of hosts by altering environmental conditions, which in turn affect host-parasite interactions. For parasites with complex life cycles, a strategy known as "hitchhiking" is sometimes employed when direct manipulation is difficult. In this strategy, parasites that can manipulate hosts may coexist with nonmanipulative parasites, targeting the same host to increase their chances of successful transmission [98, 99].

Recent research suggests that parasites can also perceive and respond to ecological variables in a state-dependent manner, optimizing their reproductive success over their lifetime [100–102]. This compensatory response pathway involves short-term behavioral or life-history adjustments that affect the parasite's exposure to environmental conditions or fitness outcomes. For example, in poor environmental conditions, parasites may trigger a shift toward earlier reproductive efforts, such as increased fecundity compensation. In the presence of predatory fish, Cladocera crustaceans may produce larger clutches of smaller offspring earlier in life to maximize reproductive success [90, 103].

The impact of manipulation on host ecology is multifaceted, influencing populations, habitats, and food webs. The complex interactions between parasites, predators, and prey significantly drive infection dynamics and population fluctuations in ecological communities. Some parasites have been shown to impair their hosts' antipredatory behaviors, which can have substantial consequences for predator-prey interactions. Predators, in turn, can acquire pathogens from their prey, making it advantageous for them to recognize and avoid consuming infected individuals [104].

For example, the trematode *Gynaecotyla adunca* alters the distribution of its snail host on sandbars [105]. By modifying the phenotypes of their hosts, manipulative parasites can create new habitats for other species or alter habitat parameters, thus acting as ecosystem engineers [106]. Infected by the parasite *Sacculina carcini*, the green crab *Carcinus maenas* experiences behavioral changes that inhibit molting and reproduction, affecting its metabolism [107].

Host modifications induced by manipulative parasites can significantly alter host populations. Certain fungi, known as "enslaver" fungi, manipulate their insect hosts—such as flies and ants—to position themselves near the tops of plants, enhancing spore dispersal by wind [108]. Tropically transmitted parasites frequently manipulate their intermediate hosts to increase the likelihood of predation by definitive hosts. For instance, killifish (*Fundulus parvipinnis*) infected with the trematode *Euhaplorchis californiensis* are up to 31 times more likely to be preyed upon than uninfected individuals [109].

Author details

Ali Idan Al-Musaedi
Department of Medical Laboratories Techniques, Technical Institute of Amarah, Southern Technical University, Maysan, Iraq

*Address all correspondence to: alialmaliky004@gmail.com

References

[1] Dobson A, Lafferty KD, Kuris AM, Hechinger RF, Jetz W. Colloquium paper: Homage to Linnaeus: How many parasites? How many hosts? Proceedings of the National Academy of Sciences of the United States of America. 2008;**105**(Suppl. 1):11482-11489. DOI: 10.1073/pnas.0803232105

[2] Brown SP. Do all parasites manipulate their hosts? Behavioural Processes. 2005;**68**(3):237-240. DOI: 10.1016/j.beproc. 2004.08.01

[3] Poulin R. Parasite manipulation of host personality and behavioral syndromes. The Journal of Experimental Biology. 2012;**216**(1):18-26. DOI: 10.1242/jeb.073353

[4] Poulin R. Parasite manipulation of host behavior: An update and frequently asked questions. In: Brockmann HJ, Roper T, Naguib M, Wynne-Edwards K, Mitani J, Simmons L, editors. Advances in the Study of Behavior. Academic Press; 2010. pp. 151-186. DOI: 10.1016/S0065-3454(10)41005-0

[5] Cozzarolo CS, Glaizot O, Christe P, Pigeault R. Enhanced attraction of arthropod vectors to infected vertebrates: A review of empirical evidence. Frontiers in Ecology and Evolution. 2020;**8**:568140. DOI: 10.3389/fevo.2020.568140

[6] Sánchez M, Biron D. Host manipulation by parasites. Frontiers in Ecology and Evolution. 2019;7:369. DOI: 10.3389/fevo.2019.00369

[7] Ingwell LL, Eigenbrode SD, Bosque-Pérez NA. Plant viruses alter insect behavior to enhance their spread. Scientific Reports. 2012;**2**:578. DOI: 10.1038/srep00578

[8] Werren JH, Baldo L, Clark ME. Wolbachia: Master manipulators of invertebrate biology. Nature Reviews Microbiology. 2008;**6**(10):741-751. DOI: 10.1038/nrmicro1969

[9] Poulin R, Thomas F. Phenotypic variability induced by parasites: Extent and evolutionary implications. Parasitology Today. 1999;**15**(1):28-32. DOI: 10.1016/s0169-4758(98)01357-x

[10] Brown SP, Loot G, Teriokhin A, Brunel A, Brunel C, Guégan JF. Host manipulation by *Ligula intestinalis*: A cause or consequence of parasite aggregation? International Journal for Parasitology. 2002;**32**(7):817-824. DOI: 10.1016/s0020-7519(02)00013-9

[11] Moore J. Parasites and the Behavior of Animals. Oxford: Oxford University Press; 2002

[12] Poulin R, Maure F. Host manipulation by parasites: A look back before moving forward. Trends in Parasitology. 2015;**31**(11):563-570. DOI: 10.1016/j.pt.2015.07.002

[13] Doherty JF. When fiction becomes fact: Exaggerating host manipulation by parasites. Proceedings of the Royal Society B. 2020;**287**(1936):20201081. DOI: 10.1098/rspb.2020.1081

[14] Hernandez-Caballero I, Garcia-Longoria L, Gomez-Mestre I, Marzal A. The adaptive host manipulation hypothesis: Parasites modify the behaviour, morphology, and physiology of amphibians. Diversity. 2022;**14**(9):739. DOI: 10.3390/d14090739

[15] Johnson PT, Lunde KB, Thurman EM, Ritchie EG, Wray SN, Sutherland DR, et al. Parasite

(*Ribeiroia ondatra*) infection linked to amphibian malformations in the western United States. Ecological Monographs. 2002;**72**(2):151-168. DOI: 10.1890/0012-9615(2002)072[0151:PROILT]2.0.CO;2

[16] Andersen Sandra B, Gerritsma S, Yusah Kalsum M, Mayntz D, Hywel-Jones Nigel L, Billen J, et al. The life of a dead ant: The expression of an adaptive extended phenotype. The American Naturalist. 2009;**174**(3):424-433. DOI: 10.1086/603640

[17] Hindsbo O. Effects of polymorphus (Acanthocephala) on color and behavior of *Gammarus lacustris*. Nature. 1972;**238**(5363):333-333. DOI: 10.1038/238333a0

[18] Goodman BA, Johnson PT. Disease and the extended phenotype: Parasites control host performance and survival through induced changes in body plan. PLoS ONE. 2011;**6**(5):20193. DOI: 10.1371/journal.pone.0020193

[19] Berdoy M, Webster JP, Macdonald DW. Fatal attraction in rats infected with *Toxoplasma gondii*. Proceedings of the Royal Society of London. Series B. 2000;**267**(1452):1591-1594. DOI: 10.1098/rspb.2000.1182

[20] Flegr J. Host manipulation by *Toxoplasma gondii*. In: Mehlhorn H, editor. Encyclopedia of Parasitology. Berlin, Heidelberg: Springer; 2015. pp. 1-6. DOI: 10.1007/978-3-642-27769-6_3464-1

[21] Flegr J, Hrdý I. Influence of chronic toxoplasmosis on some human personality factors. Folia Parasitologica. 1994;**41**(2):122-126

[22] Hari Dass SA, Vyas A. *Toxoplasma gondii* infection reduces predator aversion in rats through epigenetic modulation in the host medial amygdala. Molecular Ecology. 2014;**23**(24):6114-6122. DOI: 10.1111/mec.12888

[23] Lafferty KD. The evolution of trophic transmission. Parasitology Today. 1999;**15**(3):111-115. DOI: 10.1016/s0169-4758(99)01397-6

[24] Yanoviak SP, Kaspari M, Dudley R, Poinar G. Parasite-induced fruit mimicry in a tropical canopy ant. The American Naturalist. 2008;**171**(4):536-544. DOI: 10.1086/528968

[25] Harvey PH, Pagel M. The Comparative Method in Evolutionary Biology. Oxford: Oxford University Press; 1991. DOI: 10.1093/oso/9780198546412.001.0001. Available from: https://academic.oup.com/book/53162

[26] Reeve HK, Sherman PW. Adaptation and the goals of evolutionary research. The Quarterly Review of Biology. 1993;**68**(1):1-32. Available from: https://www.jstor.org/stable/2832133

[27] Poulin R. 'Adaptive' changes in the behavior of parasitized animals: A critical review. International Journal for Parasitology. 1995;**25**(2):1371-1383. DOI: 10.1016/0020-7519(95)00100-x

[28] Thomas F, Adamo S, Moore J. Parasitic manipulation: Where are we and where should we go? Behavioural Processes. 2005;**68**(3):185-199. DOI: 10.1016/j.beproc.2004.06.010

[29] Dawkins R. The Extended Phenotype. Oxford: Oxford University Press; 1999

[30] Heil M. Host manipulation by parasites: Cases, patterns, and remaining doubts. Frontiers in Ecology and Evolution. 2016;**4**:80. DOI: 10.3389/fevo.2016.00080

[31] Namias A, Delph LF, Lively CM. Parasitic manipulation or by-product of infection: An experimental approach using trematode-infected snails. Journal of Helminthology. 2022;**96**:e2. DOI: 10.1017/S0022149X21000699

[32] Poulin R. The rise of ecological parasitology: Twelve landmark advances that changed its history. International Journal for Parasitology. 2021;**51**(13-14):1073-1084

[33] Adamo SA, Webster JP. Neural parasitology: How parasites manipulate host behavior. The Journal of Experimental Biology. 2013;**216**(1):1-2. DOI: 10.1242/jeb.082511

[34] Poulin R. Are there general laws in parasite ecology? Parasitology. 2007;**134**(6):763-776. DOI: 10.1017/S0031182 006002150

[35] Schmid-Hempel P. Evolutionary Parasitology: The Integrated Study of Infections, Immunology, Ecology, and Genetics. 2nd ed. Oxford: Oxford University Press; 2021. DOI: 10.1093/oso/9780198832140.001.0001

[36] Andrews PW, Gangestad SW, Matthews D. Adaptationism—How to carry out an exaptationist program. The Behavioral and Brain Sciences. 2002;**25**(04):489-553. DOI: 10.1017/s0140525x02000092

[37] Lagrue C, McEwan J, Poulin R, Keeney DB. Co-occurrences of parasite clones and altered host phenotype in a snail–trematode system. International Journal for Parasitology. 2007;**37**(13):1459-1467. DOI: 10.1016/j.ijpara.2007.04.022

[38] van Houte S, Ros VID, van Oers MM. Walking with insects: Molecular mechanisms behind parasitic manipulation of host behavior. Molecular Ecology. 2013;**22**(13):3458-3475. DOI: 10.1111/mec.12307

[39] Lafferty KD, Kuris AM. Trophic strategies, animal diversity, and body size. Trends in Ecology & Evolution. 2002;**17**(11):507-513. DOI: 10.1016/S0169-5347(02)02615-0

[40] Wesołowska W, Wesołowski T. Do *Leucochloridium sporocysts* manipulate the behavior of their snail hosts? Journal of Zoology. 2014;**292**(3):151-155. DOI: 10.1111/jzo.12094

[41] Kagan IG. Aspects in the Life History of *Neoleucochloridium problematicum* (Magath, 1920) New Comb. and *Leucochloridium cyanocittae* McIntosh, 1932 (Trematoda: Brachylaemidae). Transactions of the American Microscopical Society. 1951;**70**(4):281

[42] Aeby GS. Trade-offs for the butterflyfish *Chaetodon multicinctus* when feeding on coral prey infected with trematode metacercariae. Behavioral Ecology and Sociobiology. 2002;**52**(2):158-165. DOI: 10.1007/s00265-002-0490-2

[43] Hernandez-Caballero I, Garcia-Longoria L, Gomez-Mestre I, Marzal A. The adaptive host manipulation hypothesis: Parasites modify amphibians' behavior, morphology, and physiology. Diversity. 2022;**14**(9):739. DOI: 10.3390/d1 4090739

[44] Libersat F, Delago A, Gal R. Manipulation of host behavior by parasitic insects and insect parasites. Annual Review of Entomology. 2009;**54**(1):189-207. DOI: 10.1146/annurev.ento.54.110807.090556

[45] Leroux L, Dasanayake D, Rommereim LM, Fox BA, Bzik DJ, Jardim A, et al. Secreted *Toxoplasma gondii* molecules interfere with the

expression of MHC-II in interferon gamma-activated macrophages. International Journal for Parasitology. 2015;**45**(5):319-332. DOI: 10.1016/j.ijpara.2015.01.003

[46] Biron DG, Marché L, Ponton F, Loxdale HD, Galéotti N, Renault L, et al. Behavioral manipulation in a grasshopper harboring hairworm: A proteomics approach. Proceedings of the Royal Society B. 2005;**272**(1577):2117-2126. DOI: 10.1098/rspb.2005.3213

[47] Flegr J, Markoš A. Masterpiece of epigenetic engineering—How *Toxoplasma gondii* reprogrammes host brains to change fear to sexual attraction. Molecular Ecology. 2014;**23**(24):5934-5936. DOI: 10.1111/mec.13006

[48] Parlog A, Schlüter D, Dunay IR. *Toxoplasma gondii*-induced neuronal alterations. Parasite Immunology. 2015;**37**(3):159-170. DOI: 10.1111/pim.12157

[49] Bakker TCM, Mazzi D, Zala SM. Parasite-induced changes in behavior and color make gammarus pulex more prone to fish predation. Ecology. 1997;**78**(4):1098-1104. DOI: 10.1890/0012-9658(1997)078[1098:PICIBA]2.0.CO;2

[50] Vyas A, Kim SK, Giacomini N, Boothroyd JC, Sapolsky RM. Behavioral changes induced by Toxoplasma infection of rodents are highly specific to aversion to cat odors. Proceedings of the National Academy of Sciences of the United States of America. 2007;**104**(15):6442-6447. DOI: 10.1073/pnas.0608310104

[51] Dass SAH, Vasudevan A, Dutta D, Soh LJT, Sapolsky RM, Vyas A. Protozoan parasite *Toxoplasma gondii* manipulates mate choice in rats by enhancing attractiveness of males. PLoS ONE. 2011;**6**(11):e27229. DOI: 10.1371/journal.pone. 0027229

[52] Flegr J. How and why *Toxoplasma* makes us crazy. Trends in Parasitology. 2013;**29**(4):156-163. DOI: 10.1016/j.pt.2013.01.007

[53] Weinersmith K, Faulkes Z. Parasitic manipulation of hosts' phenotype, or how to make a Zombie—An introduction to the symposium. Integrative and Comparative Biology. 2014;**54**:93-100

[54] Poirotte C, Kappeler PM, Ngoubangoye B, Bourgeois S, Moussodji M, Charpentier ME. Morbid attraction to leopard urine in *Toxoplasma* infected chimpanzees. Current Biology. 2016;**26**:R98-R99. DOI: 10.1016/j.cub.2015.12.020

[55] Ponton F, Otálora-Luna F, Lefèvre T, Guerin P, Lebarbenchon C, Duneau D, et al. Water-seeking behavior in worm-infected crickets and reversibility of parasitic manipulation. Behavioral Ecology. 2011;**22**(2):392-400. DOI: 10.1093/beheco/arq215

[56] Sánchez MI, Ponton F, Schmidt-Rhaesa A, Hughes DP, Misse D, Thomas F. Two-steps to suicide in crickets harboring hairworms. Animal Behaviour. 2008;**76**:1621-1624. DOI: 10.1016/j.anbehav.2008.07.018

[57] Thomas F, Poulin R, Brodeur J. Host manipulation by parasites: A multi-dimensional problem. Oikos. 2010;**119**(8):1217-1223. DOI: 10.1111/j.1600-0706.2009.18077.x

[58] Bakker TCM, Mazzi D, Zala S. Parasite-induced changes in behavior and color make *Gammarus pulexmore* prone to fish predation. Ecology. 1997;**78**(4):1098-1104

[59] Sánchez MI, Thomas F, Perrot-Minnot MJ, Biron DG, Bertrand-Michel J, Missé D. Neurological and physiological disorders in artemia harboring

manipulative cestodes. The Journal of Parasitology. 2009;**95**(1):20-24. DOI: 10.1645/GE-1550.1

[60] Thomas F, Rigaud T, Brodeur J. Evolutionary Routes Leading to Host Manipulation by Parasites. Oxford University Press; 2012. pp. 16-33

[61] Lafferty KD, Shaw JC. Comparing mechanisms of host manipulation across host and parasite taxa. The Journal of Experimental Biology. 2012;**216**(1):56-66. DOI: 10.1242/jeb.073668

[62] Hughes DP, Libersat F. Parasite manipulation of host behavior. Current Biology. 2019;**29**(2):R45-R47. DOI: 10.1016/j.cub.2018.12.001

[63] Adamo SA. Parasites: Evolution's neurobiologists. The Journal of Experimental Biology. 2013;**216**(1):3-10. DOI: 10.1242/jeb.073601

[64] Dheilly NM, Maure F, Ravallec M, Galinier R, Doyon J, Duval D, et al. Who is the puppet master? Replication of a parasitic wasp-associated virus correlates with host behavior manipulation. Proceedings of the Biological Sciences. 2015;**282**(1803):20142773. DOI: 10.1098/rspb.2014.2773

[65] Herbison REH. Lessons in Mind Control: Trends in research on the molecular mechanisms behind parasite-host behavioral manipulation. Frontiers in Ecology and Evolution. 2017;**5**:102. DOI: 10.3389/fevo.2017.00102

[66] Hart BL. Biological basis of the behavior of sick animals. Neuroscience and Biobehavioral Reviews. 1988;**12**(2):123-137. DOI: 10.1016/s0149-7634(88)80004-6

[67] Dantzer R. Cytokine-induced sickness behavior: A neuroimmune response to activation of innate immunity. European Journal of Pharmacology. 2004;**500**(1-3):399-411. DOI: 10.1016/j.ejphar.2004.07.040

[68] Dantzer R, O'Connor JC, Freund GG, Johnson RW, Kelley KW. From inflammation to sickness and depression: When the immune system subjugates the brain. Nature Reviews. Neuroscience. 2008;**9**(1):46-56. DOI: 10.1038/nrn2297

[69] Adamo SA. The strings of the puppet master: How parasites change host behaviour. In: Hughes D, Thomas F, editors. Host Manipulation by Parasites. Oxford: Oxford University Press; 2012. pp. 36-51

[70] Henriquez SA, Brett R, Alexander J, Pratt J, Roberts CW. Neuropsychiatric disease and *Toxoplasma gondii* infection. Neuroimmunomodulation. 2009;**16**(2):122-133. DOI: 10.1159/000180267

[71] Rozenfeld C, Martinez R, Figueiredo RT, Bozza MT, Regina F, Pires A, et al. Soluble factors released by *Toxoplasma gondii* -Infected astrocytes down-modulate nitric oxide production by gamma interferon-activated microglia and prevent neuronal degeneration. Infection and Immunity. 2003;**71**(4):2047-2057. DOI: 10.1128/iai.71.4.2047-2057.2003

[72] Adamo SA. Comparative psychoneuroimmunology: Evidence from the insects. Behavioral and Cognitive Neuroscience Reviews. 2006;**5**:128-140. DOI: 10.1177/1534582306289580

[73] Adamo SA. Bidirectional connections between the immune system and the nervous system in insects. In: Beckage NE, editor. Insect Immunology. San Diego: Academic Press; 2008. pp. 129-149. DOI: 10.1016/B978-012373976-6.50008-2

[74] Helluy S, Thomas F. Parasitic manipulation and neuroinflammation: Evidence from the system *Microphallus papillorobustus* (Trematoda) - *Gammarus* (Crustacea). Parasites & Vectors. 2010;**3**(1):38. DOI: 10.1186/1756-3305-3-38

[75] Helluy S. Parasite-induced alterations of sensorimotor pathways in gammarids: Collateral damage of neuroinfla mmation? The Journal of Experimental Biology. 2012;**216**(Pt1):67-77. DOI: 10.1242/jeb.073213

[76] Klein SL. Parasite manipulation of the proximate mechanisms that mediate social behavior in vertebrates. Physiology and Behavior. 2003;**79**(3):441-449. DOI: 10.1016/s0031-9384(03)00163-x

[77] Kavaliers M, Colwell DD, Choleris E. Parasites and behavior: An ethnopharmacological analysis and biomedical implications. Neuroscience and Biobehavioral Reviews. 1999;**23**(7):1037-1045. DOI: 10.1016/s0149-7634(99)00035-4

[78] Kristensson K, Mhlanga JD, Bentivoglio M. Parasites and the brain: Neuroinvasion, immunopathogenesis and neuronal dysfunctions. Current Topics in Microbiology and Immunology. 2002;**265**:227-257. DOI: 10.1007/978-3-662-09525-6_12

[79] Duvaux-Miret O, Stefano GB, Smith EM, Dissous C, Capron A. Immunosuppression in the definitive and intermediate hosts of the human parasite *Schistosoma mansoni* by releasing immunoreactive neuropeptides. Proceedings of the National Academy of Sciences of the United States of America. 1992;**89**(2):778-781. DOI: 10.1073/pnas.89.2.778

[80] Kamita SG, Nagasaka K, Chua JW, Shimada T, Mita K, Kobayashi M, et al. A baculovirus-encoded protein tyrosine phosphatase gene induces enhanced locomotory activity in a lepidopteran host. Proceedings of the National Academy of Sciences of the United States of America. 2005;**102**(7):2584-2589. DOI: 10.1073/pnas.0409457102

[81] Lefèvre T, Adamo SA, Biron DG, Missé D, Hughes D, Thomas F. Invasion of the body snatchers: The diversity and evolution of manipulative strategies in host-parasite interactions. Advances in Parasitology. 2009;**68**:45-83. DOI: 10.1016/S0065-308X(08)00603-9

[82] Hoover K, Grove M, Gardner M, Hughes DP, McNeil J, Slavicek J. A gene for an extended phenotype. Science. 2011;**333**(6048):1401. DOI: 10.1126/science.1209199

[83] van Houte S, Ros VI, Mastenbroek TG, Vendrig NJ, Hoover K, Spitzen J, et al. Protein tyrosine phosphatase-induced hyperactivity is a conserved strategy of a subset of baculoviruses to manipulate lepidopteran host behavior. PLoS ONE. 2012;**7**(10):e46933. DOI: 10.1371/journal.pone.0046933

[84] Venken Koen JT, Simpson Julie H, Bellen HJ. Genetic manipulation of genes and cells in the nervous system of the fruit fly. Neuron. 2011;**72**(2):202-230. DOI: 10.1016/j.neuron.2011.09.021

[85] Will I, Das B, Trinh T, Brachmann A, Ohm RA, de Bekker C. Genetic underpinnings of host manipulation by *Ophiocordyceps* as revealed by comparative transcriptomics. G3: Genes, Genomes, Genetics. 2020;**10**(7):2275-2296. DOI: 10.1534/g3.120.401290

[86] O'Reilly DR, Brown M, Miller LK. Alteration of ecdysteroid metabolism due to baculovirus infection of the fall armyworm *Spodoptera frugiperda*:

Host ecdysteroids are conjugated with galactose. Insect Biochemistry and Molecular Biology. 1992;**22**(4):313-320. DOI: 10.1016/0965-1748(92)90069-Q

[87] Poulin R, Thomas F. Epigenetic effects of infection on the phenotype of host offspring: Parasites reaching across host generations. Oikos. 2008;**117**(3):331-335. DOI: 10.1111/j.2007.0030-1299.16435.x

[88] Gómez-Díaz E, Jordà M, Peinado MA, Rivero A. Epigenetics of host–pathogen interactions: The road ahead and the road behind. PLoS Pathogens. 2012;**8**(11):e1003007. DOI: 10.1371/journal.ppat.1003007

[89] Bhattarai UR, Doherty JF, Dowle E, Gemmell NJ. The adaptiveness of host Behavioural manipulation assessed using tinbergen's four questions. Trends in Parasitology. 2021;**37**(7):597-609. DOI: 10.1016/j.pt.2021.01.006

[90] Lefèvre T, Roche B, Poulin R, Hurd H, Renaud F, Thomas F. Exploiting host compensatory responses: The 'must' of manipulation? Trends in Parasitology. 2008;**24**(10):435-439. DOI: 10.1016/j.pt.2008.06.006

[91] Poulin R, Brodeur J, Moore J. Parasite manipulation of host behavior—Should hosts always lose. Oikos. 1994;**70**:479-484

[92] Lefèvre T, Thomas F. Behind the scenes, something else is pulling the strings: Emphasizing parasitic manipulation in vector-borne diseases. Infection, Genetics and Evolution. 2008;**8**(4):504-519. DOI: 10.1016/j.meegid.2007.05.008

[93] Poulin R. Evolutionary Ecology of Parasites. 2nd ed. Princeton: Princeton University Press; 2007. DOI: 10.1515/9781400840809

[94] Zahavi A. Parasitism and nest predation in parasitic cuckoos. The American Naturalist. 1979;**113**(1):157-159

[95] Soler M, Soler JJ, Martinez JG, Moller AP. Magpie host manipulation by great spotted cuckoos: Evidence for an avian mafia? Evolution. 1995;**49**(4):770-775. DOI: 10.1111/j.1558-5646.1995.tb02312.x

[96] Hoover JP, Robinson SK. Retaliatory mafia behavior by a parasitic cowbird favors the host's acceptance of parasitic eggs. Proceedings of the National Academy of Sciences of the United States of America. 2007;**104**(11):4479-4483. DOI: 10.1073/pnas.0609710104

[97] Hatcher MJ, Dick JT, Dunn AM. Diverse effects of parasites in ecosystems: Linking interdependent processes. Frontiers in Ecology and the Environment. 2012;**10**(4):186-194

[98] Thomas F, Mete K, Helluy S, Santalla F, Verneau O, De Meeüs T, et al. Hitch-hiker parasites or how to benefit from the strategy of another parasite. Evolution. 1997;**51**(4):1316-1338. DOI: 10.1111/j.1558-5646.1997.tb03978.x

[99] Thomas F, Renaud F, Poulin R. Exploitation of manipulators: "Hitch-hiking" as a parasite transmission strategy. Animal Behaviour. 1998;**56**(1):199-206. DOI: 10.1006/anbe.1998.0758

[100] Hasik AZ, de Angeli DD, Doherty JF, Duffy MA, Poulin R, Siepielski AM. Resetting our expectations for parasites and their effects on species interactions: A meta-analysis. Ecology Letters. 2023;**26**(1):184-199. DOI: 10.1111/ele.14139

[101] Davies CM, Fairbrother E, Webster JP. Mixed strain schistosome infections of snails and the evolution

of parasite virulence. Parasitology. 2002;**124**(Pt 1):31-38. DOI: 10.1017/s0031182001008873

[102] Pfennig KS. Evolution of pathogen virulence: The role of variation in host phenotype. Proceedings of the Royal Society B: Biological Sciences. 2001;**268**(1468):755-760

[103] Sakwińska O. Response to fish kairomone in *Daphnia galeata* life history traits rely on shift to earlier instar at maturation. Oecologia. 2002;**131**(3):409-417

[104] Han BA, Searle CL, Blaustein AR. Effects of an infectious fungus, *Batrachochytrium dendrobatidis*, on amphibian predator-prey interactions. PLoS ONE. 2011;**6**(2):e16675. DOI: 10.1371/journal.pone.0016675

[105] Curtis LA. Vertical distribution of an estuarine snail altered by a parasite. Science. 1987;**235**(4795):1509-1511. DOI: 10.1126/science.3823901

[106] Thomas F, Poulin R, de Meeüs T, Guégan JF, Renaud F, Thomas F, et al. Parasites and ecosystem engineering: What roles could they play? Oikos. 1999;**84**(1):167-171

[107] Thresher RE, Werner M, Høeg JT, Svane I, Glenner H, Murphy NE, et al. Developing the options for managing marine pests: Specificity trials on the parasitic castrator, *Sacculina carcini*, against the European crab, *Carcinus maenas*, and related species. Journal of Experimental Marine Biology and Ecology. 2000;**254**(1):37-51. DOI: 10.1016/s0022-0981(00)00260-4

[108] Maitland DP. A parasitic fungus infecting yellow dungflies manipulates host perching behavior. Proceedings of the Royal Society of London. Series B. 1994;**258**:187-193. DOI: 10.1098/rspb.1994.0161

[109] Lafferty KD, Morris AK. Altered behavior of parasitized killifish increases susceptibility to predation by bird final hosts. Ecology. 1996;**77**(5):1390-1397. DOI: 10.2307/2265536

Chapter 2

Epidemiology of Urinary Bilharziasis in Taabo, South-Central Côte d'Ivoire

Gaoussou Coulibaly, Nana Rose Diakité, Fidèle Kouakou Bassa, Mamadou Ouattara and Eliézer Kouakou N'Goran

Abstract

Over 200 million people globally are affected by urogenital bilharziasis, which remains a significant public health concern, particularly in tropical regions. This study was conducted in the Taabo sub-prefecture following multiple intervention efforts to better assess the prevalence of *Schistosoma haematobium* infection. Urine samples from participants were analysed using reagent strips and the filtration technique. The overall prevalence of urogenital schistosomiasis was found to be relatively low (3.4%), with infections occurring across genders. Notably, individuals aged 15–24 years were disproportionately affected by urinary bilharziasis ($X^2 = 12.20$; $P = 0.032$). The extensive research and interventions have had a substantial and positive effect on reducing both the prevalence and intensity of *S. haematobium* infections in the region. To achieve the elimination of this disease, it is crucial to optimise control measures targeting adolescents and young adults while maintaining the progress already made.

Keywords: epidemiology, dams, intervention, reinfection profile, *Schistosoma haematobium*

1. Introduction

Schistosomiasis (or bilharziasis) is a disease caused by blood trematodes parasitic worms of the genus *Schistosoma*. The host becomes infected transcutaneously by swimming or wading in contaminated freshwater. The parasites infect the vessels of the digestive or genitourinary tract. Symptoms of the acute phase include dermatitis and, a few weeks later, fever, chills, nausea, abdominal pain, diarrhoea, myalgias, and a feeling of malaise [1, 2].

Globally, more than 200 million people are infected with schistosomiasis, classifying it as one of the neglected tropical diseases (NTDs). It ranks as the second most dangerous parasitic disease after malaria [3]. In 2021, an estimated 251.4 million people required preventive treatment for schistosomiasis, with more than 75.3 million individuals receiving treatment [4, 5].

In Côte d'Ivoire, intestinal schistosomiasis (*Schistosoma mansoni*) and urinary schistosomiasis (*S. haematobium*) are highly endemic and have distinct geographical distributions. However, *S. haematobium* is ubiquitous [6, 7]. Like most developing countries, Côte d'Ivoire has implemented water development projects as part of its agricultural-focused economic policy. However, these projects often contribute to the spread of water-borne diseases, posing a significant challenge to their success. This challenge is particularly evident in the infection of populations living near water bodies [8, 9]. These communities frequently come into contact with water during daily activities such as swimming, fishing, washing clothes, and farming. The availability of freshwater is a critical factor in the persistence of water-borne diseases, especially schistosomiasis, a neglected tropical disease (NTD) in Côte d'Ivoire [9]. In rural areas, particularly in the Department of Taabo, schistosomiasis has been reported by several epidemiological studies since 1995 [6, 10–12]. Despite achieving a satisfactory level of treatment coverage, the disease continues to be a public health concern. This study aims to evaluate the impact of various intervention strategies, including treatment and awareness campaigns, on the epidemiological profile of schistosomiasis, with a specific focus on urinary schistosomiasis.

2. Material and methods

2.1 Sites and study population

The study was conducted in November 2017 across 40 localities within the Taabo sub-prefecture a predominantly rural area in south-central Côte d'Ivoire [11]. In each locality, 30 households were selected along 6 axes defined from the centre of the community to the periphery. On each axis, five households with at least one child aged between 5 and 15 years were selected to participate in the study. The selected participants from each households included: (i) all school-aged children (5–15 years), (ii) one adolescent or adult (>15), and (iii) one preschool-aged child (<5 years) (**Figure 1**).

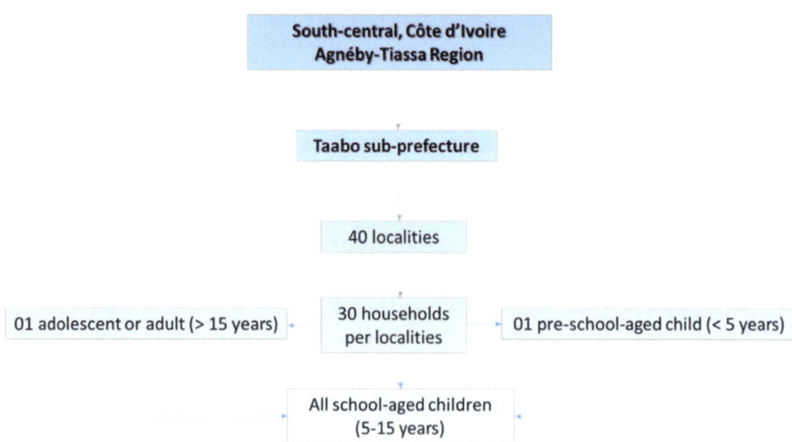

Figure 1.
Diagram showing the enrolment of study participants.

2.2 Collection of urine samples

One plastic container was given to each participant the day before the collection. Participants were asked to return the containers containing their urine samples the following morning (between 08:00 am and 12:00 pm). On the day of collection, the investigation team visited each household to collect the containers. Each container was labelled with an individual identification code and placed in racks, which were then transported to the nearest laboratory for analysis.

2.3 Laboratory procedures

The parasitological examination of the urine sample was designed to detect *S. haematobium* eggs. Collected urine samples were examined for microhaematuria, as an indicator of probable *S. haematobium* infection, using haematuria test strips (Hemastix, Siemens Healthcare, Zurich, Switzerland) (**Figure 2**). The strips were briefly dipped into the urine, and the resulting colour change was noted in accordance with the manufacturer's guidelines. The presence of blood in the urine was indicated by a colour shift from yellow to yellow with green spots, green, or dark green.

Only urine samples that were positive for microhaematuria from reagent strip testing was subjected to a filtration procedure [13] (**Figure 3a**). The urine was homogenised, and 10 mL was taken using a syringe and pressed through a 25 μm mesh filter (Sefar AG Heiden, Switzerland). The filters were placed on slides, and a drop of lugol was added before microscopic examination to identify the eggs (**Figure 3b**).

2.4 Statistical analysis

Parasitological data were double-entered into Microsoft Excel and verified using Epi Info software version 3.5.4 (Centers for Disease Control and Prevention, Atlanta, GA, USA). Statistical analyses were performed with STATA version 14.0 (Stata Corporation, College Station, TX, USA).

Schistosoma haematobium infection has been defined as the presence of at least one parasite egg on the urine filtration slide. To assess micro-haematuria in urine,

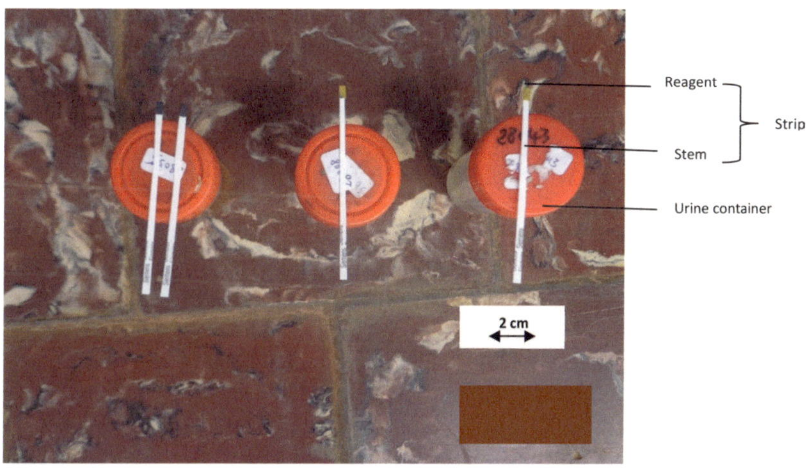

Figure 2.
Urine samples positive for microhaematuria from reagent strip testing.

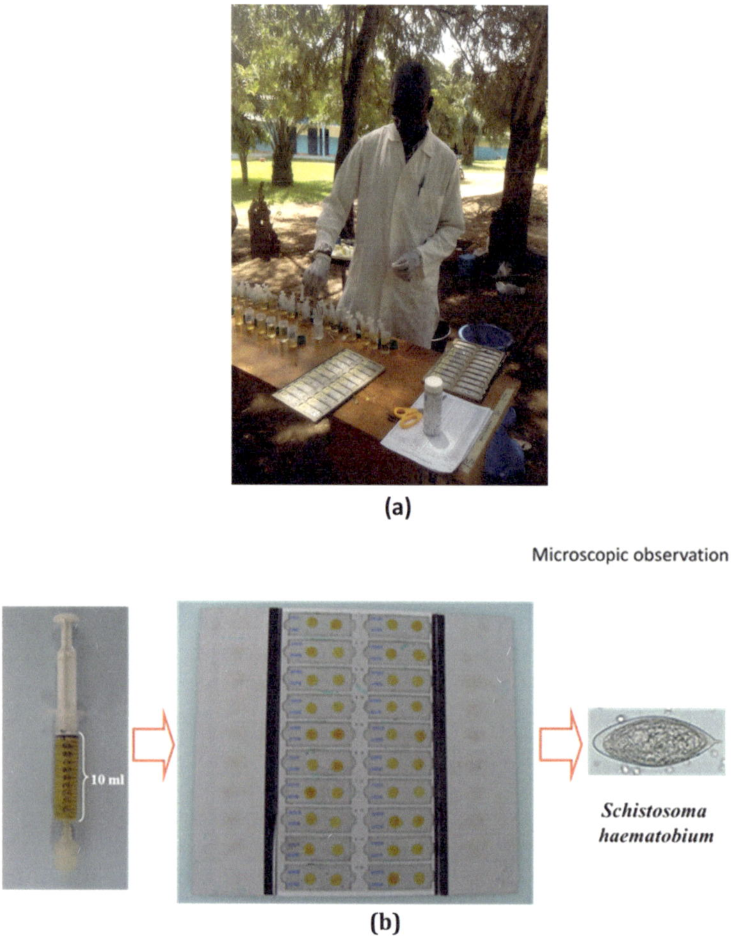

Figure 3.
Preparing urine samples for optical microscope examination.

as an indicator of bilharzian infection, the test is considered positive when the strip turns solely from yellow to green or dark green. Participants were grouped into six age groups: <5; 5–9; 10–14; 15–19; 20–24; and ≥25 years.

The prevalence of *S. haematobium* infections was calculated. Participants with a specific *S. haematobium* infection were compared with those who had not been infected by these parasites. Univariate analysis (Chi-square and Fisher exact tests) was used to compare the groups.

The probability value (p) indicated the degree of significance of the links at the 0.05 level. Fisher's exact test was used for small numbers (more than 5% of theoretical frequencies less than 5).

2.5 Ethical considerations

The study conditions have been reviewed and approved by the National Ethics and Research Committee of Côte d'Ivoire (N° 76-MSLS-CNER-dkn). Detailed explanations of the study were given to local authorities (village chiefs) and community members. Written informed consent of each participant was obtained (for children aged below 18 years, consent was given by parents or legal guardians). Participation was strictly voluntary. A single 40 mg/kg oral dose of praziquantel against schistosomiasis was administered to community members aged 5 years and above in localities where the prevalence of schistosomiasis was greater or equal to 5%, while individual case treatment was applied in localities with lower prevalences. Drug administration was implemented by the "Programme National de Lutte contre les Maladies Tropicales Négligées à Chimiothérapie Préventive" (PNLMTN-CP) in collaboration with personnel from local health districts and our research team.

3. Results

3.1 Demographic characteristics

Of the 2948 participants registered from different localities to participate in the study, 2447 individuals (1193 males and 1254 females) provided a urine sample and were considered as the final sample for the evaluation of parasitic infection. There were 205 (8.4%) preschool-aged children (<5 years), 1755 (71.7%) school-aged children (5–15 years), and 487 (19.9%) adolescents and adults (>15 years). The mean age of the participants was 14.5 years (95% CI: 13.9–15.0%).

3.2 Parasite infection status

The overall prevalence of urinary bilharziasis obtained was 3.4% (95% CI: 2.7–4.1%). However, high prevalences of schistosomiasis in the of the order of 20–27% have been noted in certain localities, namely Couradjourou (26.7%) and Kalekoua (22.2%).

Males and females were statistically equally affected by this pathology. Consequently, there was no significant difference with sex in schistosome infestation levels (3.1% vs. 3.6%; P = 0.503) (**Figure 4**).

Regarding age, participants aged 15–19 years and 20–24 years showed a significantly higher prevalence of infection (8.3% and 7.6%, respectively) (X^2 = 12.20; P = 0.032), compared with other age groups (**Figure 5**).

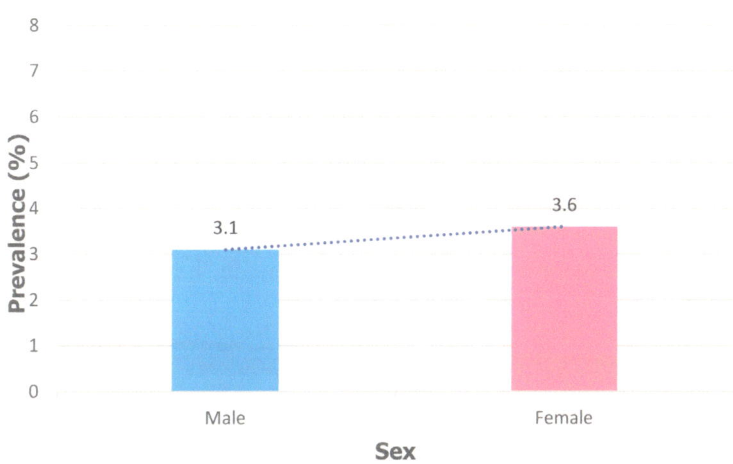

Figure 4.
Schistosoma haematobium *parasitic infection, stratified by sex, Taabo, south-central Côte d'Ivoire.*

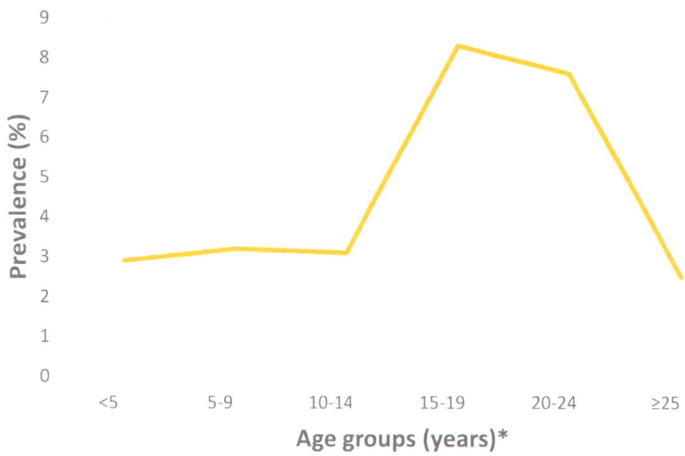

Figure 5.
Age-prevalence curve of Schistosoma haematobium *in Taabo, south-central Côte d'Ivoire *(n = 2447; < 5 years = 205, 5–9 years = 899, 10–14 years = 783, 15–19 years = 109, 20–24 years = 53, ≥25 years = 398).*

3.3 Infection intensities

Schistosoma haematobium infection intensities, determined by the arithmetic mean of eggs, were significantly low in almost all surveyed localities (1.0–4.5 eggs/10 mL of urine), except for the community of Courandjourou (27.3 eggs/10 mL urine; 95% CI: 3.5–60.0%). However, the overall intensity of infection recorded in the study area was 1.1 eggs/10 mL urine (95% CI: 1.0–1.1%).

In terms of infection intensity categories, *Schistosoma haematobium* infections were in the majority of cases of light intensity (78%; [1–49 eggs/10 mL of urine]) vs. 22% (heavy infestation, i.e. ≥50 eggs/10 mL of urine).

4. Discussion

This study aimed to reassess the prevalence of *Schistosoma haematobium* infection following multiple rounds of intervention in communities within the Taabo sub-prefecture, south-central Côte d'Ivoire. An overall prevalence of 3.4% of *S. haematobium* infection was recorded during this investigation, which significantly lower than the rates observed in previous years following the construction of the Taabo hydroelectric dam and its natural tributaries [6, 11, 14, 15]. It is conceivable that preventive chemotherapy with praziquantel, combined with Information Education Communication (IEC) and social and economic development, explains this decline [12, 16].

However, two nearby localities (Courandjourou (26.7%) and Kalekoua (22.2%)), upstream of Lake Taabo, near the Bandama river, remain "hot spots" for *S. haematobium* infection.

Historically, the prevalence of infection was much higher, with rates of up to 73% in villages surrounding Lake Taabo in the early 1990s and as high as 90% in Taabo village by the late 1990s [10, 17]. Over the past few decades, the prevalence of urinary bilharziasis has significantly decreased in the Taabo district.

Ongoing research and interventions targeting helminthiasis in the Taabo Health and Demographic Surveillance System (HDSS) have contributed to this reduction, in part by enhancing community awareness of this neglected disease. In a previous study on schistosomiasis in western Côte d'Ivoire, we found that research activities had considerably improved community knowledge [18]. Furthermore, while *S. haematobium* infection is only a problem in certain localities due to the focal distribution of the disease, it is relatively easy to tackle once these foci have been identified [14]. Elimination would not be effective without the integration of malacological control (interruption of transmission) [19–21].

One of the limitations of the study is the lack of surveys at sites where intermediate hosts of Schistosoma species are present, which would have provided a clearer understanding of transmission dynamics in relation to the environmental conditions of the various localities. The level of *Schistosoma spp*. infection was not influenced by gender in the study area. This assertion corroborates the results of a study conducted in the study area indicating that men and women are equally involved in outdoor water-related activities [22]. This is not the case in other parts of the world (significant difference between the sexes), due to social or cultural considerations that may prevent women from having access to water bodies [23, 24]. Participants aged 15–24 years were most likely to be infected with schistosomes. The lifestyles of adolescents (15–19 years) and young adults (20–24 years) expose them to the risk of helminth infection through professional activities (fishing, gardening, irrigation of crops, etc.). In addition, young adults are more mobile and more involved in farming activities that involve regular contact with infested bodies of water, which exposes them to a higher risk of bilharzia infection than the older group. This is in line with the village of Courandjourou, where adolescents and young adults are heavily involved in fishing and gardening. The higher prevalence observed in this village can therefore be attributed to the frequent contact of inhabitants with unprotected freshwater that may contain infected intermediate snail hosts. It should also be noted that this locality is located close to and upstream from Lake Taabo. This could therefore provide favourable environmental conditions for the proliferation of freshwater snails that catalyse schistosomiasis transmission.

The high level of *S. haematobium* infection observed in the village of Courandjourou (27.3 eggs/10 mL of urine) can be explained by the constant contact between the inhabitants as a result of their daily activities. The mean egg intensity found in this study is relatively equal to that found in a community-based study in Tanzania where the median intensity was 2.2 eggs/10 mL of urine [25]. This observation may be due to the fact that the community study took into account school-aged children, for whom most of the efforts to combat schistosomiasis, including annual preventive chemotherapy, are intended [25–27].

Almost a third of infections (22%) were classified as severe, according to the World Health Organisation (WHO) categorisation of *S. haematobium* infection intensities, i.e. ≥50 eggs/10 mL of urine [28]. This value is in the same order as that obtained in the same study area (25.9% of infections ≥50 eggs/10 mL of urine [14]. Categories of high intensity of *S. haematobium* infection are most often associated with multiple morbidities [29, 30].

5. Conclusion

The findings of this study are highly promising regarding the prevalence of *Schistosoma haematobium* infection. The results suggest that *S. haematobium* infection is largely under control in the Taabo area. However, adolescents and young adults engaged in agricultural work are the most affected by urinary bilharziasis. Therefore, these groups should be prioritised in awareness campaigns and mass treatment efforts to optimise disease control within the communities of the Taabo sub-prefecture, with the ultimate goal of achieving disease elimination.

6. Summary

Bilharziasis or schistosomiasis is a water-dependent parasitosis caused by the presence in human blood capillaries of a parasite (worm) called bilharzia or schistosome. Urinary bilharziasis, caused by *Schistosoma haematobium*, is common in the central part of Côte d'Ivoire. Following the construction of the hydroelectric dam in 1972, the localities of the Taabo sub-prefecture were for a long time heavily affected by bilharziasis caused by *Schistosoma haematobium*. This study has elucidated the pattern of reinfection by urinary schistosomes in this area in recent decades. This study has shown that significant progress has been made in the control of this disease in the populations of the various localities concerned. In addition, this research activities have highlighted the groups of people at risk.

Acknowledgements

We are grateful to community health workers (CHW) for their support and for facilitating the implementation of the study. We would like to thank the members of the local communities for their warm welcome and enthusiastic participation.

Conflict of interest

There is no conflict of interest.

Author details

Gaoussou Coulibaly[1,2*], Nana Rose Diakité[1,2], Fidèle Kouakou Bassa[1,2], Mamadou Ouattara[1,2] and Eliézer Kouakou N'Goran[1,2]

1 Laboratoire de Biologie et Santé, UFR Biosciences, Université Félix Houphouët-Boigny, Abidjan, Côte d'Ivoire

2 Centre Suisse de Recherches Scientifiques en Côte d'Ivoire, Abidjan, Côte d'Ivoire

*Address all correspondence to: gaoussoubrava@yahoo.fr

References

[1] Marie C, William AP. Schistosomiasis [Internet]. 2023. Available from: https://www.msdmanuals.com/professional/infectious-diseases/trematodesflukes/schistosomiasis [Accessed: 22 July 2024]

[2] Orish VN, Morhe EKS, Azanu W, Alhassan RK, Gyapong M. The parasitology of female genital schistosomiasis. Current Research in Parasitology & Vector-Borne Diseases. 2022;**2**:100093. DOI: 10.1016/j.crpvbd.2022.100093

[3] CDC. U.S. Centers for Disease Control and Prevention [Internet]. 2024. Available from: https://www.msdmanuals.com/professional/infectious-diseases/trematodes-flukes/schistosomiasis [Accessed: 22 July 2024]

[4] WHO. Schistosomiasis. 2023. Available from: https://www.who.int/news-room/fact-sheets/detail/schistosomiasis

[5] Kokaliaris C, Garba A, Matuska M, Bronzan RN, Colley DG, et al. Effect of preventive chemotherapy with praziquantel on schistosomiasis among school-aged children in sub-Saharan Africa: A spatiotemporal modelling study. The Lancet Infectious Diseases. 2022;**22**(1):136-149. DOI: 10.1016/S1473-3099(21)00090-6

[6] N'Goran EK, Diabate S, Utzinger J, Sellin B. Changes in human schistosomiasis levels after the construction of two large hydroelectric dams in Central Côte d'Ivoire. Bulletin of the World Health Organisation. 1997;**75**(6):541-545

[7] Tian-Bi YT, Ouattara M, Knopp S, Coulibaly JT, Hürlimann E, et al. Interrupting seasonal transmission of *Schistosoma haematobium* and control of soil-transmitted helminthiasis in northern and central Côte d'Ivoire: A SCORE study protocol. BMC Public Health. 2018;**18**(1):186. DOI: 10.1186/s12889-018-5044-2

[8] Diakité NR, Adja AM, von Stamm UJ, N'Goran EK. Epidemiological baseline situation before the construction of a small dam in five villages of Bouaké, central Côte-d'Ivoire. Bulletin de la Société de Pathologie Exotique. 2010;**103**:22-28. DOI: 10.1007/s13149-009-0029-4

[9] Brou AN. Knowledge of urinary schistosomiasis in rural Ivory Coast: Case study in Bamoro and N'guessan-Pokoukro (Sanitary District of Bouaké). European Scientific Journal. 2019;**15**(30):113. DOI: 10.19044/esj.2019.v15n30p113

[10] N'Goran EK, Utzinger J, N'Guessan AN, Müller I, Zamblé K, et al. Reinfection with *Schistosoma haematobium* following school-based chemotherapy with praziquantel in four highly endemic villages in Côte d'Ivoire. Tropical Medicine & International Health. 2001;**6**:817-825. DOI: 10.1046/j.1365-3156.2001.00785.x

[11] Fürst T, Silué KD, Ouattara M, N'Goran DN, Adiossan LG, et al. Schistosomiasis, soil-transmitted helminthiasis, and sociodemographic factors influence quality of life of adults in Côte d'Ivoire. PLoS Neglected Tropical Diseases. 2012;**6**:e1855. DOI: 10.1371/journal.pntd.0001855

[12] Coulibaly G, Ouattara M, Dongo K, Hürlimann E, Bassa FK, et al. Epidemiology of intestinal parasite infections in three departments of south-central Côte d'Ivoire before the

implementation of a cluster-randomised trial. Parasite Epidemiology and Control. 2018;**3**:63-76. DOI: 10.1016/j.parepi.2018.02.003

[13] Plouvier S, Leroy JC, Colette J. A propos d'une technique simple de filtration des urines dans le diagnostic de la bilharziose urinaire en enquête de masse. Médecine Tropicale. 1975;**35**(3):229-230

[14] Schmidlin T, Hürlimann E, Silué KD, Yapi RB, Houngbedji C, et al. Effects of hygiene and defecation behavior on helminths and intestinal protozoa infections in Taabo, Côte d'Ivoire. PLoS One. 2013;**8**(6):e65722. DOI: 10.1371/journal.pone.0065722

[15] Hürlimann E, Silué KD, Zouzou F, Ouattara M, Schmidlin T, et al. Effect of an integrated intervention package of preventive chemotherapy, community-led total sanitation and health education on the prevalence of helminth and intestinal protozoa infections in Côte d'Ivoire. Parasites & Vectors. 2018;**11**(1):115. DOI: 10.1186/s13071-018-2642-x

[16] Koné S, Baikoro N, N'Guessan Y, Jaeger FN, Silué KD, et al. Health & demographic surveillance system profile: The Taabo Health and Demographic Surveillance System, Côte d'Ivoire. International Journal of Epidemiology. 2015;**44**(1):87-97. DOI: 10.1093/ije/dyu221

[17] N'Goran EK, Utzinger J, Gnaka HN, Yapi A, N'Guessan NA, et al. Randomized, double-blind, placebo-controlled trial of oral artemether for the prevention of patent *Schistosoma haematobium* infections. American Journal of Tropical Medicine and Hygiene. 2003;**68**(1):24-32

[18] Acka CA, Raso G, N'goran EK, Tschannen AB, Bogoch II, et al. Parasitic worms: Knowledge, attitudes, and practices in Western Côte d'Ivoire with implications for integrated control. PLoS Neglected Tropical Diseases. 2010;**4**(12):e910. DOI: 10.1371/journal.pntd.0000910

[19] Diakité NR, N'Zi KG, Ouattara M, Coulibaly JT, Saric J, et al. Association of riverine prawns and intermediate host snails and correlation with human schistosomiasis in two river systems in south-eastern Côte d'Ivoire. Parasitology. 2018;**145**(13):1792-1800. DOI: 10.1017/S003118201800135X

[20] Assaré RK, N'Tamon RN, Bellai LG, Koffi JA, Mathieu TI, et al. Characteristics of persistent hotspots of *Schistosoma mansoni* in western Côte d'Ivoire. Parasites & Vectors. 2020;**13**(1):337. DOI: 10.1186/s13071-020-04188-x

[21] Jones IJ, Sokolow SH, Chamberlin AJ, Lund AJ, Jouanard N, et al. Schistosome infection in Senegal is associated with different spatial extents of risk and ecological drivers for *Schistosoma haematobium* and *S. mansoni*. PLoS Neglected Tropical Diseases. 2021;**15**(9):e0009712. DOI: 10.1371/journal.pntd.0009712

[22] Bassa FK, Eze IC, Assaré RK, Essé C, Koné S, et al. Prevalence of Schistosoma mono- and co-infections with multiple common parasites and associated risk factors and morbidity profile among adults in the Taabo health and demographic surveillance system, South-Central Côte d'Ivoire. Infectious Diseases of Poverty. 2022;**11**(1):3. DOI: 10.1186/s40249-021-00925-1

[23] Sady H, Al-Mekhlafi HM, Mahdy MA, Lim YA, Mahmud R, et al. Prevalence and associated factors of Schistosomiasis among children in Yemen: Implications for an effective

control programme. PLoS Neglected Tropical Diseases. 2013;7(8):e2377. DOI: 10.1371/journal.pntd.0002377

[24] Dawaki S, Al-Mekhlafi HM, Ithoi I, Ibrahim J, Abdulsalam AM, Ahmed A et al. Prevalence and risk factors of schistosomiasis among Hausa communities in Kano State, Nigeria. Revista del Instituto de Medicina Tropical. 2016;**58**:54. DOI: 10.1590/S1678-9946201658054

[25] Rite EE, Kapalata SN, Munisi DZ. Prevalence, intensity, and factors associated with urogenital Schistosomiasis among women of reproductive age in Mbogwe District Council, Geita Region, Tanzania. Biomed Research International. 2020;**2020**:5923025. DOI: 10.1155/2020/5923025

[26] Lo NC, Addiss DG, Hotez PJ, King CH, Stothard JR, et al. A call to strengthen the global strategy against schistosomiasis and soil-transmitted helminthiasis: The time is now. Lancet Infectious Diseases. 2017;**17**(2):e64-e69. DOI: 10.1016/S1473-3099(16)30535-7

[27] Lo NC, Lai YS, Karagiannis-Voules DA, Bogoch II, Coulibaly JT, et al. Assessment of global guidelines for preventive chemotherapy against schistosomiasis and soil-transmitted helminthiasis: A cost-effectiveness modelling study. Lancet Infectious Diseases. 2016;**16**(9):1065-1075. DOI: 10.1016/S1473-3099(16)30073-1

[28] WHO. Prevention and control of schistosomiasis and soil transmitted helminthiasis. WHO Technical Report Series. 2002;**912**:1-57

[29] Wiegand RE, Secor WE, Fleming FM, French MD, King CH, et al. Associations between infection intensity categories and morbidity prevalence in school-age children are much stronger for Schistosoma haematobium than for *S. mansoni*. PLoS Neglected Tropical Diseases. 2021;**15**(5):e0009444. DOI: 10.1371/journal.pntd.0009444

[30] Mott KE. Schistosomiasis. In: Murray CJL, Lopez AD, Mathers CD, editors. The Global Epidemiology of Infectious Diseases. Global Burden of Disease and Injury. IV. Geneva: World Health Organization; 2004. pp. 349-391

Chapter 3

An Update on the Control of Fasciolosis: Traditional and Alternative Treatments and Possible Future Approaches

Guillem Herrera-Torres, Diana María Barrero-Torres, José Pérez, Luis Miguel Flores-Velázquez, Álvaro Martínez-Moreno, Francisco Javier Martínez-Moreno, Leandro Buffoni, Pablo José Rufino-Moya, Verónica Molina-Hernández and María Teresa Ruiz-Campillo

Abstract

In this chapter, we aim to provide an overview of fasciolosis control, with a particular emphasis on ruminants. Controlling infections caused by *Fasciola* spp. involves implementing strategies that target both the intermediate and definitive hosts. Treating animals with anthelmintic drugs has proven to be the most effective method for managing fasciolosis. However, the emergence of drug resistance has led to the exploration of new approaches, such as the use of drug combinations and the investigation of natural compounds. While the development of a vaccine to combat this disease would be highly beneficial, varying efficacy rates have been observed, rendering current options insufficient for commercial use. Understanding the interactions between the parasite and its host is crucial, and advancements in 'omic' technologies could facilitate the identification of new therapeutic targets.

Keywords: fasciolosis, anthelmintic resistance, fasciolosis control, *F. hepatica*, *F. gigantica*, vaccines, helminthiasis, phytotherapy, anthelmintics

1. Introduction

Fasciolosis is caused by two species of trematodes: *Fasciola hepatica* and *Fasciola gigantica*. It is classified as a neglected tropical disease and a zoonosis. Neglected tropical diseases are often overlooked or ignored zoonoses that have significant social and economic impacts worldwide, primarily affecting vulnerable and marginalized communities in tropical and subtropical regions. The disease is closely associated with animal production and limited access to water, sanitation and hygiene [1, 2].

Fasciolosis is recognized as the most geographically widespread parasitic infection, with more than 180 million people at risk of infection [3, 4]. In the agricultural sector, it is responsible for economic losses estimated at USD 3.2 billion per year [5]. Triclabendazole is considered the most effective anthelmintic drug due to its efficacy against both juvenile and adult forms of the parasite [6]. However, the prevalence of fasciolosis is believed to be increasing due to rising resistance to triclabendazole and other commonly used anthelmintics [7, 8], with climate change also contributing to this trend [9, 10].

Traditionally, the effectiveness of fasciolosis control and prevention has focused on various measures aimed at reducing the population of intermediate hosts, such as lymnaeid snails like *Galba truncatula*. This includes preventing outbreaks of *Fasciola* spp. in the definitive host (ruminants) by administering the appropriate anthelmintic following early diagnosis [11]. The emergence of resistance, along with social concerns regarding drug residues in animal products and the environment, as well as the necessity for farmers to adhere to withdrawal periods, underscores the urgent need for alternative methods to control fasciolosis [12, 13].

Immunization through vaccines has been proposed as a promising strategy for controlling this disease [14]. Experimental studies have explored various vaccine formulations, including attenuated, recombinant, gene knockdown/silencing, nucleic-acid-based vaccines and cocktail vaccines, all aimed at enhancing the humoral or cell-mediated immune response to fasciolosis [15]. However, *F. hepatica* employs mechanisms to evade the host's protective immune response, such as releasing proteolytic enzymes that play crucial roles in virulence, infection, tissue migration and modulation of both innate and adaptative immune responses [16]. This complicates the development of an effective vaccine.

Additionally, the use of plants with recognized anthelmintic activity is being explored as a potential alternative. Several *in vitro* and *in vivo* trials have reported a flukicidal effect in ruminants using compounds derived from these plants [4].

The aim of this review is to provide a comprehensive and up-to-date overview of the various methods traditionally used to control fasciolosis, as well as alternative approaches. In addition, it proposes potential future methods for effectively managing this disease based on a review of the literature.

2. The control of *Fasciola* infection

In the roadmap for the sustainable and effective control of foodborne trematodiases, the World Health Organization advocates for a One Health approach that encompasses the health of people, animals and ecosystems. This approach is complemented by the implementation of a multidisciplinary strategy that includes sanitation measures and education on safe food practices [2, 17, 18].

Controlling fasciolosis in the animal health sector requires a coordinated effort involving veterinarians, farmers, rural communities, meat inspectors, authorities and policymakers [1]. It is necessary to raise awareness among local populations and farmers about the implications of fasciolosis and the issue of anthelmintic resistance and to inform them about the various existing control strategies and their effectiveness [19–21].

Furthermore, considering the impact of fasciolosis in low-income areas with traditional agricultural practices and longstanding cultural beliefs, it is crucial to explore cost-effective methods, technical and financial resources and a dialog strategy

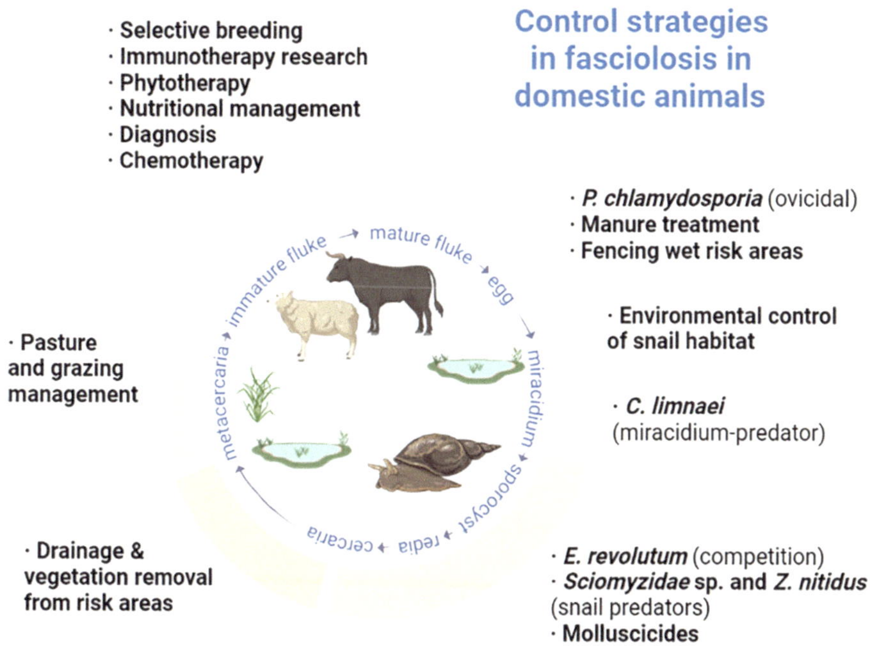

Figure 1.
Scheme of control strategies of fasciolosis targeting the intermediate host (IH), the definitive host (DH) and their habitats at key stages of the Fasciola *spp. life cycle.*

with traditional communities [1, 22]. Long-term adoption of these measures can be achieved by ensuring minimal disruption to existing agricultural practices [21, 22].

In the Northern Bolivian Altiplano [23], community engagement was prioritized, involving local leaders to help persuade other communities of the progress made. In West Java, Indonesia [22], a combination of continuous participatory learning to empower farmers, along with the provision of productive materials and financial incentives, proved to be effective.

Other factors to consider when designing control strategies include the epidemiological situation and local environmental characteristics, such as topography and meteorology [17, 20]. Utilizing computer models with this data can help predict outbreaks [11, 24].

Understanding how and under what conditions the transmission of different stages of *Fasciola* occurs will facilitate the adoption of integrated control strategies for domestic animals [22]. Accordingly, in this chapter, control strategies for domestic animals are structured around two main focuses: the intermediate host (lymnaeid snails) and the definitive host (primarily domestic ruminants), aiming to interrupt the parasite's life cycle and thereby halt disease transmission (**Figure 1**).

2.1 Control strategies targeting the intermediate host and its habitat

This encompasses a variety of biological, ecological, chemical and environmental control methods designed to alter the conditions for snail development and modify their ecological habitat. The primary goals are to eliminate or reduce snail populations and to prevent their infection by *Fasciola* miracidia. This preventive approach would decrease pasture contamination, lower medical expenses in livestock production and limit the development of drug resistance [25].

The first step is to assess the presence of snails on the farm. Since they thrive in wet conditions, their permanent habitats include springs, drainage ditches, pond banks, marshes, slow-moving streams and areas around drinking troughs and water pipes. Temporary habitats are created by tractor passage [20, 26]. The presence of the plant *Juncus acutiflorus* has been linked to the presence of snails [27].

Environmental factors that influence the development of *Fasciola*'s free-living stages, snail survival and infection include temperatures ranging from 10 to 30°C, humidity and slightly acidic soil. Detection methods are available for identifying environmental DNA from snails and free-living parasite stages in plants and water [28].

2.1.1 Biological and ecological control

Beginning with the disruption of the parasite's cycle before snail infection, there are various control methods targeting free-living eggs and miracidia. The saprophytic fungus *Pochonia chlamydosporia* has demonstrated ovicidal effects through hyphal colonization and specialized structures known as 'appressoria', which penetrate the egg surface, leading to external and embryological alterations [29]. Laboratory assays have been conducted using fungal isolates of strains VC1 and VC4 [30], as well as the fungus isolate Pc-10 [31, 32]. Additionally, a field experiment involving cattle has been carried out, incorporating VC1 strain fungal mycelium in pellets [33]. This biological control method does not require withdrawal periods and is compatible with organic livestock production, although determining the effective dosage is essential [34].

Furthermore, the annelid *Chaetogaster limnaei* forms a symbiotic relationship with the snail *Galba truncatula*, providing shelter and locomotion in exchange for protection against miracidia infection of *F. hepatica* through predation, a capacity that has been demonstrated *in vitro* [35]. Natural predators of snails include birds (such as mallard ducks, lapwings, starlings, thrushes and geese), other snails, flies, crustaceans, amphibians, reptiles, rodents and beetles [26, 35]. Some of these predators may also act as food competitors [36]. The introduction of free-ranging ducks and geese is proposed as a complementary strategy for controlling fasciolosis and has shown positive results in India [37] and the Philippines [22]. Since the parasite encysts into metacercariae before harvest, the introduction of ducks should occur beforehand, always considering the potential crop damage they may cause [22].

The carnivorous land snail *Zonitoides nitidus* positively impacts the control of the snail population, and its beneficial effects are enhanced by introducing the snail *Oxychilus draparnaudi* or by using cupric chloride as a molluscicide [27]. Similarly, Sciomyzidae flies have been studied as potential candidates for snail control due to their high reproductive rate and voracious appetite [38]. However, there is currently no scientific evidence supporting the efficacy of ground and water beetles against helminth parasites [39].

From another perspective, Suhardono et al. [40] conducted a study in which dung from ducks infected with *Echinostoma revolutum* was placed in rice fields fertilized with dung from cattle infected with *F. gigantica*. They concluded that snails in rice fields containing dung infected with *E. revolutum* had fewer *F. gigantica* miracidia, demonstrating the interspecific antagonism between the two trematodes.

Subsequently, the Australian Centre for International Agricultural Research (ACIAR) [22] documented practical applications on farms in Southeast Asia to limit disease transmission in two days: by allowing the simultaneous entry of cattle and ducks or chickens infected with *E. revolutum* into the rice fields, and by adding duck or chicken dung infected with *E. revolutum* to cattle dung used as fertilizer. Only a small number of ducks are required, and *E. revolutum* does not affect livestock; however, this practice does pose a risk of cercarial dermatitis for farmers.

Finally, while it has been suggested that reduced viability of snails and/or competitive interactions among snails under conditions of dual infections with other parasites, such as *Muellerius capillaris* [41] or *Calicophoron daubneyi* [27, 42], may occur, it is important to note that these parasites are significant pathogens for domestic animals, causing pulmonary verminosis and paramphistomosis, respectively. Therefore, they are not considered safe biocontrol strategies.

2.1.2 Chemical control

The use of molluscicides or chemicals to control the snail population should be approached with caution due to their low selectivity and potential negative impacts on the environment and other living organisms [19, 20]. Eradicating intermediate hosts is challenging because of their rapid reproduction, and an additional concern is the economic cost associated with repeated applications and the necessary [24, 43]. Various compounds and formulations exist [43]. Currently, authorized products in Europe [44] include spinosad, metaldehyde, ferric phosphate, diatomaceous earth and Bordeaux mixture, which consist of a blend of copper sulfates and quicklime. In rice fields, where susceptible domestic animals may coexist with *Fasciola*, one or two applications of molluscicides are recommended after rice planting [22].

2.1.3 Environmental control

There is a wide range of management measures available aimed at modifying the snail's habitat and interrupting its life cycle [19]. Draining areas with high water retention, along with removing vegetation associated with pipes, ditches, wells and any water source, have traditionally been used to prevent snails from finding refuge, thereby hindering their survival [36]. The construction of dams, the maintenance and repair of water leaks, plowing fields, or directly using snail traps are other methods of snail control [11, 19, 26, 45, 46]. Additionally, fences can be installed around wet-risk areas to limit snail contact with livestock [43].

The analysis of the environmental DNA (eDNA) has been described as a promising new tool for the epidemiological investigation of parasite infection on farms, offering the potential to implement effective control strategies [28, 47].

2.2 Control strategies targeting the definitive host and its habitat

One of the traditional methods for managing fasciolosis on dairy farms involves the early prediction of infection, allowing for the appropriate use of anthelmintics to prevent losses without the risk of overtreating animals or promoting the development of drug resistance in parasites [48]. The clinical signs of fasciolosis are nonspecific, potentially causing anemia, elevated liver enzyme levels and reduced serum albumin levels [49]. Since coprological methods, such as fecal egg count (FEC) and flotation-sedimentation techniques like Flukefinder® and mini-FLOTAC® [4], are only useful in the late stage of fasciolosis, other techniques have been developed over time.

Immunological methods offer high sensitivity in early stages of infection and are both reproducible and cost-effective. Specific antibodies can be analyzed in blood, feces and milk.

Additionally, the FAMACHA© system [50], which evaluates anemia levels through conjunctival color, is proposed as a tool for selectively treating chronic fasciolosis in sheep. Abattoir feedback on liver damage and bile examination can provide valuable insights into parasite circulation on the farm [26, 51]. Over the past decade, molecular diagnostic methods and 'omics' techniques, such as PCR, RT-PCR, PCR-RFLP and loop-mediated isothermal amplification (LAMP), have been used for faster diagnosis with greater sensitivity and specificity [4].

2.2.1 Pasture and grazing management

These practices aim to reduce the risk of infection with *Fasciola* metacercariae [1] or finding alternatives for livestock grazing in high-risk areas and periods [11], which may be challenging in certain circumstances [26]. Other management practices include pasture rotation, as described by Boray [52].

The viability of metacercariae can be reduced by drying the hay the animals will consume and ensuring proper ensiling [45]. Additionally, cutting plant stalks above the water level in irrigated rice fields and sun-drying them for 3 days, or storing them in a dry place for five weeks before use, can help reduce contamination [22].

Constructing drinking troughs at elevated levels may help minimize contamination of drinking water with infected vegetation. As for fertilizing rice fields with livestock manure, it is recommended to sun-dry the manure for 1 month or subject it to a fermentation process with temperatures above 45°C [22, 23, 45].

2.2.2 Chemotherapy

Currently, pharmaco-therapeutics remain at the forefront of strategies to control fasciolosis in livestock due to the absence of an effective commercial vaccine. As a result, they are considered the most effective method for ensuring animal welfare, maintaining productivity and preventing pasture contamination with *F. hepatica* eggs [49, 53, 54].

Raising awareness among farmers about the importance of avoiding overexposure of animals to drug treatments and the correct use of anthelmintics is essential to reduce the emergence of resistance.

Fasciolicidal products are grouped into the following families: halogenated phenols (nitroxynil), salicylanilides (oxyclozanide, rafoxanide and closantel), sulfonamides (clorsulon), benzimidazoles (albendazole and triclabendazole) and nitrophenylguanidine derivatives (netobimin) [51, 55, 56].

Because triclabendazole has a broad spectrum of efficacy, a high safety margin, a good tolerance and acts against both immature and adult forms of the parasite, it has become the most widely used anthelmintic against fasciolosis [57]. Anthelmintic efficacy depends on the developmental stage of the fluke, which is related to the physiological environment of the host and the drug's mechanism of action. Like albendazole, triclabendazole binds to β-tubulin and causes microtubule depolymerization. Additionally, triclabendazole inhibits adenylate cyclase activity. Halogenated phenols and salicylanilides target the uncoupling of oxidative phosphorylation in the mitochondrial membrane, while sulfonamides inhibit phosphoglycerate kinase and phosphoglyceromutase enzymes involved in glycolysis [55].

Except for triclabendazole, the rest of the anthelmintics are not effective against all life stages of *Fasciola*. Clorsulon and nitroxinil have been reported to act against 7-week post-infection flukes and closantel and rafoxanide are effective against 6-week post-infection flukes. Nevertheless, variable efficacy against early immature flukes is reported for closantel and rafoxanide, and their efficacy is lower compared to that of triclabendazole [56].

The administration routes include subcutaneous, topical (pour-on) and oral, with the oral route being the most commonly used. Administering the correct dosage according to authorized therapeutic guidelines is critical [1]. To avoid under-dosing, it is necessary to weigh animals [58] or at least sample and group them, ensuring proper administration, particularly with the oral route. If feasible, it is desirable to restrict feeding beforehand. Grooming, a dirty coat, or adverse weather conditions could lead to under-dosing using the pour-on route [59].

Ruminant species exhibit pharmacokinetic variability. For example, sheep metabolize anthelmintics, especially benzimidazoles, more rapidly than other species [60]. Buffalo requires a double dose of triclabendazole compared to cattle due to differences in pharmacokinetics [22]. Similarly, the high efficacy of oxyclozanide against adult forms in sheep is not observed in cattle [1], and rafoxanide is ineffective against 6-week-old flukes in cattle but effective in sheep [55].

The appropriate use of fasciolicides should rely on selective and strategic treatments supported by prior diagnosis and evaluation of treatment efficacy. The aim of targeted selective treatment (TST) is not to treat all animals en masse but rather to target the group suffering from severe parasitism, while preserving susceptible worms on the farm through *refugia*-based control. This approach helps delay the evolution of resistance [26, 61].

Monitoring the pharmacological efficacy of a treatment is crucial to prevent resistance. A treatment is considered effective if there is a 95% reduction in FEC 14–28 days post-treatment, or if *Fasciola* coproantigens are undetectable by the coproantigen reduction test (CPR) 14 days post-treatment [62].

Sequential use (rather than rotation) or combining fasciolicides with different mechanisms of action is recommended to delay the development of resistance [48]. The most effective combination without triclabendazole in *F. hepatica*-infected cattle consisted of nitroxynil, clorsulon and ivermectin [63]. Additionally, as mixed infections are common in livestock, broad-spectrum formulations combining fasciolicides with drugs targeting cestodes or nematodes are available [55, 56]. The main mechanisms of resistance to triclabendazole described so far, as well as possible strategies to combat fasciolosis, are summarized in **Figure 2**.

2.2.3 Nutritional management

The availability and balance of nutrients in an animal significantly influence physiological processes, including immune system function. Therefore, nutritional strategies should be considered as a complement to antimicrobial use [64].

Studies have examined how nutrition affects the host–parasite relationship in parasitic nematode infections, demonstrating that optimized nutrition enhances the host's ability to manage pathogenic effects, control disease progression and recover more effectively from infections [58, 65].

It has been shown that a high-protein diet, including cottonseed or cottonseed oil cake, reduces the impact of *F. gigantica* infection in cattle and sheep. This protective effect is reflected in improved daily weight gain and blood parameters

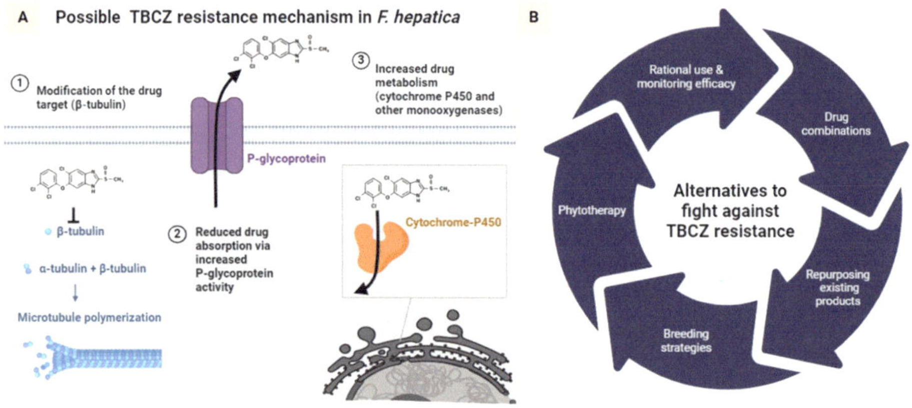

Figure 2.
A. Possible mechanisms of triclabendazole (TCBZ) resistance in F. hepatica*: (1) altered drug target (β-tubulin); (2) activation of P-glycoproteins that enhance the expulsion of the drug from its site of action and (3) increased drug metabolism* via *cytochrome P450 and other monooxygenases. Adapted from Fairweather et al. [48]. B. Alternatives to fight against TCBZ resistance: promoting rational drug use and monitoring efficacy, exploring new combination therapies, investigating the fasciolicidal properties of preexisting drugs, elucidating the genetic basis of resistance to develop breeding strategies and exploring phytotherapy options.*

[66, 67]. Additionally, dietary urea as a source of degradable nitrogen, helps mitigate the effects of gastrointestinal nematode infections in sheep. In developing countries, urea offers a valuable alternative to high-quality protein supplements due to its lower cost [65].

Vitamins have been reported to enhance antibody production and the activity of lymphocytes, NK cells and neutrophils. Dietary supplementation with antioxidant vitamins, such as vitamin E, helps neutralize reactive oxygen species (ROS), thereby reducing cellular damage under oxidative stress conditions [64]. Oxidative stress plays a crucial role in the pathogenesis of parasitic infections like fasciolosis [68]. A study by Martínez-Pérez et al. [69] showed that vitamin E supplementation in sheep experimentally infected with *F. hepatica* reduced parasite burden and liver lipid oxidation. Similarly, *F. hepatica*-infected rats supplemented with dietary zinc showed improved antioxidant status, as evidenced by hepatic biomarkers, alongside an increase in body weight [70].

2.2.4 Selective breeding

Selective breeding of resistant and resilient livestock offers a complementary, sustainable approach to the control of fasciolosis. Furthermore, understanding the mechanisms of resistance could provide new tools in the field of immunity against the disease [71].

Among sheep, the immune-mediated response described in Indonesian Thin-tailed sheep against the early stages of *F. gigantica* is particularly noteworthy [71–73]. Other breeds showing resistance to *F. hepatica* include St. Croix sheep (compared to Barbados Blackbelly sheep), Romanov sheep (compared to Merino sheep) [74], Salt Range sheep (compared to Afghani sheep) [75] and Horro breed (compared to Arsi and Menz breeds) [76]. In goats, Nubian goats exhibit acquired resistance, with a lower fluke burden of *F. gigantica* after initial exposure [77]. The Local Hairy and Beetal breeds show a lower prevalence of *F. hepatica* infection compared to crossbred goats [75].

2.2.5 Alternative control strategies based on plant extracts (phytotherapy)

Given growing consumer concern about chemical residues in food, the significant demand for animal products derived from organic livestock, and the development of helminth resistance to commercially available anthelmintic drugs, there has been increased interest in the development of natural compounds derived from plants with potential activity in fasciolosis control, particularly over the last decade [4, 78]. Active compounds with reported fasciolicidal activity are summarized in **Figure 3**.

2.2.5.1 In vitro *studies*

In vitro studies have reported high ovicidal activity against *F. hepatica* eggs studies using *Peganum harmala* seeds [79] and methanolic extracts of *Zingiber officinale* [80]. Similarly, extracts from *Momordica charantia* leaves extracts have been shown to reduce larval formation in *F. hepatica* eggs due to the presence of flavonoids, such as quercetin [81], and methanolic extracts of *Moringa oleifera* seeds decreased the vitality and hatchability of *F. hepatica* eggs [82].

Phenolic compounds, tannins and terpenes found in a variety of plant extracts (*Eugenia uniflora*, *Harpagophytum procumbens*, *Psidium guajava* and *Stryphnodendron adstringens*) are also linked to ovicidal activity in fasciolosis by preventing miracidium hatching [83]. Similar findings have been observed with extracts from the *Commiphora molmol* commercially recognized as Mirazid®, where decreased egg production and damage to adult parasites have been reported. However, the required concentration for proper use of this product is controversial and needs further research [84].

Curcumin and thymoquinone, active components of *Curcuma longa* and *Nigella sativa*, have been shown to significantly disrupt the tegument and provoke erosion of the spines of *F. gigantica*, decreasing its motility and migration functions [85]. Likewise, the flukicidal effect of *Etlingera elatior* ethanolic extract on egg and adult stages of *F. gigantica* has been confirmed, with evidence of damaged skin and spine, inner membrane erosion and detached syncytium from the tegument [86]. Methanolic extracts of *Cymbopogon jwarancusa* and *Conyza canadensis* were tested on *F. gigantica* adults, resulting in inhibited motility and eventual parasite death [87].

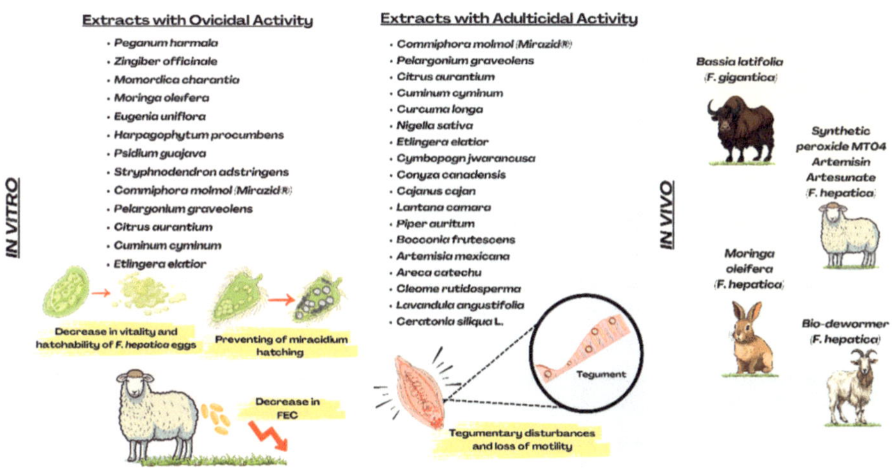

Figure 3.
Plant extracts used for the control of fasciolosis.

The anthelmintic effects of 15 tropical plant extracts were evaluated on newly excysted juveniles (NEJs) of *F. hepatica*, with five showing promising effects (*Cajanus cajan*, *Lantana camara*, *Piper auritum*, *Bocconia frutescens* and *Artemisia mexicana*). These extracts showed over 80% efficacy against motility and tegument alterations of *F. hepatica in vitro*, 72 hours post-exposure [88].

The anthelmintic effects of betel nut (*Areca catechu*) and neem (*Azadirachta indica*) leaf extracts were tested *in vitro* against *Fasciola* spp., with betel nut extract reducing parasite movement post-exposure compared to albendazole-treated parasites. Nevertheless, neem leaf extract did not reduce parasitic movement [89]. Similarly, increasing concentrations of ethanolic leaf extract of fringed spiderflower (*Cleome rutidosperma*) led to decreased motility of *Fasciola* spp. and structural alterations of the parenchyma and tegument [90].

The ovicidal and adulticidal activity of *Pelargonium graveolens* (geranium) and *Citrus aurantium* (sour orange) essential oils were evaluated on *F. hepatica*, with both oils proving 100% effective in inactivating trematode eggs and causing disruptive changes within the tegument and spines of adult forms, demonstrating potent ovicidal and adulticidal activity [91]. Another study also evaluated the efficacy of *Cuminum cyminum* (cumin) essential oil against *F. hepatica* eggs and adults. All concentrations tested in the ovicidal assay were 100% effective, and histological examination of adults revealed severe vacuolization, suggesting that cumin oil could be a promising compound for fasciolosis control [92].

In vitro evaluation of the anthelmintic activity of lavender (*Lavandula angustifolia*) and carob (*Ceratonia siliqua* L.) essential oils against *F. hepatica* revealed disruption within the parasite's DNA along with oxidative stress and an increase in ROS levels [93].

Although these compounds show promising potential for the control of fasciolosis, further studies are needed to evaluate their safety and potential side effects on treated animals, as they could lead to long-term metabolic disturbances.

2.2.5.2 In vivo *studies*

Several *in vivo* studies have been conducted to evaluate the efficacy of plant extracts against fasciolosis.

The condensed tannins and saponins present in deoiled mahua seed cake (*Bassia latifolia*) have been shown to possess significant anti-fasciolic activity, reducing the intensity of infection with *F. gigantica* in buffaloes when used at a concentration of 10% in a concentrated mixture [94].

In vivo studies in sheep naturally infected with *F. hepatica* have been carried out to assess the effectiveness of synthetic peroxides OZ78 and MTP4. The results indicated that MT04 led to a significant reduction in egg count and worm burden [95].

Artemether, an artemisinin derivate, produced a significant reduction in both egg count and worm burden in sheep when administered intramuscularly. However, episodes of abortion occurred, suggesting a potential embryotoxic effect [96]. Artesunate, another semisynthetic artemisin derivate, was tested in *F. hepatica*-infected sheep through intravascular and intramuscular injections. Both administration routes resulted in significant reductions in egg count and worm burden [97].

The effects of methanolic extract from *Moringa oleifera* seeds were tested *in vivo* in rabbits orally infected with *F. hepatica*. A 100% reduction in fecal egg count (FEC) was observed 7 days post-treatment. In addition, postmortem examination revealed the absence of flukes and fewer liver lesions in histopathological evaluations [82]. Finally, the efficacy of feeding goats naturally infected with *F. hepatica* with a herbal mixture (bio-dewormer) has been supported, as reductions in *F. hepatica* egg counts and positive effects on hematologic parameters and weight gain were observed [98].

2.2.6 Immunotherapy and vaccine development against fasciolosis

The discovery of individual and recombinant antigens of *Fasciola* spp. excretory-secretory products (ESPs) have been crucial in the development of vaccines against fasciolosis. The formulation of vaccines based on antigens that induce protective immunity in the host remains a key challenge for the scientific community. It is estimated that a vaccine inducing 50–60% efficacy in fluke reduction could significantly reduce economic losses in many countries, while also minimizing egg shedding on pastures, leading to a positive impact on the disease's epidemiology [99].

Proteases such as cathepsins, leucine aminopeptidase and peroxiredoxin are among the primary molecules used as active ingredients in vaccine preparations due to their role in proteolytic activity during parasite penetration, migration and feeding [100]. Additionally, the use of cathepsins in combination with high molecular weight proteins, such as hemoglobin, has been shown to significantly reduce fecal egg count (FEC) [12, 101]. Vaccine formulations are usually made with adjuvants, being aluminum, Freund's, Montanide and Alhydrogel, the most commonly used, as they have been shown to help induce protective immune responses in the host [13, 102].

The use of polyvalent vaccines, which include multiple antigens or proteins, has demonstrated a synergistic effect when combined with a single vaccine. For example, a vaccine combining recombinant pro-proteins of cathepsin L1H and B3 was tested in mice infected with *F. gigantica* [102], and a cocktail vaccine including *F. hepatica* recombinant CL1, peroxiredoxin, helminth defense molecules and leucine aminopeptidase resulted in a reduced parasite burden and less liver damage [13]. Similarly, two major proteins involved in the digestive process of *F. gigantica* were tested in mice, revealing a synergistic effect with protection rates of around 80% [103].

The variability observed in the results from numerous vaccine trials over the years, along with differences in immune responses across species and the unknown mechanism by which vaccines induce protection, make it difficult to establish an effective vaccine [4]. It has been suggested that vaccine protection depends on vaccine-induced antibodies targeted against cathepsins [104].

In the search for alternative vaccination routes that do require injections, a recent study showed that oral vaccination using freeze-dried transgenic lettuce expressing the cysteine proteinase from *F. hepatica* helped reduce infection intensity, liver damage and *F. hepatica* fecundity in cattle and sheep [105]. The release of the active components in the stomach and intestine stimulates both local (mucosal) and systemic immune responses [105, 106]. Other research has focused on using mimotopes of *F. hepatica* [107, 108], which induced a mixed Th1/Th2 response and reduced fluke burden.

In the early stages of fasciolosis, the immune response typically involves a mixed Th1/Th2 type with expression of cytokines such as IFN-γ, IL-4, IL-10 and TGF-β. With the course of infection, the Th1 response is suppressed, leading to a Th2-dominated response that facilitates parasite survival within the host [99]. In sheep and goats that show protection against fasciolosis, the vaccine promotes a mixed Th1/Th2 response with higher levels of IFN-γ and lower levels of IL-4. It has also been suggested that a lower increase in IFN-γ may correlate with fewer hepatic lesions [109].

Proteomic approaches are being used to identify new vaccine candidates targeting NEJs to help develop protective immune responses at early stages of infection [99, 110].

Vaccine development has primarily focused on proteins located in the parasite's tegument and gut. Recently, extracellular vesicles (EVs), which are present in the parasite's secretome, have been identified as playing a key role in host invasion, immune modulation and parasite survival. However, 'omics' studies should also focus on the affected liver to understand the host's perspective [111].

The analysis of EVs enriched with different protein molecules and RNA that aid in parasite survival during the migration within the host [112, 113], as well as the discovery of small non-coding RNAs (sncRNAs), such as microRNAs (miRNAs), has revealed the mechanisms by which *Fasciola* manipulates host immune cells [114, 115]. The study of sncRNAs is paving the way for improved detection and diagnostic methods for fasciolosis [116], and it will help develop new vaccine formulations with higher levels of immunization, inducing a mixed Th1/Th2 response by blocking the various parasite ESPs that regulate the host's immune response.

Moreover, the development of peptide-based vaccines against *F. gigantica* using immune bioinformatic tools to construct *in silico* vaccines, and the synthesis of new compounds derived from known drugs are currently under investigation [117, 118].

Future vaccination strategies should focus on different adjuvants, formulations and delivery methods. Furthermore, a comprehensive analysis of vaccine efficacy and the immune responses generated is crucial. To achieve this, relevant host species (ruminants) should be used in experimental studies, with an appropriate number of animals and repeated experiments to ensure statistical robustness [111].

3. Conclusions

Fasciolosis is becoming an increasingly significant emerging issue due to resistance phenomena and limited resources for effective infection control. Epidemiological studies based on up-to-date data could help implement modern and specific control strategies on farms. Forecasting systems based on past and current data could serve as a tool to predict outbreaks, although technical and financial support is needed, especially in resource-limited communities. The future of chemotherapy lies in early diagnosis, combined with the study of the effects of different anthelmintics combinations and the fasciolicidal properties of existing drugs. Additionally, the validation of the anthelmintic activity of plant-based compounds is essential for their use alone or in combination with other anti-fasciolicide techniques. Finally, high-throughput 'omic' technologies have provided unprecedented insights, and further studies on miRNAs and EVs involved in fasciolosis could reveal therapeutic targets for vaccine development.

Acknowledgements

G.H.T.: Writing original draft and design of the work; D.M.B.T.: Participation in drafting; J.P.; Work revision; A.M.M.: Work revision; F.J.M.M.: Work revision; L.M.F.V.: Work revision; L.B.: Work revision; P.J.R.M.: Work revision; V.M.H.: Work revision; M.T.R.C.: Design of the work and work revision.

The authors thank the websites BioRender.com and Canva.com for their help in performing parts of **Figures 1–3**.

Author details

Guillem Herrera-Torres[1], Diana María Barrero-Torres[1], José Pérez[1], Luis Miguel Flores-Velázquez[1], Álvaro Martínez-Moreno[2], Francisco Javier Martínez-Moreno[2], Leandro Buffoni[2], Pablo José Rufino-Moya[2], Verónica Molina-Hernández[1] and María Teresa Ruiz-Campillo[1*]

1 Departament of Anatomy, Pathological Anatomy and Toxicology, Competitive Research Unit: Zoonosis and Emerging Diseases (ENZOEM), University of Córdoba, Córdoba, Spain

2 Departament of Animal Health (Parasitology), Competitive Research Unit: Zoonosis and Emerging Diseases (ENZOEM), University of Córdoba, Córdoba, Spain

*Address all correspondence to: v42rucam@uco.es

References

[1] FAO, OIE, WHO. A Key Role for Veterinary Authorities and Animal Health Practitioners in Preventing and Controlling Neglected Parasitic Zoonoses: A Handbook with Focus on *Taenia Solium*, *Trichinella*, *Echinococcus* and *Fasciola*. Rome, Paris & Geneve: FAO, OIE & WHO; 2021

[2] World Health Organization. Tripartite and UNEP Support OHHLEP's Definition of "One Health" [Internet]. 2021. Available from: https://www.who.int/news/item/01-12-2021-tripartite-and-unep-support-ohhlep-s-definition-of-one-health [Accessed: September 20, 2024]

[3] Nyindo M, Lukambagire A. Fascioliasis: An ongoing zoonotic trematode infection. BioMed Research International. 2015;**2015**:786195. DOI: 10.1155/2015/786195

[4] Rufino-Moya PJ, Zafra R, Martínez-Moreno A, Buffoni L, Valderas E, Pérez J, et al. Advancement in diagnosis, treatment, and vaccines against *Fasciola hepatica*: A comprehensive review. Pathogens. 2024;**13**:669. DOI: 10.3390/pathogens13080669

[5] Mehmood K, Zhang H, Sabir AJ, Abbas RZ, Ijaz M, Durrani AZ, et al. A review on epidemiology, global prevalence and economical losses of fasciolosis in ruminants. Microbial Pathogenesis. 2017;**109**:253-262. DOI: 10.1016/j.micpath.2017.06.006

[6] Flores-Ramos M, Leyva-Gómez G, Rojas-Campos T, Cruz-Mendoza I, Hernández-Campos A, Vera-Montenegro Y, et al. Fosfatriclaben, a prodrug of triclabendazole: Preparation, stability, and fasciolicidal activity of three new intramuscular formulations. Veterinary Parasitology. 2024;**327**:110113. DOI: 10.1016/j.vetpar.2024.110113

[7] Novobilský A, Amaya Solis N, Skarin M, Höglund J. Assessment of flukicide efficacy against *Fasciola hepatica* in sheep in Sweden in the absence of a standardised test. International Journal for Parasitology: Drugs and Drug Resistance. 2016;**6**:141-147. DOI: 10.1016/j.ijpddr.2016.06.004

[8] Kamaludeen J, Grahan-Borwn J, Stephens N, Miller J, Howell A, Beesley NJ, et al. Lack of efficacy of triclabendazole against *Fasciola hepatica* is present on sheep farms in three regions of England, and Wales. The Veterinary Record. 2019;**184**:502. DOI: 10.1136/vr.105209

[9] Fox NJ, White PCL, McClean CJ, Marion G, Evans A, Hutchings MR. Predicting impacts of climate change on *Fasciola hepatica* risk. PLoS One. 2011;**6**:16126-16126. DOI: 10.1371/journal.pone.0016126

[10] Haydock LAJ, Pomroy WE, Stevenson MA, Lawrence KE. A growing degree-day model for determination of *Fasciola hepatica* infection risk in New Zealand with future predictions using climate change models. Veterinary Parasitology. 2016;**228**:52-59. DOI: 10.1016/j.vetpar.2016.05.033

[11] Rojo-Vázquez FA, Meana A, Valcárcel F, Martínez-Valladares M. Update on trematode infections in sheep. Veterinary Parasitology. 2012;**189**:15-38. DOI: 10.1016/j.vetpar.2012.03.029

[12] Molina-Hernández V, Mulcahy G, Pérez J, Martínez-Moreno Á, Donnelly S, O'Neill S, et al. *Fasciola hepatica* vaccine:

We may not be there yet by we're on the right road. Veterinary Parasitology. 2015;**208**:101-111. DOI: 10.1016/j.vetpar.2015.01.004

[13] Zafra R, Buffoni L, Pérez-Caballero R, Molina-Hernández V, Ruiz-Campillo MT, Pérez J, et al. Efficacy of a multivalent vaccine against *Fasciola hepatica* infection in sheep. Veterinary Research. 2021;**52**:13. DOI: 10.1186/s13567-021-00895-0

[14] Beesley NJ, Williams DJL, Paterson S, Hodgkinson J. *Fasciola hepatica* demonstrates high levels of genetic diversity, a lack of population structure and high gene flow: Possible implications for drug resistance. International Journal for Parasitology. 2017;**47**:11-20. DOI: 10.1016/j.ijpara.2016.09.007

[15] Rehman T, Elsaid FG, Garijo-Toledo MM, Gentile A, Gul RA, Rashid M, et al. Fasciolosis: Recent update in vaccines development and their efficacy. Pakistan Veterinary Journal. 2023;**43**:224-231. DOI: 10.29261/pakvetj/2023.034

[16] Cwiklinski K, Donnelly S, Drysdale O, Jewhurst H, Smith D, De Marco Verissimo C, et al. The cathepsin-like cysteine peptidases of trematodes of the genus *Fasciola*. Advances in Parasitology. 2019;**104**:113-164. DOI: 10.1016/bs.apar.2019.01.001

[17] Mas-Coma S, Valero MA, Bargues MD. One health for fascioliasis control in human endemic areas. Trends in Parasitology. 2023;**39**:650-667. DOI: 10.1016/j.pt.2023.05.009

[18] Tidman R, Kanankege KS, Bangert M, Abela-Ridder B. Global prevalence of 4 neglected foodborne trematodes targeted for control by WHO: A scoping review to highlight the gaps. PLoS Neglected Tropical Diseases. 2023;**17**:e0011073. DOI: 10.1371/journal.pntd.0011073

[19] Alba A, Vazquez AA, Hurtrez-Boussès S. Towards the comprehension of fasciolosis (re-)emergence: An integrative overview. Parasitology. 2021;**148**:385-407. DOI: 10.1017/S0031182020002255

[20] Knubben-Schweizer G, Rössier AS, Schade-Weskott E, Torgerson PR. Epidemiology and control. In: Dalton JP, editor. Fasciolosis. Vol. 6. Cambridge (UK): CABI Publishing; 2022. pp. 180-210. DOI: 10.1079/9781789246162.0006

[21] Calvani NED, Šlapeta J. *Fasciola gigantica* and *Fasciola* hybrids in Southeast Asia. In: Dalton JP, editor. Fasciolosis. Vol. 13. Cambridge (UK): CABI Publishing; 2022. pp. 423-460. DOI: 10.1079/9781789246162.0013

[22] Copland RS, Skerratt LF. Options for the control of liver fluke. In: Gray GD, Copland RS, Copeman DB, editors. Overcoming Liver Flike as a Constraint to Ruminant Production in South-East Asia. Vol. 133. Australian Centre of International Agriculture Research (ACIAR). Australian Government. Monograph; 2008. p. 55

[23] Angles R, Buchon P, Valero MA, Bargues MD, Mas-Coma S. One health action against human fascioliasis in the Bolivian Altiplano: Food, water, housing, behavioural traditions, social aspects, and livestock management linked to disease transmission and infection sources. International Journal of Environmental Research and Public Health. 2022;**19**:1120. DOI: 10.3390/ijerph19031120

[24] Mas-Coma S, Valero MA, Bargues MD. Fascioliasis. In: Toledo R, Fried B, editors. Digenetic Trematodes.

Springer Nature; 2024. pp. 157-201. DOI: 10.1007/978-3-031-60121-7

[25] Robles-Pérez D. Nuevas técnicas para el estudio de cepas ovinas de *Fasciola hepatica* con diferente origen y grado de resistencia a fármacos antihelmínticos [thesis]. Dialnet. Universidad de León (Spain); 2015

[26] Liver Fluke Control in Grazing Livestock. Agriculture and Horticulture Development Board [Internet]. Stubbings L (LSSC Limited), Skuce P (Moredun Research Institute) and Williams D (University of Liverpool); 2022. Available from: https://www.scops.org.uk/workspace/pdfs/ahdb-liver-fluke-manual-2022_1.pdf [Accessed: October 10, 2024]

[27] Rondelaud D, Vignoles P, Dreyfuss G, Mage C. The control of *Galba truncatula* (Gastropoda: Lymnaeidae) by the terrestrial snail *Zonitoides nitidus* on acid soils. Biological Control. 2006;**3**:290-299. DOI: 10.1016/j.biocontrol.2006.07.015

[28] Jones RA, Brophy PM, Davis CN, Davies TE, Emberson H, et al. Detection of *Galba truncatula, Fasciola hepatica* and *Calicophoron daubneyi* environmental DNA within water sources on pasture land, a future tool for fluke control? Parasites & Vectors. 2018;**11**:342. DOI: 10.1186/s13071-018-2928-z

[29] Araújo JV, Braga FR, Mendoza-de-Gives P, Paz-Silva A, Vilela VLR. Recent advances in the control of helminths of domestic animals by helminthophagous fungi. Parasitologia. 2021;**1**:168-176. DOI: 10.3390/parasitologia1030018

[30] Braga FR, Araújo JV, Campos AK, Araújo JM, Carvalho RO, Silva AR, et al. *In vitro* evaluation of the action of the nematophagous fungi *Duddingtonia flagrans*, *Monacrosporium sinense* and *Pochonia chlamydosporia* on *Fasciola hepatica* eggs. World Journal of Microbiology and Biotechnology. 2008;**24**:1559-1564. DOI: 10.1007/s11274-007-9643-9

[31] Castro LS, Martins IV, Tunholi VM, Araújo JV, Tunholi-Alves VM, Bittencourt VR. Ovicidal potential of *Pochonia chlamydosporia* isolate Pc-10 (Ascomycota: Sordariomycetes) on egg masses of the snail *Pseudosuccinea columella* (Mollusca: Gastropoda). Journal of Invertebrate Pathology. 2019;**166**:107212. DOI: 10.1016/j.jip.2019.107212

[32] Castro LS, Martins IVF, Alves VMT, Vieira FDPR, Tavares GP, Araújo JV. Effect of the enzymatic fungal extract of *Pochonia chlamydosporia* on the viability of *Fasciola hepatica* eggs. Journal of Advances Veterinary Research. 2020;**10**:135-140

[33] Dias AS, Araújo JV, Braga FR, Puppin AC, Perboni WR. *Pochonia chlamydosporia* in the biological control of *Fasciola hepatica* in cattle in Southeastern Brazil. Parasitology Research. 2013;**112**:2131-2136. DOI: 10.1007/s00436-013-3372-9

[34] Meissner MV. Control biológico de infecciones parasitarias mediante hongos en rumiantes autóctonos del País Vasco [thesis]. Dialnet. Universidad de Santiago de Compostela (Spain); 2022

[35] Muñiz-Pareja FC, Iturbe-Espinoza PA. Effectiveness of *Chaetogaster limnaei* as a controller of *Fasciola hepatica* in experimental infections of *Galba truncatula*. Tropical Parasitology. 2018;**8**:88-93. DOI: 10.4103/tp.TP_24_15

[36] Morales GA, Pino de Morales L. *Fasciola hepatica* y Distomatosis Hepática Bovina en Venezuela. II: Diagnóstico, Tratamiento y Control. CENIAP HOY 2017

[37] Rai RB, Senai S, Ahlawat SPS, Kumar BV. Studies on the control of fascioliasis in Andaman and Nicobar Islands. The Indian Veterinary Journal. 1996;**73**:822-825

[38] Murphy WL, Knutson LV, Chapman EG, Mc Donnell RJ, Williams CD, Foote BA, et al. Key aspects of the biology of snail-killing *Sciomyzidae* flies. Annual Review of Entomology. 2012;**57**:425-447. DOI: 10.1146/annurev-ento-120710-100702

[39] Forbes AB, Scholtz CH. The impact of dung beetles on the free-living stages of ruminant parasites in faeces and their role as biological control agents in grazing livestock. Veterinary Parasitology. 2024;**331**:110267. DOI: 10.1016/j.vetpar.2024.110267

[40] Suhardono RJA, Copeman DB. Biological control of *Fasciola gigantica* with *Echinostoma revolutum*. Veterinary Parasitology. 2006;**140**:166-170. DOI: 10.1016/j.vetpar.2006.02.028

[41] Hourdin P, Rondelaud D, Cabaret J. The development of *Fasciola hepatica* parthenitae in *Lymnaea truncatula* by modification of *Muellerius capillaris* infection. International Journal for Parasitology. 1993;**23**:235-243. DOI: 10.1016/0020-7519(93)90146-p

[42] Jones RA, Williams HW, Dalesman S, Ayodeji S, Thomas RK, Brophy PM. The prevalence and development of digenean parasites within their intermediate snail host, *Galba truncatula*, in a geographic area where the presence of *Calicophoron daubneyi* has recently been confirmed. Veterinary Parasitology. 2017;**240**:68-74. DOI: 10.1016/j.vetpar.2017.03.021

[43] Rizwan HM, Sajid MS, Abbas H, Ghazanfer S, Arshad M. An insight into different strategies for control and prophylaxis of Fasciolosis: A review. Journal of Advances in International Veterinary Research. 2022;**4**:5-14. DOI: 10.30564/jaivr.v4i1.4665

[44] European Medicines Agency [Internet]. Available from: https://www.ema.europa.eu/en/documents/scientific-guideline/reflection-paper-anthelmintic-resistance_en.pdf-0 [Accessed: October 10, 2024]

[45] Pedreira-García J, Díaz-Fernández P, Arias-Vázquez MS. In: Servet, editor. Guías prácticas en producción bovina. Zaragoza: Parasitología y enfermedades parasitarias; 2017

[46] Hernández-Malagón JA, Fl A-B, Bonilla-Quintero R, Sanchez-Andrade-Fernandez R, Arias-Vázquez MS. Control biológico de parásitos en la ganadería. Hongos del suelo. Zoociencia. 2015;**2**:3-11

[47] Rathinasamy V, Tran L, Swan J, Kelley J, Hosking C, Williamson G, et al. Towards understanding the liver fluke transmission dynamics on farms: Detection of liver fluke transmitting snail and liver fluke-specific environmental DNA in water samples from an irrigated dairy farm in Southeast Australia. Veterinary Parasitology. 2021;**291**:109373. DOI: 10.1016/j.vetpar.2021.109373

[48] Fairweather I, Brennan GP, Hanna REB, Robinson MW, Skuce PJ. Drug resistance in liver flukes. International Journal for Parasitology: Drugs and Drug Resistance. 2020;**12**:39-59. DOI: 10.1016/j.ijpddr.2019.11.003

[49] Lalor R, Cwiklinski K, Calvani NED, Dorey A, Hamon S, Corrales JL, et al. Pathogenicity and virulence of the liver flukes *Fasciola hepatica* and *Fasciola gigantica* that cause the zoonosis Fasciolosis. Virulence. 2021;**12**:2839-2867. DOI: 10.1080/21505594.2021.1996520

[50] Olah S, van Wyk JA, Wall R, Morgan ER. FAMACHA©: A potential tool for targeted selective treatment of chronic fasciolosis in sheep. Veterinary Parasitology. 2015;**212**:188-192. DOI: 10.1016/j.vetpar.2015.07.012

[51] Alba A, Grech-Angelini S, Vázquez AA, Alda P, Blin Q, Lemmonier L, et al. Fasciolosis in the Mediterranean island of Corsica (France): Insights from epidemiological and malacological investigations. Food and Waterborne Parasitology. 2023;**30**:e00188. DOI: 10.1016/j.fawpar.2023.e00188

[52] Boray JC. Fortschritte in der Bekämpfung der Fasciolose. Schweizer Archivfür Tierheilkunde. 1971;**113**:361-386

[53] John BC, Davies DR, Howell AK, Williams DJL, Hodgkinson JE. Anaerobic fermentation results in loss of viability of *Fasciola hepatica* metacercariae in grass silage. Veterinary Parasitology. 2020;**285**:109218. DOI: 10.1016/j.vetpar.2020.109218

[54] Madsen H, Stauffer JR. Zoonotic trematode infections; their biology, intermediate hosts and control. In: Morales-Montor J, Del Río-Araiza VH, Hernandéz-Bello R, editors. Parasitic Helminths and Zoonoses: From Basic to Applied Research. Vol. 16. London, UK, London (UK): BoD–Books on Demand. IntechOpen; 2022. pp. 291-326. DOI: 10.5772/intechopen.102434

[55] Castro-Hermida JA, Gonzalez-Warleta M, Martinez SV, Ubeira FM, Mezo M. Current challenges for fasciolicide treatment in ruminant livestock. Trends in Parasitology. 2021;**37**:430-444. DOI: 10.1016/j.pt.2020.12.003

[56] Álvarez LI, Lanusse CE, Williams DJL, Fairweather I, Hodgkinson JE. Flukicidal drugs: Pharmaco- therapeutics and drug resistance. In: Dalton JP, editor. Fasciolosis. Vol. 7. Cambridge (UK): CABI Publishing; 2022. p. 211, 272. DOI: 10.1079/9781789246162.0006

[57] Boray JC, Crowfoot P, Strong M, Allison J, Schellenbaum M, von Orelli M, et al. Treatment of immature and mature *Fasciola hepatica* infections in sheep with Triclabendazole. The Veterinary Record. 1983;**113**:315-317. DOI: 10.1136/vr.113.14.315

[58] Maqbool I, Wani ZA, Shahardar RA, Allaie IM, Shah MM. Integrated parasite management with special reference to gastro-intestinal nematodes. Journal of Parasitic Diseases. 2017;**41**:1-8. DOI: 10.1007/s12639-016-0765-6

[59] European Medicines Agency (EMA). Reflection paper on anthelmintic resistance. EMA/CVMP/EWP/573536/2013. Committee of Medical Products for Veterinary use (CVMP). 2017. Available from: https://www.ema.europa.eu/en/documents/scientific-guideline/reflection-paper-anthelmintic-resistance_en.pdf-0 [Accessed: October 15, 2024]

[60] Domke AV, Chartier C, Gjerde B, Leine N, Vatn S, Østerås O, et al. Worm control practice against gastro-intestinal parasites in Norwegian sheep and goat flocks. Acta Veterinaria Scandinavica. 2011;**53**:29. DOI: 10.1186/1751-0147-53-29

[61] Hodgkinson JE, Kaplan RM, Kenyon F, Morgan ER, Park AW, Paterson S, et al. Refugia and anthelmintic resistance: Concepts and challenges. International Journal for Parasitology: Drugs and Drug Resistance. 2019;**10**:51-57. DOI: 10.1016/j.ijpddr.2019.05.001

[62] Flanagan A, Edgar HWJ, Gordon A, Hanna RE, Brennan GP, Fairweather I. Comparison of two assays, a faecal egg count reduction test (FECRT) and a coproantigen reduction test (CRT), for the diagnosis of resistance to triclabendazole in *Fasciola hepatica* in sheep. Veterinary Parasitology. 2011;**176**:170-176. DOI: 10.1016/j.vetpar.2010.10.057

[63] Hutchinson GW, Dawson K, Fitzgibbon CC, Martin PJ. Efficacy of an injectable combination anthelmintic (nitroxynil+clorsulon+ivermec tin) against early immature *Fasciola hepatica* compared to triclabendazole combination flukicides given orally or topically to cattle. Veterinary Parasitology. 2009;**162**(3-4):278-284. DOI: 10.1016/j.vetpar.2009.03.032

[64] Carroll JA, Forsberg NE. Influence of stress and nutrition on cattle immunity. The Veterinary Clinics of North America. Food Animal Practice. 2007;**23**:105-149. DOI: 10.1016/j.cvfa.2007.01.003

[65] Coop RL, Kyriazakis I. Influence of host nutrition on the development and consequences of nematode parasitism in ruminants. Trends in Parasitology. 2001;**17**:325-330. DOI: 10.1016/s1471-4922(01)01900-6

[66] Graber M. Role of diet in bovine and ovine fascioliasis caused by *Fasciola gigantica*. Bulletin of Epizootic Disease of Africa. 1971;**19**:45-60

[67] Nour AM, Abou-Akkada AR, Badr MF, El-Shazly K. The effect of type of ration on some blood components and daily gain of sheep infected with *Fasciola gigantica*. Alexandria Journal of Agricultural Research. 1979;**27**:52

[68] Pawłowska M, Mila-Kierzenkowska C, Szczegielniak J, Woźniak A. Oxidative stress in parasitic diseases—Reactive oxygen species as mediators of interactions between the host and the parasites. Antioxidants. 2023;**13**:38. DOI: 10.3390/antiox13010038

[69] Martínez-Pérez JM, Robles-Pérez D, Rojo-Vázquez FA, Martínez-Valladares M. Effect of dietary supplementation with flaxseed oil or 192 vitamin E on sheep experimentally infected with *Fasciola hepatica*. Research in Veterinary Science. 2014;**97**:71-79. DOI: 10.1016/j.rvsc.2014.05.009

[70] Gabrashanska M, Teodorova SE, Anisimova M. Oxidative-antioxidant status of *Fasciola hepatica*-infected rats supplemented with zinc. A mathematical model for zinc bioaccumulation and host growth. Parasitology Research. 2008;**104**:69-78. DOI: 10.1007/s00436-008-1160-8

[71] Piedrafita D, Spithill TW, Smith RE, Raadsma HW. Improving animal and human health through understanding liver fluke immunology. Parasite Immunology. 2010;**32**(8):572-581. DOI: 10.1111/j.1365-3024.2010.01223.x

[72] Piedrafita D, Estuningsih E, Pleasance J, Prowse R, Raadsma HW, Meeusen EN, et al. Peritoneal lavage cells of Indonesian thin-tail sheep mediate antibody-dependent superoxide radical cytotoxicity *in vitro* against newly excysted juvenile *Fasciola gigantica* but not juvenile *Fasciola hepatica*. Infection and Immunity. 2007;**75**:1954-1963. DOI: 10.1128/IAI.01034-06

[73] Pleasance J, Raadsma HW, Estuningsih SE, Widjajanti S, Meeusen E, Piedrafita D. Innate and adaptive resistance of Indonesian thin tail sheep to liver fluke: A comparative analysis of *Fasciola gigantica* and *Fasciola hepatica* infection. Veterinary Parasitology. 2011;**178**(3-4):264-272. DOI: 10.1016/j.vetpar.2011.01.037

[74] Gruner L, Bouix J, Cabaret J, Boulard C, Cortet J, Sauve C, et al. Effect of genetic type, lactation and management on helminth infection of ewes in an intensive grazing system on irrigated pasture. International Journal for Parasitology. 1992;**22**(7):919-925. DOI: 10.1016/0020-7519(92)90048-P

[75] Afshan K, Qayyum M, Rizvi SSR, Mukhtar M, Mushtaq M, Miller JE. Serological and coprological comparison for rapid diagnosis of *Fasciola hepatica* infection in small ruminants from sub-tropical area of Pakistan. Small Ruminant Research. 2013;**113**(1):267-272. DOI: 10.1016/j.smallrumres.2013.01.020

[76] Eguale T, Mekonnen GA, Chaka H. Evaluation of variation in susceptibility of three Ethiopian sheep breeds to experimental infection with *Fasciola hepatica*. Small Ruminant Research. 2009;**82**(1):7-12. DOI: 10.1016/j.smallrumres.2008.12.017

[77] Haroun E, Elsanhouri A, Gameel A. Response of goats to repeated infections with *Fasciola gigantica*. Veterinary Parasitology. 1989;**30**:287-296. DOI: 10.1016/0304-4017(89)90098-8

[78] Mulcahy G, Dalton JP. Cathepsin L proteinases as vaccines against infection with *Fasciola hepatica* (liver fluke) in ruminants. Research in Veterinary Science. 2001;**70**:83-86. DOI: 10.1053/rvsc.2000.0425

[79] Moazeni M, Ardakani ZSS, Saharkhiz MJ, Jalaei J, Khademolhoseini AA, Abad SSE, et al. *In vitro* ovicidal activity of *Peganum harmala* seeds extract on the eggs of *Fasciola hepatica*. Journal of Parasitic Diseases. 2017;**41**:467-472. DOI: 10.1007/s12639-016-0830-1

[80] Moazeni M, Khademolhoseini AA. Ovicidal effect of the methanolic extract of ginger (*Zingiber officinale*) on *Fasciola hepatica* eggs: An *in vitro* study. Journal of Parasitic Diseases. 2016;**40**:662-666. DOI: 10.1007/s12639-014-0554-z

[81] Pereira CAJ, Oliveira LLS, Coaglio AL, Santos FSO, Cezar RSM, Mendes T, et al. Anti-helminthic activity of Momordica charantia L. against *Fasciola hepatica* eggs after twelve days of incubation *in vitro*. Veterinary Parasitology. 2016;**228**:160-166. DOI: 10.1016/j.vetpar.2016.08.025

[82] Kandil OM, Hassan NM, Sedky D, Ata EB, Nassar SA, Shalaby HA, et al. Anthelmintic efficacy of *Moringa oleifera* seed methanolic extract against *Fasciola hepatica*. Journal of Parasitic Diseases. 2018;**42**:391-401. DOI: 10.1007/s12639-018-1014-y

[83] Marques LT, Guedes RA, Rodrigues WD, Archanjo AB, Severi JA, Martins IVF. Chemical composition of various plant extracts and their *in vitro* efficacy in control of *Fasciola hepatica* eggs. Ciencia Rural. 2020;**50**:5. DOI: 10.1590/0103-8478cr20190363

[84] Abdelaal MMO, Brennan GP, Abdel-Aziz A, Fairweather I. Ultrastructural changes to the tegumental system and gastrodermal cells of adult *Fasciola hepatica* following treatment *in vivo* with a commercial preparation of myrrh (Mirazid). Journal of Helminthology. 2017;**62**:336-347. DOI: 10.1017/S0022149X16000705

[85] Ullah R, Rehman A, Zafeer MF, Rehman L, Khan YA, Khan MAH, et al. Anthelmintic potential of Thymoquinone and curcumin on *Fasciola gigantica*. PLoS One. 2017;**12**:e0171267. DOI: 10.1371/journal.pone.0171267

[86] Wulandari AR, Nurlaelasari A, Nugroho HA, Cahyadi M, Kurniawan W, Hamid PH. Ethanolic extract of *Etlingera*

elatior flower exhibits anthelmintic properties to *Fasciola gigantica in vitro*. Open Veterinary Journal. 2023;**13**:576-587. DOI: 10.5455/OVJ.2023.v13.i5.10

[87] Shaquif A, Ranwal R, Qureshi RU, Chaudhry FR. *In vitro* screening of *Cymbopogon jwarancusa* and *Conyza canadensis* against liver flukes. Tropical Biomedicine. 2015;**32**:407-412

[88] Álvarez-Mercado J, Ibarra-Velarde F, Alonso-Díaz MA, Vera-Motenegro Y, Ávila-Acevedo JG, García-Bores AM. *In vitro* anthelmintic effect of fifteen tropical plant extracts on excysted flukes of *Fasciola hepatica*. BMC Veterinary Research. 2015;**11**:45. DOI: 10.1186/s12917-015-0362-4

[89] Yamson EC, Tubalinal GASP, Viloria VV, Mingala CN. Anthelmintic effect of betel nut (*Areca catechu*) and neem (*Azadirachta indica*) extract against liver fluke (*Fasciola* spp.). Journal of Advanced Veterinary and Animal Research. 2019;**6**:44-49. DOI: 10.5455/javar.2019.e310

[90] Luis HC, Matias FBR, Tubalinal GAS, Mingala CN. *In vitro* anthelminthic activity of friend spiderflower (*Cleome rutidosperma*) ethanolic leaf extract against *Fasciola* spp. Annals of Parasitology. 2021;**67**:243-248. DOI: 10.17420/ap6702.335

[91] de Mello AB, Fruet-Baccega B, Obelar-Martins F, da Rosa-Farias NA, de Giacometi M, da Fonseca RN, et al. Microscopic alterations in *Fasciola hepatica* treated with the essential oils in *Pelargonium graveolens* and *Citrus aurantium*. Veterinary Parasitology. 2023;**314**:109863. DOI: 10.1016/j.vetpar.2022.109863

[92] de Mello AB, Baccega B, Martins FO, de Santi II, Islabão YW, de Giacometi M, et al. Activity of cumin essential oil to control fascioliasis: Efficacy and changes in the tegument of *Fasciola hepatica*. Experimental Parasitology. 2023;**252**:108587. DOI: 10.1016/j.exppara.2023.108587

[93] Allahyari M, Malekifard F, Yakhchali M. Anthelmintic effects of some medicinal plants on different life stages of *Fasciola hepatica*: Evidence of oxidative stress biomarkers, and DNA damage. PLOS Neglected Tropical Diseases. 2024;**18**:e0012251. DOI: 10.1371/journal.pntd.0012251

[94] Singh P, Verma AK, Jacob AB, Gupta SC, Mehra RU. Hematological and biochemical changes in *Fasciola gigantica* infected buffaloes fed on diet containing deoiled mahua (*Bassia latifolia*) seed cake. Journal of Applied Animal Research. 2011;**39**:185-188. DOI: 10.1080/09712119.2011.607703

[95] Meister I, Duthaler U, Huwyler J, Rinaldi L, Bosco A, Cringoli G, et al. Efficacy and pharmacokinetics of OZ78 and MT04 against a natural infection with *Fasciola hepatica* in sheep. Veterinary Parasitology. 2013;**198**:102-110. DOI: 10.1016/j.vetpar.2013.08.007

[96] Keiser J, Rinaldi L, Veneziano V, Mezzino L, Tanner M, Utzinger J, et al. Efficacy and safety of artemether against a natural *Fasciola hepatica* infection in sheep. Parasitology Research. 2008;**103**:517-522. DOI: 10.1007/s00436-008-0998-0

[97] Keiser J, Veneziano V, Rinaldi L, Mezzino L, Duthaler U, Cringoli G. Anthelmintic activity of artesunate against *Fasciola hepatica* in naturally infected sheep. Research in Veterinary Science. 2010;**88**:107-110. DOI: 10.1016/j.rvsc.2009.05.007

[98] Abbas RZ. Anthelmintic effects and toxicity analysis of herbal Dewormer

against the infection of *Haemonchus contortus* and *Fasciola hepatica* in goat. Pakistan Veterinary Journal. 2020;**40**:455-460. DOI: 10.29261/pakvetj/2020.083

[99] Flores-Velázquez LM, Ruiz-Campillo MT, Herrera-Torres G, Martínez-Moreno Á, Martínez-Moreno FJ, Zafra R, et al. Fasciolosis: Pathogenesis, host-parsite interactions, and implication in vaccine development. Frontiers in Veterinary Science. 2023;**11**:1270064. DOI: 10.3389/fvets.2023.1270064

[100] Dominguez MF, González-Miguel J, Carmona C, Dalton JP, Cwiklinski K, Tort J, et al. Low allelic diversity in vaccine candidates genes from different locations sustain hope for *Fasciola hepatica* immunization. Veterinary Parasitology. 2018;**258**:46-52. DOI: 10.1016/j.vetpar.2018.06.011

[101] Spithill TW, Toet H, Rathinasamy V, Zerna G, Swan J, Cameron T, et al. Vaccines for *Fasciola*: New thinking for an old problem. In: Dalton JP, editor. Fasciolosis. 2nd ed. Cambridge: CABI Publishing; 2022. pp. 379-422. DOI: 10.1079/9781789246162.0012

[102] Kueakhai P, Changklungmoa N, Cheukamud W, Osotprasit S, Chantree P, Preyavichyapugdee N, et al. The combined recombinant cathepsin L1H and cathepsin B3 vaccine against *Fasciola gigantica* infection. Parasitology International. 2021;**83**:102353. DOI: 10.1016/j.parint.2021.102353

[103] Changklungmoa N, Cheukamud W, Jaikua W, Meemon K, Sobhon P, Kueakhai P. Combination vaccines of *Fasciola gigantica* Saposin-like Protein-2 and leucine aminopeptidase. Tropical Medicine and Infectious Disease. 2023;**8**:334. DOI: 10.3390/tropicalmed8070334

[104] Wesołowska A, Basałaj K, Norbury LJ, Sielicka A, Wędrychowicz H, Zawistowska-Deniziak A. Vaccination against *Fasciola hepatica* using cathepsin L3 and B3 proteases delivered alone or in combination. Veterinary Parasitology. 2018a;**250**:15-21. DOI: 10.1016/j.vetpar.2017.12.007

[105] Kesik-Brodacka M, Lipiec A, Kozak Ljunggren M, Jedlina L, Miedzinska K, Mikolajczak M, et al. Immune response of rats vaccinated orally with various plant-expressed recombinant cysteine proteinase constructs when challenged with *Fasciola hepatica* metacercariae. PLoS Neglected Tropical Diseases. 2017;**11**:E0005451. DOI: 10.1371/journal.pntd.0005451

[106] Wesołowska A, Kozak Ljunggren M, Jedlina L, Basałaj K, Legocki A, Wedrychowicz H, et al. A preliminary study of a lettuce-based edible vaccine expressing the cysteine proteinase of *Fasciola hepatica* for Fasciolosis control in livestock. Frontiers in Immunology. 2018b;**9**:2592. DOI: 10.3389/fimmu.2018.02592

[107] Villa-Mancera A, Olivares-Pérez J, Olmedo-Juárez A, Reynoso-Palomar A. Phage display-based vaccine with cathepsin L and excretory-secretory products mimotopes of *Fasciola hepatica* induces protective cellular and humoral immune responses in sheep. Veterinary Parasitology. 2021;**289**:109340. DOI: 10.1016/j.vetpar.2020.109340

[108] Villa-Mancera A, Alcalá-Canto Y, Olivares-Pérez J, Molina-Mendoza P, Hernández-Guzmán K, Utrera-Quintana F, et al. Vaccination with cathepsin L mimotopes of *Fasciola hepatica* in goats reduces worm burden, morphometric measurements, and reproductive structures. Microbial Pathogenesis. 2021;**155**:104859. DOI: 10.1016/j.micpath.2021.104859

[109] Ruiz-Campillo MT, Pacheco IL, Abril N, Bautista MJ, Martínez-Moreno Á, Martínez-Moreno FJ, et al. Evaluation of Th1/Th2, regulatory cytokines and transcriptional factor FoxP3 in sheep immunized with a partially protective and non-protective vaccine and challenged with *Fasciola hepatica*. Veterinary Research. 2024;**55**:53. DOI: 10.1186/s13567-024-01308-8

[110] Cwiklinski K, Dalton JP, Dufresne PJ, La Course J, Williams DJ, Hodgkinson J, et al. The *Fasciola hepatica* genome: Gene duplication and polymorphism reveal adaptation to the host environment and the capacity for rapid evolution. Genome Biology. 2015;**16**:71. DOI: 10.1186/s13059-015-0632-2

[111] Cwiklinski K, Dalton JP. Exploiting comparative omics to understand the pathogenic and virulence-associated protease: Anti-protease relationships in the zoonotic parasites *Fasciola hepatica* and *Fasciola gigantica*. Genes (Basel). 2022;**13**:1854. DOI: 10.3390/genes13101854

[112] Trelis M, Sánchez-López CM, Sánchez-Palencia LF, Ramírez-Toledo V, Marcilla A, Bernal D. Proteomic analysis of extracellular vesicles from *Fasciola hepatica* hatching eggs and juveniles in culture. Frontiers in Cellular and Infection Microbiology. 2022;**12**:903602. DOI: 10.3389/fcimb.2022.903602

[113] Sheng ZA, Wu CL, Wang DY, Zhong SH, Yang X, Rao GS, et al. Proteomic analysis of exosome-like vesicles from *Fasciola gigantica* adult worm provides support for new vaccine targets against fascioliasis. Parasites & Vectors. 2023;**16**:62. DOI: 10.1186/s13071-023-05659-7

[114] Tran N, Ricafrente A, To J, Lund M, Marques TM, Gama-Carvalho M, et al. *Fasciola hepatica* hijacks host macrophage miRNA machinery to modulate early innate immune responses. Scientific Reports. 2021;**11**:6712. DOI: 10.1038/s41598-021-86125-1

[115] Sais D, Chowdhury S, Dalton JP, Tran N, Donnelly S. Both host and parasite non-coding RNAs co-ordinate the regulation of macrophage gene expression to reduce pro-inflammatory immune responses and promote tissue repair pathways during infection with *Fasciola hepatica*. RNA Biology. 2024;**21**:62-77. DOI: 10.1080/15476286.2024.2408706

[116] Chowdhury S, Ricafrente A, Cwiklinski K, Sais F, Dalton JP, Tran N, et al. Exploring the utility of circulating miRNAs as diagnostic biomarkers of fasciolosis. Scientific Reports. 2024;**14**:7431. DOI: 10.1038/s41598-024-57704-9

[117] Das KC, Konhar R, Biswal DK. *Fasciola gigantica* vaccine construct: An *in silico* approach towards identification and design of a multi-epitope subunit vaccine using calcium binding EF-hand proteins. BMC Immunology. 2023;**24**:1. DOI: 10.1186/s12865-022-00535-y

[118] Valderas-García E, Castilla-Gómez de Agüero V, González Del Palacio L, Galli G, Escala N, Ruiz-Somacarrera M, et al. New benzimidazole derivative compounds with *in vitro* fasciolicidal properties. Parasites & Vectors. 2024;**17**:173. DOI: 10.1186/s13071-024-06224-6

Chapter 4

Evolutionary Lineage of Invasive Anisakidae of Zoonotic Significance under Environmental Influence

Sandeep K. Malhotra and Anita Yadav

Abstract

The search for the ancestors of roundworms with zoonotic significance that cause diseases in humans has faced obstacles because nematodes have evolved multiple times over the course of evolution. Biogeographical evidence traces the drainage pathways of streams leading to the Tethys Ocean, which formed 65 million years ago, and as it receded over time, it drained into what became the Arabian Sea 100 million years ago. The dispersal of species, therefore, contributed additional inputs to the marine ecosystem, while riverine connectivity along a stretch of 2000 km from the Himalayas was effectively maintained. The simple filamentous *Rhabdochona* represented the initial fauna that exclusively parasitized the family Cyprinidae in the Garhwal Himalaya riverine ecosystem, and climate change-induced characteristics caused significant alterations in the fauna. The turning point led to the emergence of *Tridentocamallanus indica* n.gen., n.sp., and Pronakid n.gen., the latter of which possessed both camallanine and anisakid characteristics. The differentiation of buccal capsule, with or without complete or incomplete sclerotized striations, was recorded in *T. indica* regardless of sexual dimorphism. To address erroneous interpretations arising from severe mixing of taxonomic characters, 10 genera under *T. indica* n.gen., n.sp. have been synonymized. Due to adaptations from evolution, newer advanced characteristics, such as intestinal ceca, ventriculus, and ventricular appendix, were acquired, leading to the development of a robust anisakid, that is, *Rotundocollarette capoori*.

Keywords: Tethys Ocean, Arabian Sea, Garhwal Himalayas, anisakidae, zoonotic, *Rotundocollarette capoori*, anisakid evolution

1. Introduction

Admittedly, the evidence of *Rhabdochona* having spread from Asia, thereby giving rise to all American species, was clearly illustrated [1]. It is strongly emphasized that "nematodes of this genus most probably originated in the region of present southern Asia at the beginning of the Tertiary." This means that the focus of current investigations has essentially been on Southern Asia. From here, the spread and adaptation of *Rhabdochona*, along with members of Leuciscinae that originated from Asia, remains a mystery, as they adapted effectively to associated fish groups and spread across South and Central, as well as North America. In the situation outlined in Ref. [1], due to the lack of molecular analysis and insufficient cladistics data, it is very difficult to draw conclusions about the phylogeny of members of Rhabdochonidae members. Therefore, conclusions about the origin and evolution of Rhabdochonidae members can only be drawn from the morphology and distribution of available species, their interacting relationships, the types of obligatory hosts, and their phylogeny. This investigation aims to provide a detailed analysis and interpretation of morphometric data from freshly collected organisms and on the overlapping structural organization of newer taxa in comparative terms. This will help determine the evolutionary pathways originating from drainages along the Tethys Sea, influenced by the varied environments of the Himalayas, Gangetic plains, and Arabian Sea.

2. Materials and methods

The map-covering area of investigations in Garhwal Himalayas, as well as Arabian Sea and other parts of the country, include recently discovered *Ilhe Grande* Island, 19 kms. Away from Panaji (Goa). Forty-seven fishes of Family Cyprinidae*, viz. Nemacheilus rupicola* collected at 525–575 meters above sea level, yielded 18 roundworms of *Rhabdochona* sp., which were identified to be *Rhabdochona nemacheli* [2] from river Alakhnanda, examined at Pauri (Garhwal), U.P., India. Its phylogeny was difficult to be established on account of non-availability of sophisticated techniques in those years. However, details of their origin and biogeographical association helped elaborate the existing host-parasite interactions and morphometric assessment, which were used to critically differentiate the newly established species [2] from congeneric species in the Garhwal Himalayas.

The details of other nematodes investigated during this study are available [3] illustrating methodology of *Rotundocollarette capoori*.

3. Results and discussion

The nematodes are known to have evolved after their origin several times during the course of evolution [4]. The possibility of *Rhabdochona*'s origin being associated with the extinct basins that once flowed across the Tethys Sea cannot be ruled out [5].

The first representative of the genus *Rhabdochona* from India, *that is, R. nemacheli* was first reported (**Figure 1**) in a hill-stream fish, *Nemacheilus rupicola* [2]. The cold water streams of Garhwal Himalayas in the Northern State of Uttar Pradesh in India were actually a part of ancient streams of Tethys Ocean that receded to contribute to the aquatic reservoir of Arabian Sea 100 M.Y.A.

The biogeographical changes following the onset of tectonic movements of the Earth's plates indicated a noticeable connectivity between the Atlantic and Indian Oceans through the Tethys Ocean link 65 million years ago, during the Late

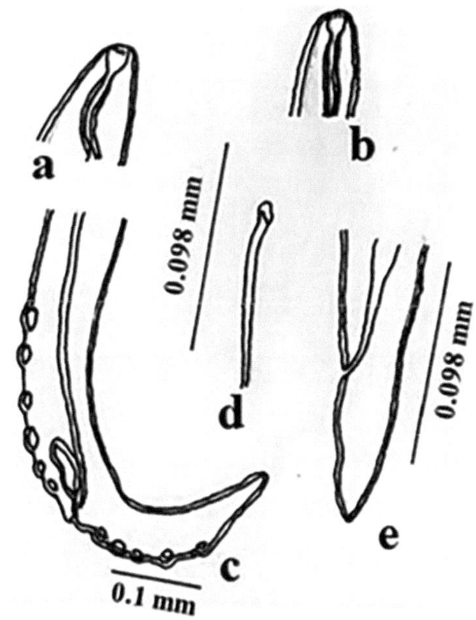

Figure 1.
Rhabdochona nemacheli *(Rautela and Malhotra [2]). (a) Male—anterior end of worm; (b) female—anterior end of worm; (c) posterior end of worm to show spicules in male; (d) terminal part of left larger spicule; (e) posterior end of body of female worm.*

Cretaceous period (**Figure 2a**) [6]. To counter the effect of vicariance, biologically induced dispersal was more noticeable in segregating the South African stock of sardine fishes, which was influenced by the climate change. These fishes were impacted by warm waters from the western Indian Ocean (Agulhas Current) and cold waters from the Benguela Current, flowing from the South Atlantic Ocean (**Figure 1a-e**). These characteristics were considered indicative of potential bioindicators. The association of *Rhabdochona*'s origin with the flow of streams into the Tethys Sea has also been emphasized [5]. The family Cyprinidae has played a primary role in this association, as it includes the most favored hosts of *Rhabdochona* spp. across various biogeographical regions worldwide. However, their dispersal in the South American region was limited due to the absence of cyprinid fish populations in that area [5].

The association of species of *Rhabdochona* within America also did not reflect monophyly. This too verified the multiple point origin of species under this genus. The Australasian region was deprived of the spurt of origin of *Rhabdochona* spp. The chief affiliation of *Rhabdochona* was encountered with their cyprinid fish host and their distribution within basins in the stretches of northern segment was linked to the drainages of the erstwhile Tethys Ocean. This illustrated the dispersal pathways of the worms.

The genus *Rhabdochona* is a member of subfamily Rhabdochoninae [7, 8], under family Rhabdochonidae, under the superfamily Thelazioidea [9, 10]. It is usually characterized by the presence or absence of rudimentary pseudolabia; a hexagonal or spherical oral aperture; frequent presence of buccal teeth in the anterior end of the vestibule, the absence of caudal alae along with sessile caudal papillae. A raised proportion of host-specificity assigned to *Rhabdochona* was concluded [8]. The most frequent parasitization of a variety of *Rhabdochona* was encountered in the fish

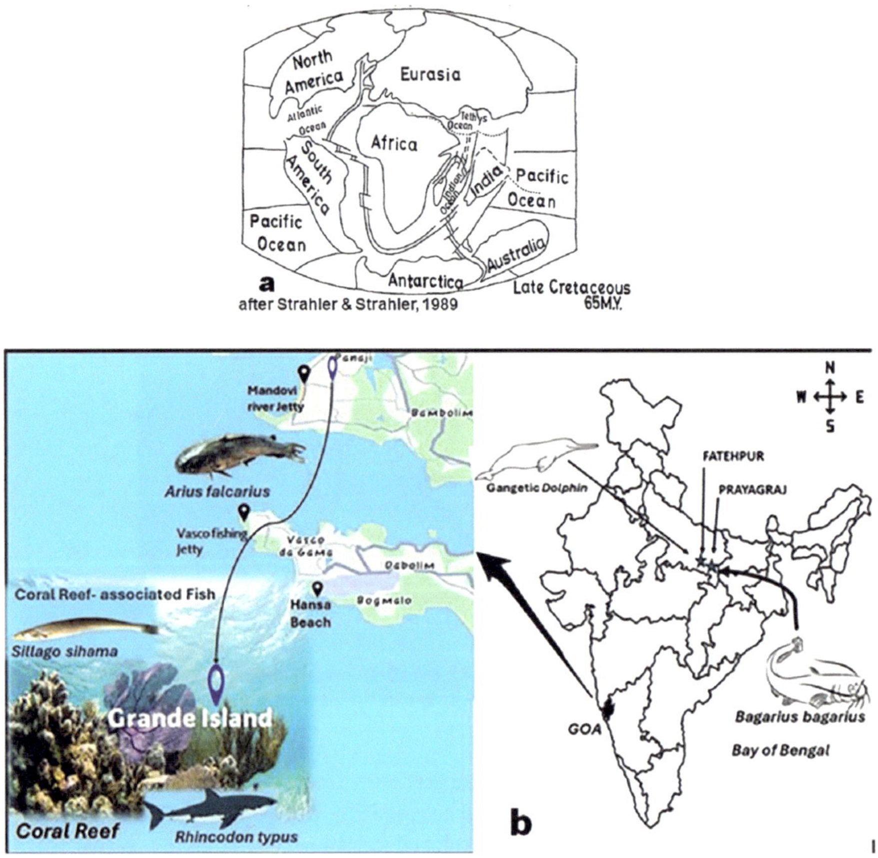

Figure 2.
(a) Biogeographic connectivity of subcontinents (schematic) (after Strahler and Strahler [6]). (b) Sites of investigation at Grande Island (19Kms from Panaji, Goa) at the Central West coast of India).

hosts encompassed under monophyletic lineages (e.g., 43 species in cyprinids, five in salmonids, three in catostomids, two in goodeids). The adoption of consistent co-evolution was, however, a striking characteristic, mainly because of such lineage restrictions. But excessive host-switching coupled with unrestricted ecological host extensions was adopted by *Rhabdochona* spp. during its long evolutionary history, mainly because of diversified host-parasite associations as well as the distribution advancements.

Rhabdochona has been strongly characterized as monophyletic based on the analyzed phylogeny [5]. The evolutionary lineage of the group that did not comprise monophyletic assemblages, for instance, other than Cyprinidae family of host fishes of *Rhabdochona*, commonly adopted exhaustive host-switching and did not conform to co-speciation. *Rhabdochona*, after its origin in the Tethys Ocean region, therefore, evolved further to give rise to organisms bearing identical buccal capsule structure, particularly to the worms of Camallanidae (Super order: Camallanoidea) [11], *Camallanid* genera *Camallanus* and *Procamallanus*, as well as the subgenera *Procamallanus* and *Spirocamallanus* are confirmed to be paraphyletic. Paraphyly has also been found within Filarioidea, Habronematoidea, and Thelazioidea and in Cystidicolidae, Physalopteridae, and Thelaziidae. The results of the analyses also show that *Neoascarophis*, *Spinitectus*, and *Rhabdochona* are monophyletic, in contrast to the paraphyletic genus *Ascarophis*. This further confirms the independence of two subgenera, *Rhabdochona* and *Globochona*, in the genus *Rhabdochona*. Evidently, host-switching played a crucial role in the evolution of Camallanidae from *Rhabdochonidae* inasmuch as that the colder stream from Himalayas, as they traversed down to the Bay of Bengal, traversing across 2000kms downstream in the Ganga Basin (**Figure 2b**), several accompanying events evolved, among which the emergence of first-connecting link, *that is*, *Indospinezia* (Tribe: Indospineziinea) (**Figure 3**) [12] between Camallanidae and Anisakidae was a critical discovery. During the prior evolutionary events, when *Procamallanus chauhanensis* [13] and *Paracamallanus tridenti* [14] (**Figure 4**) along with a host of other worms reported under Camallanoidea [11] with typical characteristics of subfamily Camallaninae emerged, the development of specific features of sclerotization in the buccal capsule of camallanid nematodes, as an advancement from rhabdochonid's funnel-shaped buccal capsule, noticeably explained the linkage characteristics. The last significant introduction to the evolutionary lineage under family Camallanidae was apparently *Tridentocamallanus indica* n.gen., n.sp. (**Figure 5**), apparently studded with a prominent sclerotized buccal capsule, a pair of tridents placed dorsally and ventrally, combined with typical physalopterid characters exemplified by the unique heavily papillated body surface and the unique muscularized/sclerotized cephalic collarette.

The following text summarized morphometric characteristics of *Tridentocamallanus indica* n.gen., n.sp. as published by Yadav *et al.*, (accepted):-A sturdy architecture of roundworms comprised multiple papillations in varied patterns all over the body of the worm. Worms (male, 1.76–3.09 (2.80) x 0.21–0.28 (0.28)mm; female, 2.86–4.31 (3.90) x 0.15–0.19 (0.17)mm) in size. A set of specialized papillae on circumoral flange is shown in **Figure 5**). The cuticularized labial flange comprised four sensory pits. A prominent cephalic collarette with a unique terminal frill was present in the anterior part of body of the worm. The thick cuticularized striations on inner wall of buccal capsule, 11–13 in females, though incomplete spiral striations were encountered on the inner walls of males. A typically bifid and papillated mucron was present at the tail tip of female (**Figure 6**) as well as male. Male worms were with

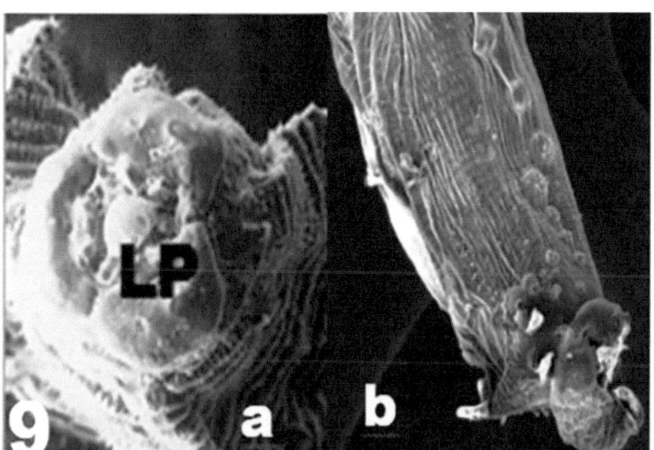

Figure 3.
Indospinezia multispinatum *from freshwater riverine ecosystems at Prayagraj, U.P., India. 9) Scanning electron micrographs to show—(a) triangular lid on oral aperture atop cephalic complex. (b) Posterior part of worm to show sunflower papillae and foliate papilla.*

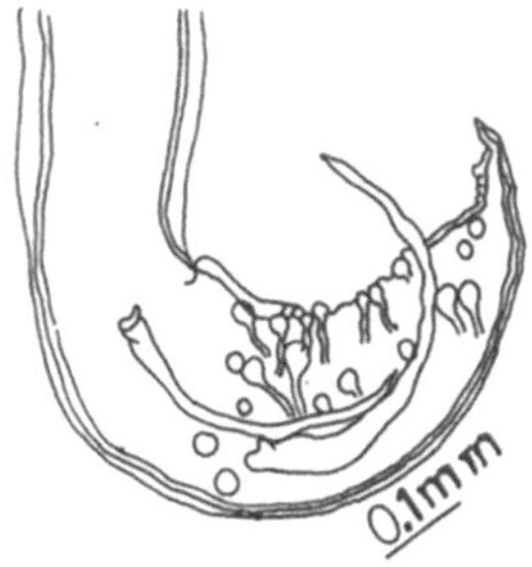

Figure 4.
Paracamallanus tridenti *(Jaiswal and Malhotra [12])—posterior end to show spicules (Not to scale).*

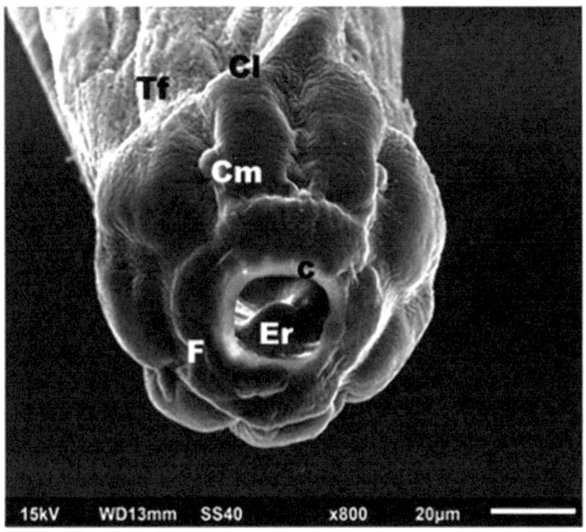

Figure 5.
Tridentocamallanus indica *n.gen., n.sp. Scanning electron micrograph of anterior part of body to show buccal capsule (x800).*

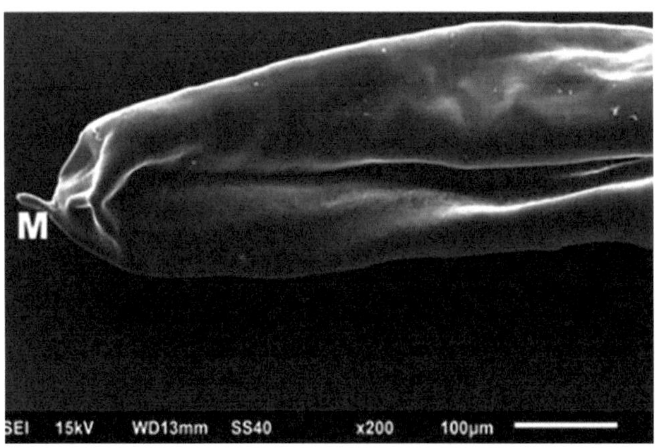

Figure 6.
Tridentocamallanus indica *n.gen., n.sp. Scanning electron micrograph of posterior part of body of female to show mucron (x100).*

area rugosa on the body of male worm, as well as two unequal spicules that were dissimilar (**Figure 7**). Vulva pre-equatorial was at 3.09–4.26 (3.84) from posterior end in female (**Figure 8**). The caudal alae were prominent (**Figure 9**) at the terminal end of body of male. Left longer spicule, 0.682–0.784 (0.692) long, and right shorter spicule, 0.421–0.501 (0.473) in length. Gubernaculum, 0.14–0.25 (0.188) long.

Family	Tridentocamallanidae n.fam.
Subfamily	Tridentocamallaniinae n. subfam.
Genus	*Tridentocamallanus* n.gen.
Species	*Tridentocamallanus indica* n.gen., n. sp.
Type-host	Sincroaker, *Johnius dussumieri* (Teleostei:Belonidae)
Type-locality:	Panjim, Central west coast of India, Goa, India.
Site of infection:	Small intestine.
Mean intensity:	2.40
Prevalence:	66.60%
Specimens deposited	Holotype, Male- IV-1393; Allotype, Female- IV-1396; Zoological Survey of India, Jabalpur, M.P.
Etymology	The Order, Vireshwararida n.ord. is named after the name of Professor Vireshwar Nath Capoor, the eminent Parasitologist from the University of Allahabad, Prayagraj, U.P., India.

The SubOrder, Vireshwararina n.subord. is named after the name of Professor Vireshwar Nath Capoor, the eminent Parasitologist from the University of Allahabad, Prayagraj, U.P., India.

The superfamily Tridentocamallanoidea n.supfam. is named after the characteristics of trident in Tridentocamallanid worms.

The family Tridentocamallanidae n.fam. is named after the characteristics of trident in Tridentocamallanid worms.

The family Tridentocamallaniinae n.subfam. is named after the characteristics of trident in Tridentocamallanid worms.

The genus is named after the characteristics of trident in Tridentocamallanid worms.

The species is named after the country of its origin, *that is,* India.

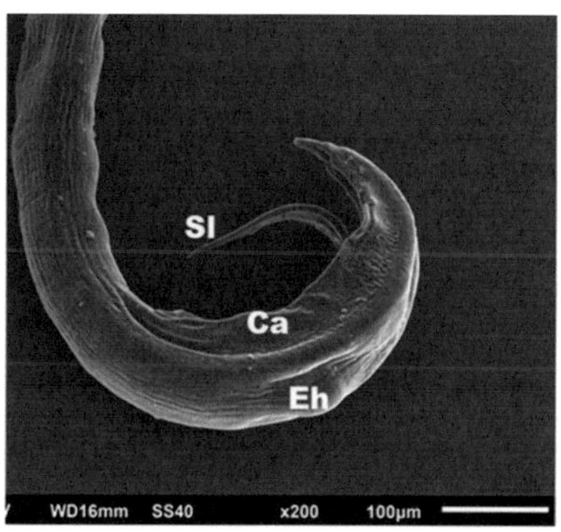

Figure 7.
Tridentocamallanus indica *n.gen., n.sp. Scanning electron micrographs of area rugosa on the body of male to show raised cloaca and spicule (x200).*

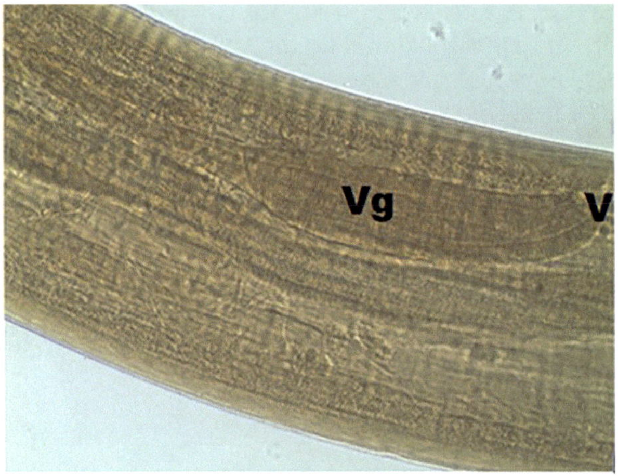

Figure 8.
Tridentocamallanus indica *n.gen., n.sp. LM of mid-body of female to show vagina.*

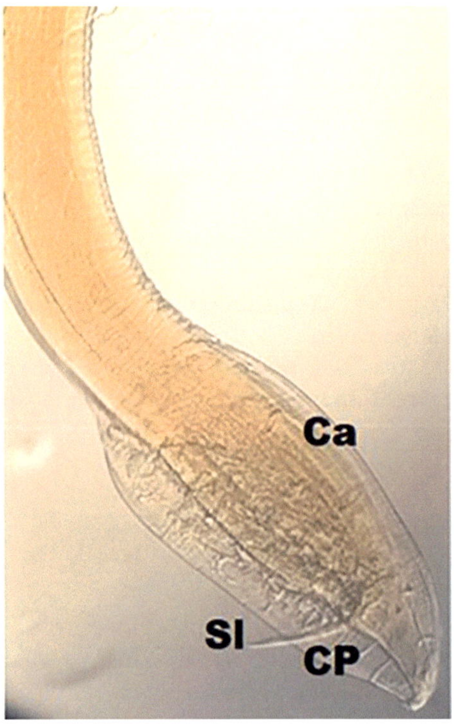

Figure 9.
Tridentocamallanus indica *n.gen., n.sp. LM of posterior end of body of male to show caudal alae.*

3.1 Remarks

It is remarkable that the enumeration of buccal teeth, including the distribution of denticles of various sizes and shapes, teeth at the anterior end, at the basal ring, and numerous ridges on sclerotized spiral thickenings, as well as their distribution inside and outside the buccal capsule, which have been described in various genera and subgenera under Camallanidae, are, in some form, part of the morphology of the now established Tridentocamallanoid worms [15]. It is obvious that a considerable overlap of morphological features has been dominant, as various authors over the years have found it difficult to explain the inexplicable complexities in the systematic placement of various taxa, such as subgenera, genera, under the superfamily Camallanoidea and related groups. The synthesis of morphological and molecular data available from studies to date has yet to resolve the issue.

The two independent genera, *Camallanus* and *Paracamallanus* under the newly revised classification of order Spirurida [16], based on their unique morphological infrastructure, are upheld as valid. In the recently revised classification of nematoda [17], superfamily Camallanoidea [18, 19] kept under order Spirurida [16] comprised Genera *Malayocamallanus*, *Neoparacamallanus*, *Oncophora*, *Platocamallanus*, *Procamallanus* with subgenera *Aspiculus, Denticamallanus, Procamallanus syn. Procamallanides, Punctocamallanus, Spirocamallanus*, Genus *Serpinema* [20]. The current investigation has also upheld the validity of synonymy of *Monospiculus* [21] (Subgenus [11]) n.comb., *Isospiculus* [21] (subgenus [11]) n.comb., *Spirocamallanus* (genus [22]; genus [23]) (subgenus [11]) n.comb., *Spirocamallanoides* (subgenus [23]) (subgenus [11]) n.comb., *Punctocamallanus* (subgenus [24]) (subgenus [11]) n.comb., *Denticamallanus* (subgenus [25]) (subgenus [11]) n.comb., *Onchocamallanus* (subgenus [26]) (subgenus [11]) n.comb., Genus*: Malayocamallanus* (subgenus [27]) (subgenus [11]) n.comb., *Platocamallanus* (subgenus [28]) (subgenus [11]) n.comb., *Batrachocamallanus* (subgenus [29]) (subgenus [11]) n.comb. under genus *Tridentocamallanus* n.gen. of the family *Tridentocamallan*idae [15].

3.2 Key to orders of class chromadorea

Chitinized buccal capsule with cavity behind valves [11], longitudinal beaded bands absent on buccal capsule, worms with cephalic collarette or not, caudal collarette absent, tridents absent, Trilaminate-layered sunflower papillae absent, Mucron non-bifid… …Spirurida [16, 17].

Chitinized buccal capsule without cavity behind valves, longitudinal beaded bands drop down from the rim of buccal flange. Cephalic or caudal collarette present or not, tridents present or not, paired or single, trilaminate-layered sunflower papillae present, mucron bifid… … Vireshwararida n.ord.

The detailed taxonomic interpretations, based on specific diagrams to validate the newer taxa proposed herein, are beyond the scope of this chapter due to space limitations.

The parallel emergence of roundworms retained though the essential characters of family Camallanidae *viz*. a sclerotized cup in buccal capsule with typical pair of tridents, one dorsal and another ventral to the opening of buccal capsule, along with unique emergence of anisakid characters *viz*. a ventriculus with ventricular appendix, and intestinal ceca. A unique structure had developed at the tip of spicule in male worms giving it a spoon-like appearance was an advanced feature too.

3.3 Conclusive evidence of genetic support

The closeness of the new genus, *Tridentocamallanus* with *I. multispinatum* (*p* distance, 0.0–0.0172) was remarkably established, as these specimens were also the closest (*p* distance, 0.0–0.0447) to *R. capoori* (both Raphidascarididae, now transferred to Tridentocamallanidae n.fam.). The characters common between all the three genera, *Tridentocamallanus* n.gen., *Indospinezia*, and *Rotundocollarette* were cephalic collarette and a heavily papillate body, which were the physalopteran features. The genetic support to tridents in *T. indica* and *I. multispinatum* was more consistent than buccal cavity in these two genera. Mucron – spiny, non-bifid in *I. multispinatum*; papillate and bifid in *T. indica* n.gen., n.sp., and non-papillate, non-bifid in *R. capoori* were genetically supported in the three genera. A ventriculus with ventricular appendix and an intestinal caecum in *I. multispinatum* and *R. capoori* were the morphological features that corroborated with the genetic analysis. Although contrary to a strong genetic support between *Tridentocamallanus* n.gen. and *I. multispinatum,* the similarity in characteristics of buccal capsule, its teeth and denticulated ridges were varied. Typically, the oral cavity with a cover, which replaced the true buccal capsule, was a characteristic of *I. multispinatum*, while a typical buccal capsule with denticles on the internal and external walls, and denticulated ridges and teeth on the internal walls, was found in *Tridentocamallanus* n.gen. Additionally, the presence of six teeth around three pores in the oral apparatus, along with denticles and dentigerous ridges on the cephalic region in *R. capoori*, received heterologous support.

3.4 The critical evidence of cephalic tooth in second-stage larva of *Indospinezia*

Genus *Indospinezia* [12] discovered from the Ganga Basin area encompassing Gangetic freshwater riverine ecosystem at Parayagraj was the first diversification in the line of evolution, in which the connecting features of the most advanced family, Anisakidae developed. Specifically, with two non-indented lips of camallanid worms, the characters, like paired tridents on dorsal and ventral side of oral aperture (**Figures 10** and **11a**), were remarkably developed in *Indospinezia*. Simultaneously, anisakid characters like ventriculus, ventricular appendix, and intestinal ceca were also encountered in *Indospinezia*. However, it is unique that no anisakid worm has ever been reported from a freshwater habitat worldwide, except for the worms of Raphidascarididae (e.g., *Rostellascaris spinicaudatum* [30]) and Anisakidae (e.g., *Anisakis typica*), which were recorded in the Ganga Basin and are believed to have emerged from the former Tethys Ocean.

Anisakid worms have exclusively been reported from marine habitats worldwide, except from Indian wetlands.

The first bioinvasive raphidascaridoid roundworm, *Rostellascaris spinicaudatum* [30] was recorded from Gangetic riverine ecosystem. It showed effective transmission from Arabian Sea sharks, *Rhincodon typus* and catfishes, *Arius maculatus*. The strengthening modifications in interlabia and emergence of sunflower papillae thus far seen only in the roundworms that inhabited the streams associated with Gangetic riverine ecosystem have given reasons to conclude specific environmental interventions due to which distinctly different morphotypes have evolved.

One of the major events that demonstrated significant environmental intervention during the appearance of bioinvasive nematodes into the freshwater riverine body from Arabian Sea was a sudden environmental upheaval, *that is*, Tsunami in December, 2004 in the area of long-term investigations for three decades by the authors and coworkers [31]. Initially, two camallanid worms, *that is, Procamallanus* and *Paracamallanus*, occurred primarily in the Indian part of Tethys Ocean area in fish of marine habitat during 2003–2005, in the two host fishes, *that is,* the reef fish namely, *Lutjanus malabaricus* and reef-associated, *Johnius dussumieri*. But after sudden environmental upheaval, *that is*, Tsunami in December, 2004, the fish *L. malabaricus* disappeared suddenly [32], and the second one, *that is*, *J. dussumeri* continued

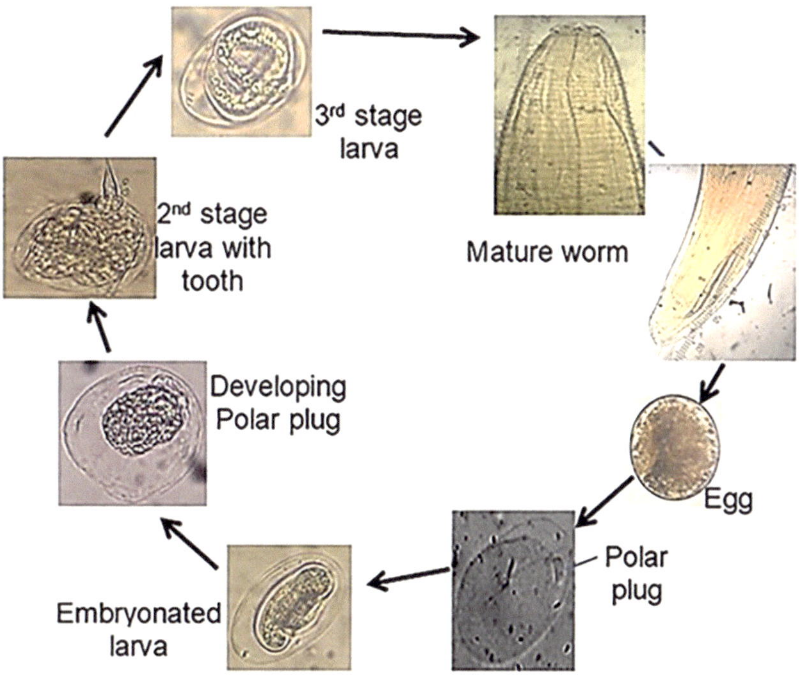

Figure 10.
Indospinezia multispinatum *from freshwater riverine ecosystems at Prayagraj, U.P., India: Life cycle stages to show cephalic tooth on second stage larva.*

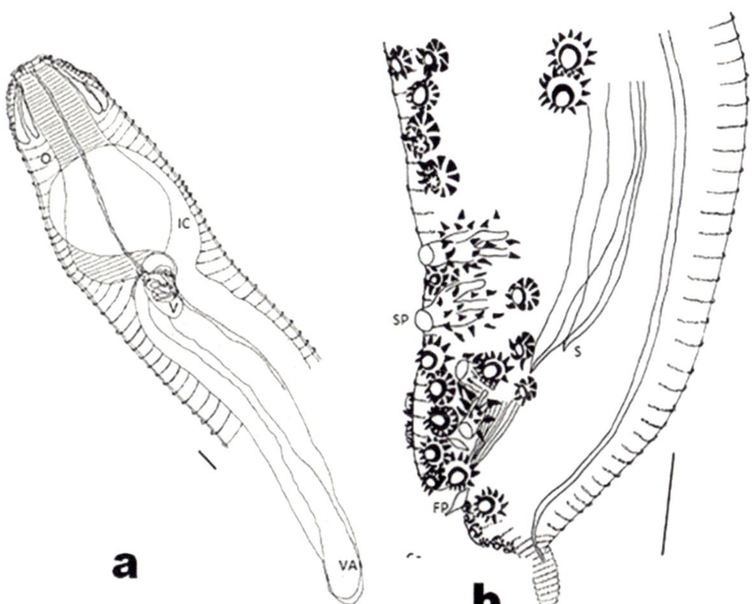

Figure 11.
Indospinezia multispinatum. *(a) Tridents, bifid ventricular appendix and intestinal ceca. (b) Pre- and post-caudal sun-flower papillae on posterior part of body of the worm.*

to remain infested by *Paracamallanus tridenti* [33]. However, thereafter during post-Tsunami period, its distribution was not restricted only to these two fishes, *J. dussumieri* and *L. malabaricus*, but its host range was enhanced after the major climatic change *viz.* Tsunami (December 2004) [32]. Thus, this nematode now occurred in at least eight other additional fishes in Goan coastal zone during the post-Tsunami period. However, this roundworm also began recurring with the reappearance of *L. malabaricus* in 2022 around Goan coastal waters.

4. The *Pronakid goai* n.gen., n.sp. connectivity

The medium to large worms with weaker buccal flange (**Figure 12a, b**) around large, sclerotized buccal capsule possessed 14–16 sclerotized dentigerous striations in female, which lacked in males. Eight minute sensory pits (**Figure 13a, b**) present, a pair on each of the four corners, two each on dorsal as well as two on ventral side of buccal flange. In addition, 3–5 sensory pits were observed in the mid-region of buccal flange on dorsal side. A pair of these was also present on ventro-lateral margin. These sensory pits were the sedentary constituents that played role in copulation. Four small sessile papillae on dorsal as well as ventral margin of buccal flange present. Cephalic collar distinct (**Figure 12b**) extends well beyond hinder part of head and terminates into a frill. Teeth in buccal cavity two pairs on the upper dorso-lateral sides at the periphery of buccal capsule. Three teeth were present at the basal ring of buccal capsule. A pair of muscular, sucker-like organ was present attached to the buccal flange, one each on dorso-lateral and ventro-lateral side. These are interrupted in between by the two paired apical lobes, each of which is extended by two hanging large lobes. A medial lobe (**Figure 12a** and **13a**) hangs further in the middle of the two apical lobes. Single trident (**Figure 12**) was present on each dorsal and ventral side of oral aperture. Deirids two in number, the first one near the base of head in the hinder part,

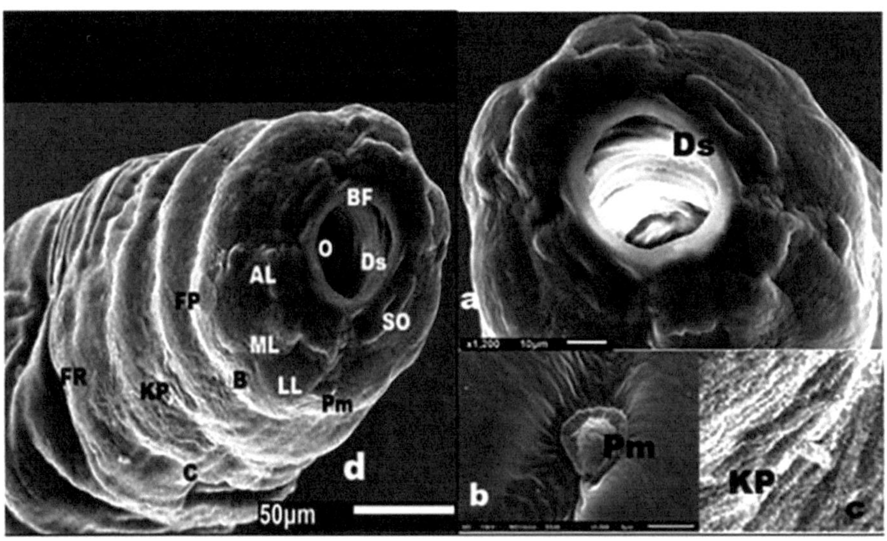

Figure 12.
Pronakid goai *n.gen., n.sp. Scanning electron micrograph of anterior part of worm to show (a) Incomplete and complete sclerotized ridges in buccal capsule. (b) Sclerotized cephalic collarette and incomplete and complete sclerotized ridges in buccal capsule.*

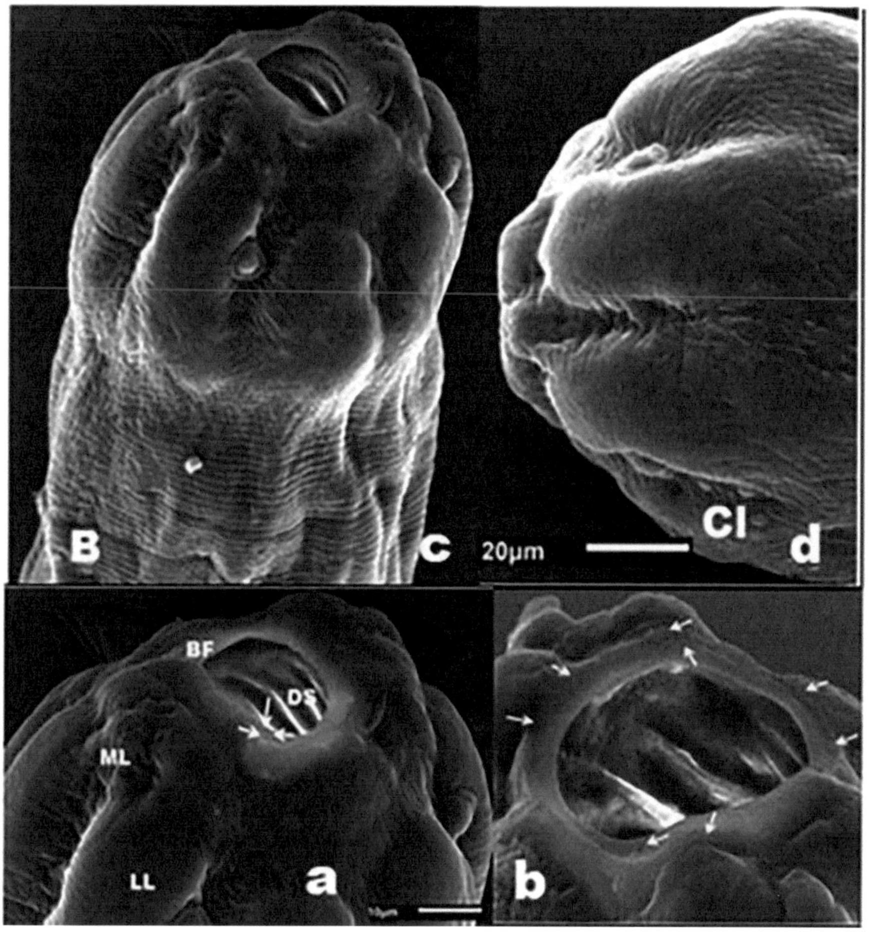

Figure 13.
Pronakid goai *n.gen., n.sp. (a) Weak buccal flange with sensory pits; (b) buccal capsule with sclerotized teeth and buccal flange possessing sensory pits; (c) cephalic collarette and typical cephalic papillae; and (d) unique cluster papillae at the base of buccal capsule.*

and the second one at a short distance away from the base of head. For certain minute sessile papillae were seen at the anterior end adjacent to first deirid (**Figure 13d** and **14a, b**). Esophagus divided into two- with an anterior elongate muscular esophagus and a glandular part that finally joined a small ventriculus (**Figure 15c**). An intestinal caecum and ventricular appendix were observed at the esophageo-intestinal junction. Button-shaped papillae were located anteriorly. A cluster of minute sessile papillae were also seen near mid-circle papilla at the cephalic complex. One pair of phasmids, one after the other, was present ventro-laterally in the post-anal part of tail, while single phasmid was located dorso-laterally in the pre-anal region as well.

4.1 Male

There is a cluster of 16–20 minute sessile cephalic papillae at the dorso-lateral margin of buccal flange. A pair of lingual cephalic papillae is at the hinder part of cephalic region, one each on dorsal as well as on the ventral side. Mid-circle papillae prominent, large, 6 in number, was present on the outer wall of buccal capsule

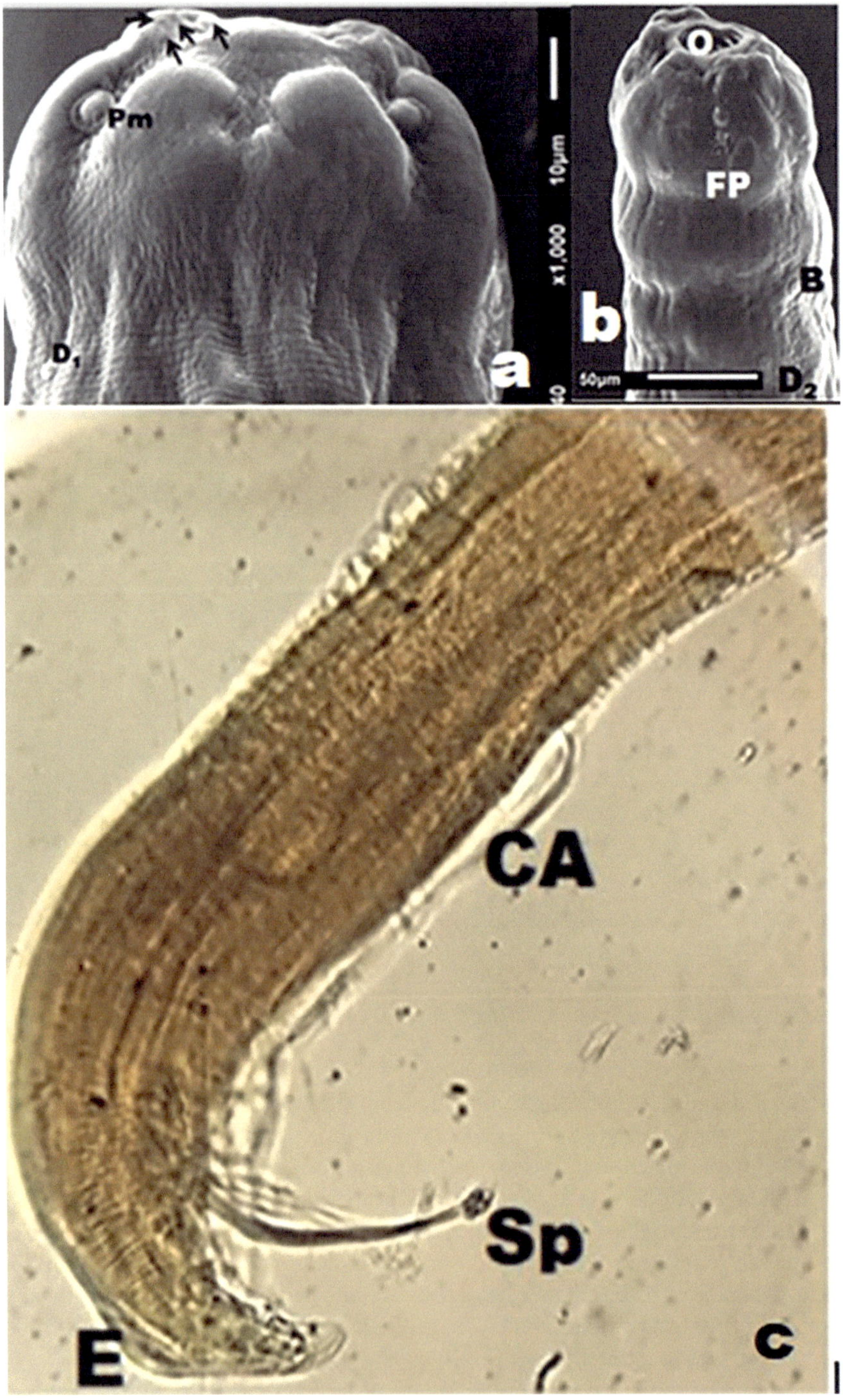

Figure 14.
Pronakid goai *n.gen., n.sp. (a) Deirid and cephalic papillae besides labial lobes on the wall of buccal capsule; (b) button-shaped papillae besides labial lobes on the wall of buccal capsule; (c) caudal alae, anus at elevated hump and spicule with spoon-shaped extremity at the posterior end of body of male.*

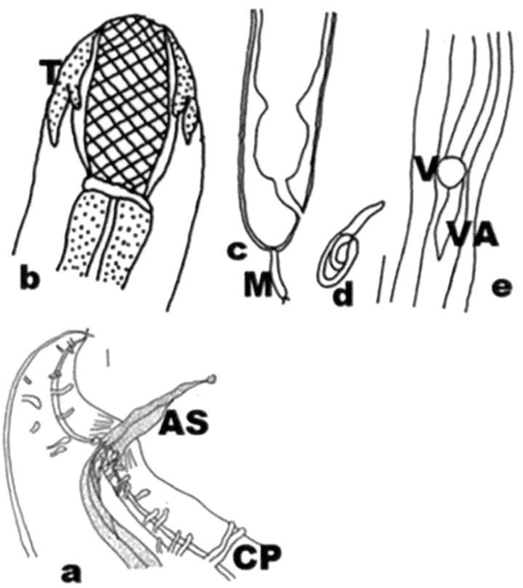

Figure 15.
Pronakid goai *n.gen., n.sp. (a) Caudal alae in the posterior part of the worm with costiform papillae. (b) Anterior part of worm to show tridents. (c) Cloacal association with anal pore identical to that reported in* Procamallanus chauhanensis. *(d) Coiled larva recovered from female. (e) Ventriculus with ventricular appendix.*

(**Figure 12a, d,** and **13c**). Four hanging beaded strings extend from the margin of buccal flange, at the point where the key chain ring head was located, from the latero-dorsal as well as latero-ventral side of apical plate. Each of this beaded string encircled mid-circle papillae to join leaf-like foliate papilla, on way to its joining another foliate papilla in the vicinity of the next mid-circle papilla on the external surface of buccal capsule. The structure of mid-circle papilla is unique in that its heart-shaped body is placed over a flat disc (**Figure 12b** and **13c**), that is, located between the two lateral lobes hanging down attached proximally with the twin apical lobes around buccal flange. Spicules 2, dissimilar, unequal; the left longer being almost double of the other right smaller spicule. The distal tip of longer left spicule has a spoon-like extremity prominently projected out of anus (**Figure 14c**). Gubernaculum present. Costiform papillae provide support to caudal alae posteriorly. A weakly muscular, caudal sucker without rim was present at the level of anus. An elevated hump in the region of *area rugosa* was distinctly visible externally at the hinder region of the tail of male worm. Caudal alae prominent, wide extending up till base of the mucron, which bears a divided pointed tip showing two tiny processes (**Figure 16**).

4.2 Distribution of caudal papillae

Caudal papillae 98–99 in total. One pair button-shaped papillae on latero-ventral side in the pre-anal area and one medio-lateral row comprising 13–14 pairs, accompanied by one row of 14–16 ventro-lateral papillae; ad-anal 8 pairs of sessile papillae; post-anal 18 pairs papillae; 3 pairs of denticulated rosette papillae, of which 1 pair medio-lateral and 2 pairs of latero-ventral papillae; and additionally, 6 pairs of

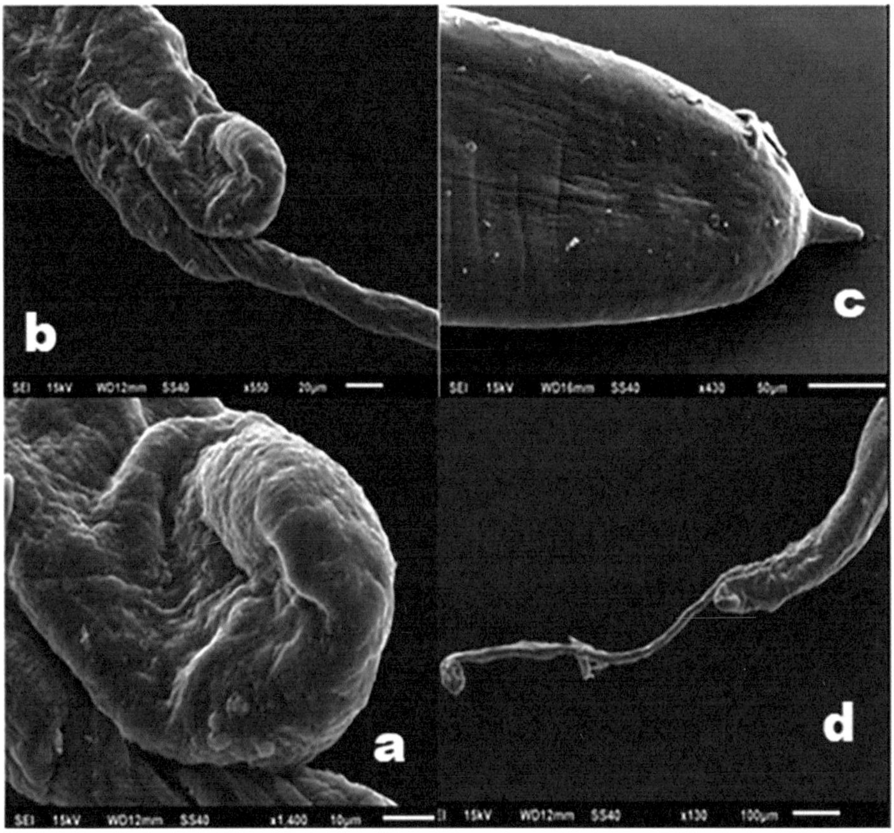

Figure 16.
Pronakid goai *n.gen., n.sp. (a, b) Base of spicule (magnified) exhibiting spoon-shaped extremity; (c) tail with mucron; (d) elected elongate spicule in male with spoon-shaped extremity.*

latero-ventral papillae in a series, and 3 pairs of sessile medio-ventral papillae parallel to the prior series.

4.3 Female

The body was sturdy and appeared slimy. It was viviparous with the vulva located post-equatorially. The vagina was muscular and long, consisting of minute brush-like hairs at the opening of the vulva.

4.4 Remarks

The present worms on account of their typical anisakid characteristics, *viz*. ventriculus, ventricular appendix, and intestinal ceca, along with the camallanine feature of a trident each on the dorsal as well as ventral side of buccal capsule, and a unique spoon-like extremity of a spicule of the newer worms were the supportive attributes to erect a new genus, *Pronakid* with a new species, namely, *goai*. Its evolution stood parallel to *Indospinezia multispinatum* emerging from worms of *T. indica* n.gen., n.sp.

The assertions on differentiation of species on the basis of incomplete vs. complete sclerotized ridges (**Figure 12a, d**) on the inner wall of buccal capsule, or the absence or presence of such ridges on the inner wall of buccal capsule being a basis due to sexual differentiation were disputed by eminent parasitologists at some stage or the other [34–36] emphasized disagreement with the diagnostic differentiation of sclerotized ridges could not stand the test on the basis of phylogenetic assessment proposed by several earlier authors. The incomplete developmental stages of camallanines were assigned the reason to discredit any diagnostic value on incomplete/complete cuticularized striations on the internal walls of buccal capsule [37] along with other assertions highlighted in the forgoing text.

Additionally the authors have reasons to assert significant value to be attached to the structural differentiation in mucron as well as the adaptation of physalopteran features of cephalic and/or post-caudal collarette. The appearance of papillated configuration of Physalopteridae in worms that possessed significant characteristics of Camallaninae also provided reasonable issues to be discussed from the point of view of connecting links during the course of evolution. The ambiguities being raised due to the unavoidable overlap in features of taxonomic value under subfamily Camallaniinae were also highlighted in the recent years [38].

The investigations [20], to illustrate division of family Camallanidae into Camallaninae [18] and Procamallaninae [20] with twin halves in buccal capsule in the former as well as possessing single buccal capsule in the latter, in the six genera that he proposed, were analyzed phylogenetically to elaborate on the phylogeny of genera of Camallaninae [39].

The main characteristics of the newer roundworms include a typical single buccal capsule, not split into two buccal valves, and a unique feature of a fully formed collarette in the cephalic region, which has traditionally been a physalopteran characteristic.

Additionally, the unique key-chain head papillae on buccal flange as well as parts of body were noticeable features.

The most intriguing feature of the current worms in difference from *Tridentocamallanus indica* n.gen., n.sp., was the typical anisakid characteristics, ventriculus, ventricular appendix as well as intestinal caecum that were lacking in *T. indica*. Nevertheless, the paired tridents (**Figure 11a**), a camallanine characteristic, brought the newly proposed genus, closer to the genus *Indospinezia* [12], which progressively emerged to attain next level. But the stout spines [40] all over its body surface placed these at the higher pedestal in the evolutionary lineage. The characteristic sharp and larger spines of *Indospinezia* were lacking in *Pronakid* n.gen.,n.sp., and the truly anisakid feature like ventricular appendix was present in both *Indospinezia* [40] and *Pronakid* n.gen, n.sp. On the other hand, evidently both *Pronakid* n.gen. and *I. multispinatum* were at a higher ladder than *T. indica*, and *Pronakid* evolved to give rise to the spine-studded *I. multispinatum* [40], which finally was a predecessor to *Rostellascaris* that comprised significantly evolved oral armature as part of cephalic armature with strengthening by newly evolved interlabia in *Rostellascaris* [30].

On the other hand, the major difference between *Pronakid* n.gen.,n.sp. and *Tridentocamallanus* was a highly developed bifid mucron in the latter genus that was distinctly like a simple spine in *Pronakid* n.gen. However, both of these worms possessed cephalic collarette, which was similar to *Indospinezia*, but the body of both lacked spines unlike *Indospinezia*. It was remarkable that both *Pronakid* n.gen.,n.sp. and *Tridentocamallanus* n.gen.,n.sp. were exclusively marine, while *Indospinezia* was exclusively freshwater parasite, with 98–99 papillae on body of the former than up to >140 in the latter.

An appraisal of phylogenetic analysis of the newer worms based on 18S rDNA gene (**Figure 17**) distinctly revealed, on one hand, the alignment of *Pronakid* n.gen. With *T. indica*, with three other species of genus *Procamallanus*, while on the other hand, another sequence of *Pronakid* n.gen. Fell into the larger clade comprising two anisakids, *Hysterothylocium pelagicum* and *Goezia spinulosa* as well as three sequences of genus *Indospinezia*, the worms of whom possessed characteristics of Camallanoidea and Anisakidae. Therefore, conclusively, since the stronger anisakid characteristics of the proposed new genus, *Pronakid* n.gen.,n.sp. outweigh the camallanine features on which it might resemble *Tridentocamallanus* n.gen., n.sp., that have also been phylogenetically examined and verified, and the author proposes to raise a new genus *Pronakid goai* n.gen.,n.sp. on the basis of features of the newer worms investigated here.

The newer worms were also uniquely different from other camallanines as well as *I. multispinatum* in possessing features of Anisakidae that was a major point of taxonomic significance due to which the revision of Class Chromadorea has been undertaken. The author is, therefore, inclined to raise the present nematodes to a new generic level and named as *Pronakid goai* n.gen., n.sp., named after the combined characteristics of *Procamallanus* and Anisakidae; the species being named after the city, Goa, at the West coast of India, from where these worms have been discovered.

a. Family: Tridentocamallanidae n.fam.

b. Genus: *Pronakid n.gen.*

c. Species*: P. goai n.sp.*

d. Type-host: *Johnius dussumieri* (Perciformes: Scianidae)

e. Type-locality: Jetty, Goa, Central west coast of India.

f. Site of infection: Small intestine.

g. Mean intensity: 1.32 (2020–2022).

h. Prevalence: 14.28–24.85%

i. Specimens deposited: Holotype: *Pronakid n.gen.*-IV-1394; Zoological Survey of India, Jabalpur (Madhya Pradesh), India.

5. *Rostellascaris spinicaudatum*

The finding of raphidascaridoid roundworm, *R. spinicaudatum* [30] initially from the freshwater fish *Mystus seenghala*, that evidently emerged as a bioinvasive worm that invaded from marine habitats of Arabian Sea into the freshwater of Gangetic riverine ecosystem was a remarkable event. The significant characteristics of evolutionary consequence, *viz.* the three essential raphidascaridoid features, *that is,* ventriculus, ventricular appendix, and intestinal ceca, combined with a post-caudal collarette akin to family Physalopteridae provided a conclusive assertive of overlapping features of three families, namely, Raphidascarididae, Physalopteridae, and Anisakidae being present in *R. spinicaudatum*. The unique feature of nematodes, *that is,* sunflower papillae that emerged in *I. multispinatum* from the fish *Xenentodon cancila* (Teleostomi: Belonidae) of the Gangetic riverine ecosystem highlighted the significant role of environmental interactions because such distinguished sunflower

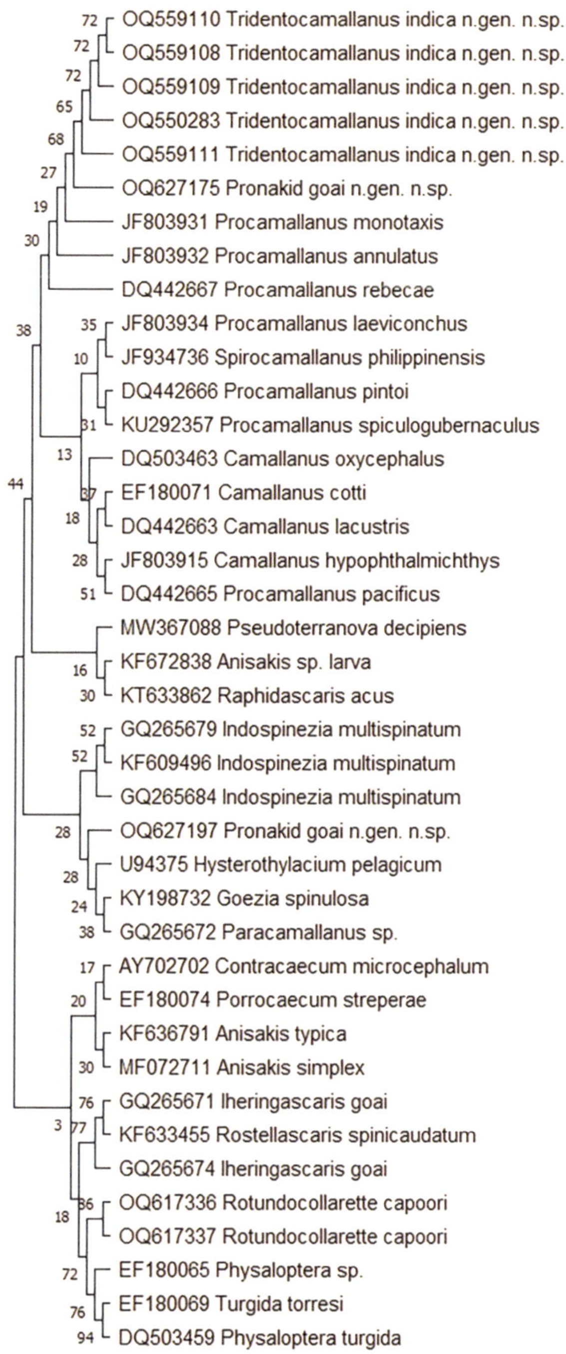

Figure 17.
Neighbor-joining tree based on nucleotide 18S rDNA sequences of Pronakid goai *n.gen, n.sp. and reference species. Nucleotide 18S rDNA sequence data are as described in the text with GenBank accession numbers. Bootstrap values based on 1000 replicates were used. Scale bar represents an interval of the Kimura two-parameter (K2P) model.*

papillae were seen for the first time in the freshwater fishes inhabiting Gangetic habitats only. Another set of sunflower papillae was recorded from *Goezia spinulosa* (now *species inquirenda* [41]) from a fish inhabiting in the tributary of river Ganges that entered Bangladesh as River Padma from India [42]. In no other specimen, such papillae have ever been observed, on which the qualitative influence of river water has been supposed to be operative within India and Bangladesh. Interestingly, these worms, equipped with remarkably advanced features, parasitized a primitive host group like Pisces in the vertebrate series, contrary to the typical pattern of co-evolution, where the parasitizing organism gradually acquires advanced features as it progresses up the evolutionary ladder (from Pisces to Mammalia). In the parasitic world, therefore, the worm like *Ancylostoma* with its occupancy in the highly evolved group, *that is,* mammals obviously exemplified "co-evolution," while on the contrary "Reverse Co-evolution" was the event that was encountered in *R. spinicaudatum*.

Although *G. bangladeshi* fell very closer morphologically to *I. multispinatum* mainly because of heavily spinated body and "sunflower" papillae yet it was strikingly different because of the presence of unique camallanid as well as physalopteran features in *I. multispinatum*. But the misidentification of *G. bangladeshi* was brought to the fore recently [41] mainly because of absence of larval tooth in the second-stage larvae of the specimens studied [42] that actually were "juveniles" and not the required second-stage larvae in their life cycle. Due to this major laxity, G. *bangladeshi* were accommodated as "species inquerendae" [41].

6. Evolution of human agents of zoonoses, *Anisakis typica*

From here onward, specific emergence of anisakid worms with sturdy cephalic complex and additional structures like buccal tooth were remarkable elements in the process of development of members of Family Anisakidae (**Figures 18–22**). The account of their evolutionary perspective along with environmental implications regulating nemic diversity in the components of their life cycles in freshwater as well as marine zones has been dealt with by the authors and coworkers [43]. With the development of a single, prominent dorsal tooth placed atop cephalic complex, the evolution of genus *Anisakis* was accomplished. A comparison of worldwide encountered specimens of *Anisakis* third-stage larvae of different species of *Anisakis*, as well as a variety of adult specimens of different species of *Anisakis* have categorically illustrated the specimens collected for the present investigation to be the smallest from all, be these larvae or adult worms. The variations in size of body parts of third-stage larvae and adult worms were summarized by authors [43]. The specific presence of rosette-shaped caudal papilla in first- and second-stage larvae of *Anisakis* sp. was observed which was absent in third-stage larvae. Sensory pits (**Figure 23b**) were short lateral invaginations, observed atop ventro-lateral lip in the cuticle of the head, and these are the cuticular lining of the lateral sense organs, *that is*, amphids [44]. The gradual adoption of technique of migration by the first- and second-stage larvae of *Anisakis* from the dolphin reservoir in river Ganges to the marine ecosystem of Arabian Sea, as against the reverse migration from marine ecosystem to the freshwater riverine habitat by the raphidascaridoid worms, *R. spinicaudatum*, added to the process of evolution of Anisakidae worms that highlighted the influence of environmental variations in the emergence of relatively sturdy roundworms (**Figures 24-30**).

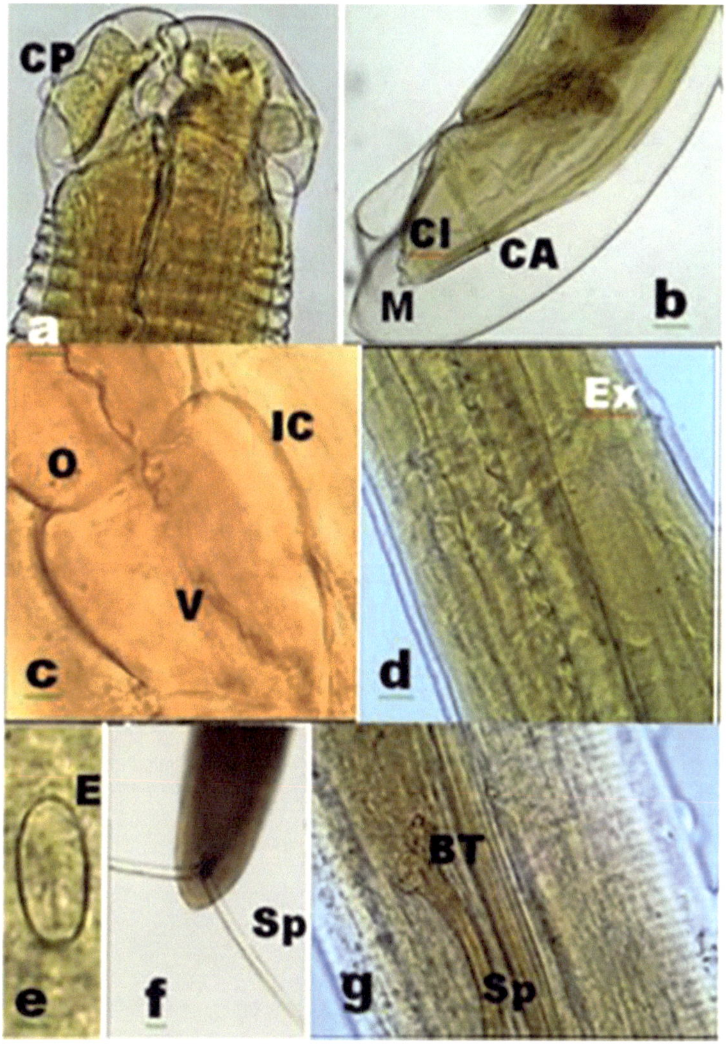

Figure 18.
Rostellascaris spinicaudatum *from Goan coast. (a) Head showing cephalic papilla; (b) posterior end to show post-caudal collarette and caudal alae; (c) anterior end of body to show ventriculus and intestinal ceca; (d) anterior end of worm to show excretory pore; (e) egg; (f) spicules in male; and (g) posterior part of body of male to show spicule.*

The occurrence of *Anisakis* larvae in the feed or in the ambient environment is most of the time accountable for the spread of anisakid infections in fish [45]. It is interesting to note that the record of present *Anisakis* larvae from freshwater riverine ecosystem of River Ganges is from the same area that has been frequently occupied by freshwater dolphins in District Fatehpur, U.P. Simultaneously, this is the same area of the stream of River Ganges, in the vicinity of District Prayagraj, up to which the bioinvasion by raphidascaridoid nematodes from Arabian Sea *via* catfishes of Indian Ocean has been concluded on the basis of molecular and phylogenetic characterization, by the authors and associates [46, 47]. The smaller invertebrates are the common intermediate hosts of anisakids in natural water bodies as well as aquaculture reservoirs.

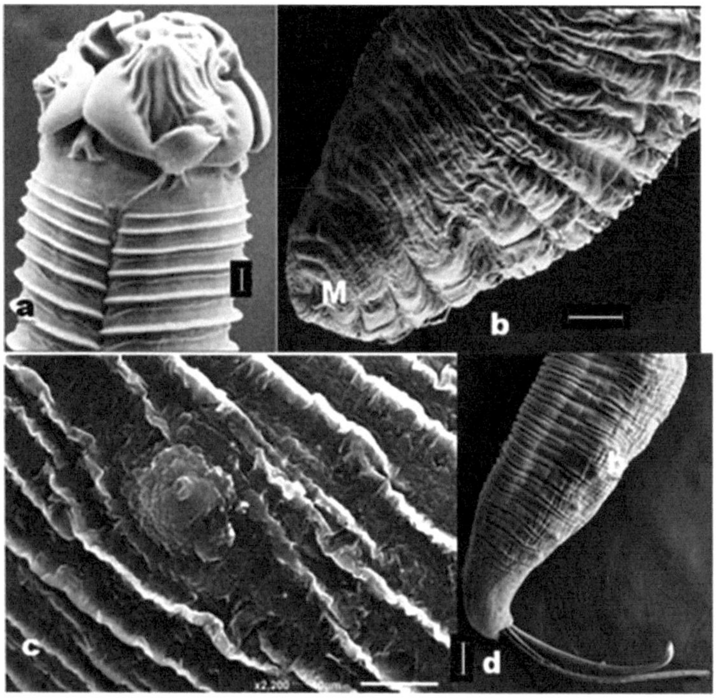

Figure 19.
Rostellascaris spinicaudatum *from Goan coast. (a) Head with strengthened cephalic armature; (b) Posterior part of body to show mucron at the tail tip; (c) sunflower papilla in the posterior part of body; (d) spicules and caudal papillae on the body of male worm.*

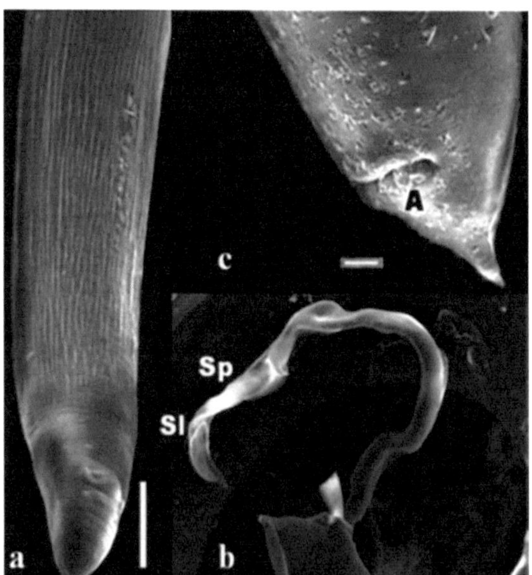

Figure 20.
Rostellascaris spinicaudatum *parasitizing* Bagarius bagarius *in freshwater river at Prayagraj. (a) Posterior part of body with caudal papillae; (b) scanning electron micrograph of spicule and mucron at the tail tip; (c) pre-anal and ad-anal papillae at the posterior part of body of worm.*

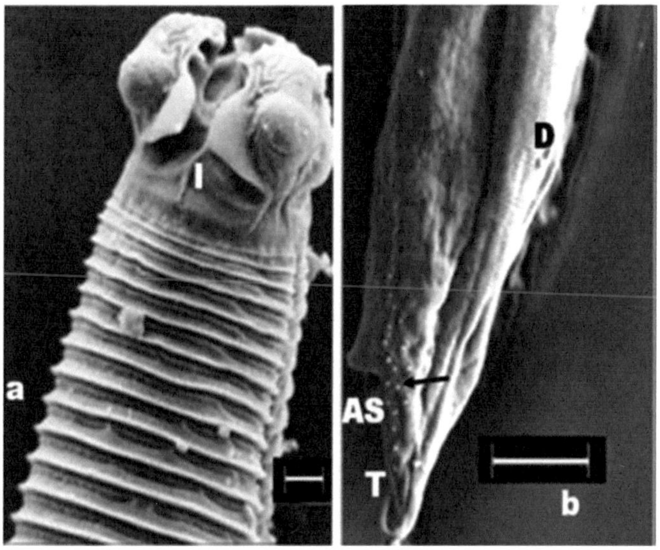

Figure 21.
Rostellascaris spinicaudatum *parasitizing* Bagarius bagarius *in freshwater river at Prayagraj. (a) Cephalic end with interlabia and (b) pre- and post-caudal papilla.*

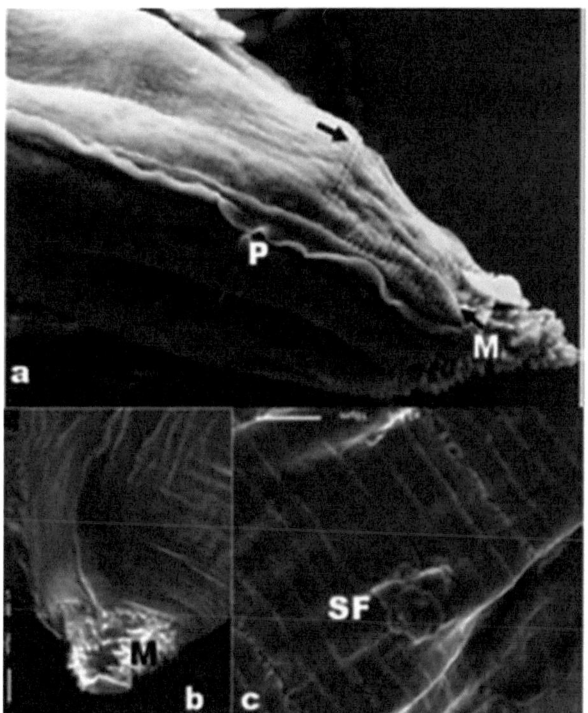

Figure 22.
Rostellascaris spinicaudatum *parasitizing* Bagarius bagarius *in freshwater river at Prayagraj. (a) Post-caudal mucron and collarette; (b) mucron (magnified at the tail tip); (c) sunflower papillae in the caudal area of the worm.*

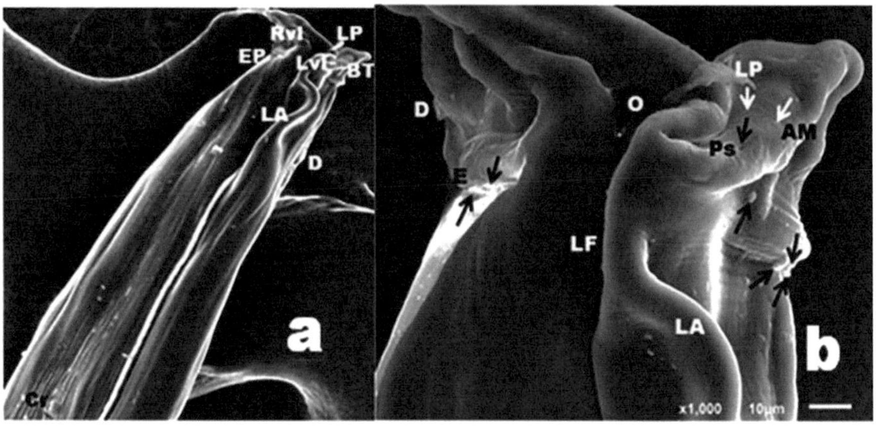

Figure 23.
Anisakis typica. *(a) Anterior end of body of worm to show linguiform papilla, dorsal tooth, and lateral alae; (b) scanning electron micrograph of head (magnified) to show sensory pits and linguiform papilla.*

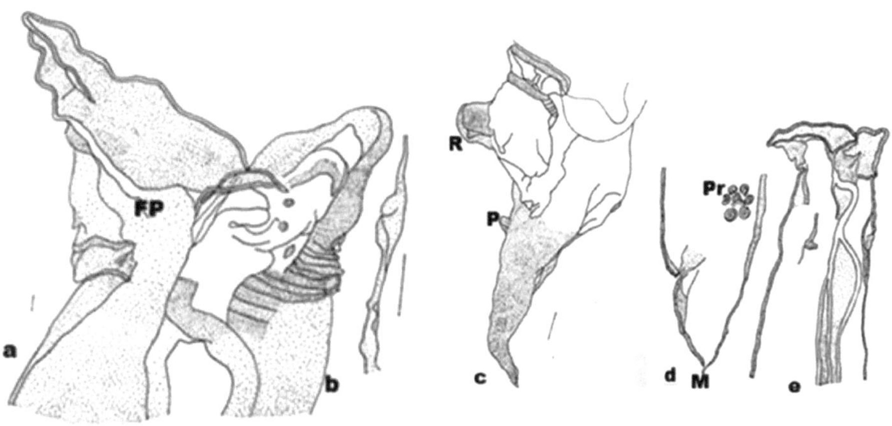

Figure 24.
Anisakis typica. *(a) Head (magnified) to show linguiform papilla and (b) lip* Anisakis typica. *(c) Posterior end of body to show tail and raised anus; (d) posterior part of body of worm to show rosette papillae and mucron; (e) anterior end of body of worm to show dorsal tooth and lateral folds.*

Finally, the authors [3] came across a newer set of roundworms, *Rotundocollarette capoori* that possessed a cephalic complex well equipped with three sets of paired teeth around each of the three sets of apertures namely, excretory pore, oral aperture and genital pore atop cephalic complex. These worms infesting pyloric ceca of marine coral reef-associated *Johnius dussumieri* inhabiting *Ilhe Grande* Island, 19Kms apart from Panaji in Arabian Sea represented climax of evolutionary process among nematodes with specialized characteristics of ventriculus, ventricular appendix, intestinal ceca in addition to the aforesaid teeth around three sets of distinguished apertures atop cephalic complex, and the typical physalopteran, sturdy cephalic, and post-caudal collarette.

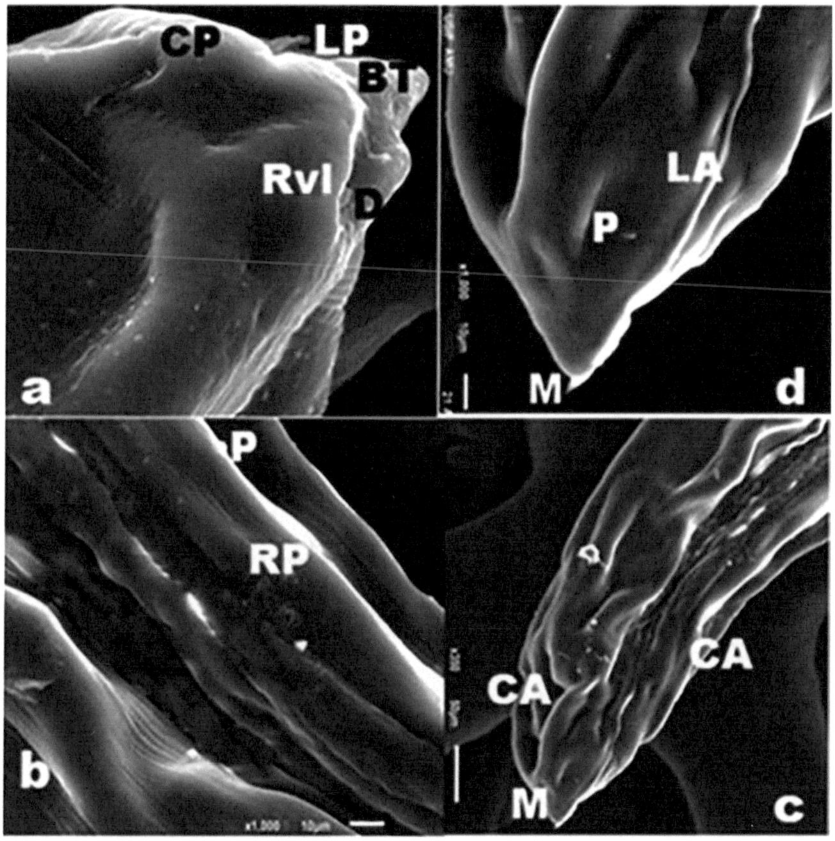

Figure 25.
Anisakis typica. *Scanning electron micrograph of (a) anterior end of worm to show linguiform papilla and dorsal buccal tooth; (b) rosette papillae on mid-body surface; (c) mucron at the terminal tip and lateral folds; (d) mucron with a spiny tip.*

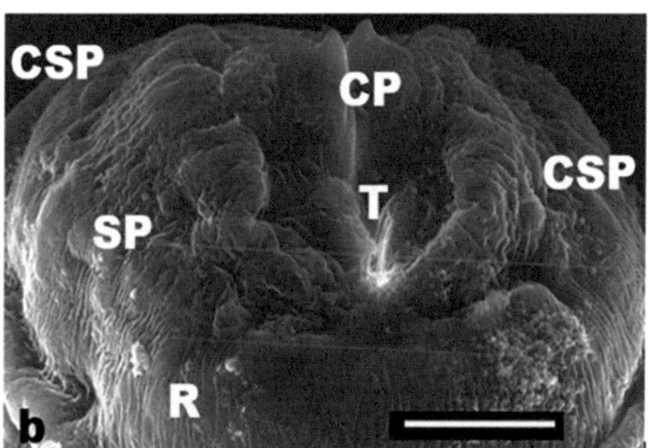

Figure 26.
Rotundocollarette capoori. *Scanning electron micrograph of head (magnified).*

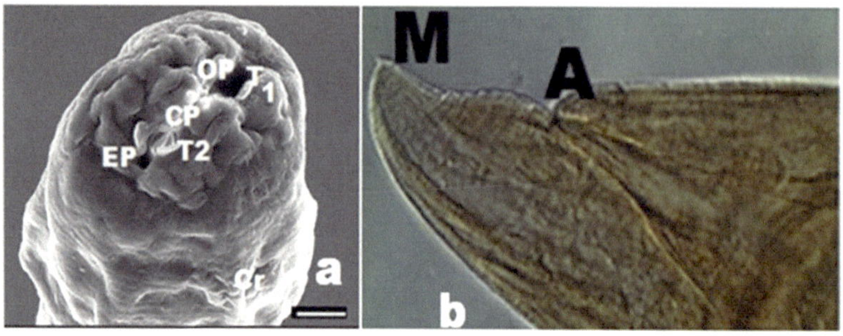

Figure 27.
Rotundocollarette capoori. *(a) Scanning electron micrograph of head to show pores and cephalic papillae atop cephalic complex; OP, oral aperture, EP, excretory pore, CP, cephalic papilla;* T_1*, first set of teeth,* T_2*, second set of teeth, Cr, cervical papilla. (b) Terminal part of body to show mucron and anus.*

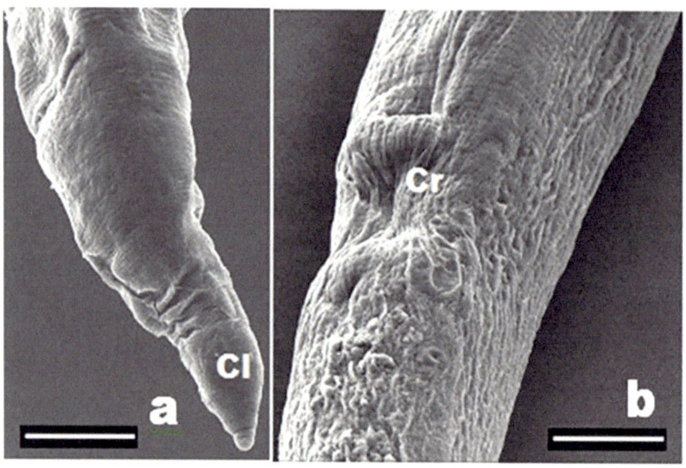

Figure 28.
Rotundocollarette capoori. *(a) Posterior part of body to show post-caudal collarette. (b) Cervical papilla on body of worm.*

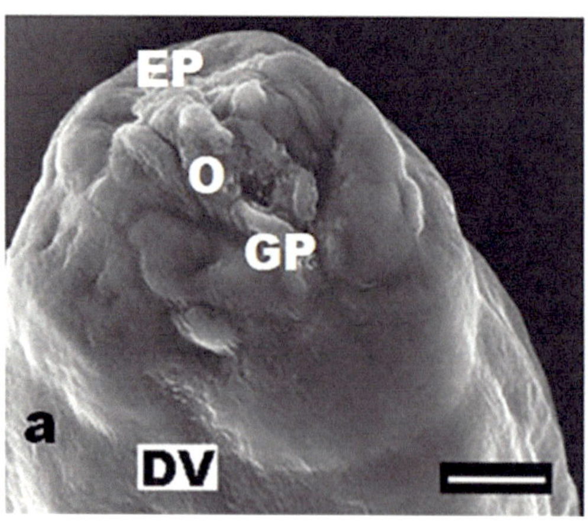

Figure 29.
Rotundocollarette capoori. *(a) Three pores atop cephalic complex* viz., *EP, excretory pore; O, oral aperture; GP, genital pore.*

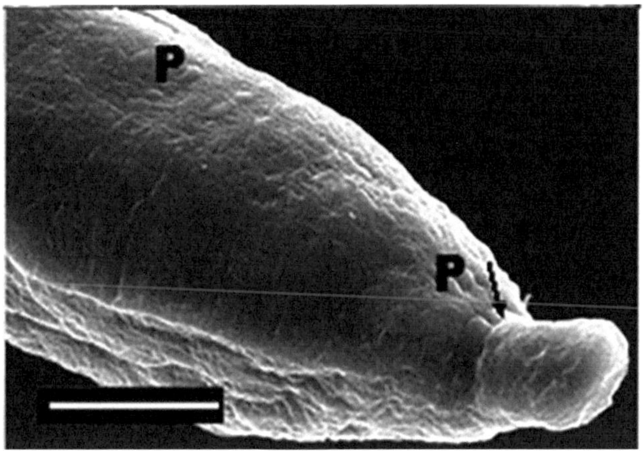

Figure 30.
Posterior end of body to show typical widened mucron.

7. The anisakid climax: *Rotundocollarette capoori*

7.1 Conclusions

The dispersal pathways of nematodes of Rhabdochonidae were linked to the drainage course of the streams of erstwhile Tethys Ocean [5]. The authors while working in the Himalayan cold water streams recorded occurrence of *Rhabdochona nemacheli* [2]. The rudimentary pseudolabia of this group, *viz.* Family Rhabdochonidae under superfamily Thelazioidea [48, 49], did undergo noticeable transformations throughout the course of evolution, while most of the time these appeared as weak buccal flanges, but for the worms attaining climax, where specific muscular formations were supported by three sets of paired teeth around oral aperture in *Rotundocollarette capoori* [3]. The host specificity along with monophyletic lineages was characterized appearance of Rhabdochindae in the fishes of Family Cyprinidae. However, the worms resorted to frequent host switching during overboard ecological host extensions. Therefore, as they crossed over through long distance course of riverine pathways in the Himalayas to reach estuarine reservoirs in the vicinity of Bay of Bengal, the nematodes have shown noticeable adaptations, while members of Anisakinae migrated from their freshwater host fish, *Bagarius bagarius*, to the intermediate host copepods, who could well receive anisakid larvae through fecal matter of fish, and finally when the latter are consumed by marine fish *S. sihama*, complete transfer of developing anisakids to marine environment could be achieved. The gradual events of emergence of *Paracamallanus tridenti* [14], and its coexistence with *Procamallanus chauhanensis* [13], *Tridentocamallanus* n.gen., n.sp. [49], *Pronakid* n.gen, n.sp. [49], *Indospinezia multispinatum* [12], *Rostellascaris spinicaudatum* [30], *Anisakis typica* [31], and *Rotundocollarette capoori* [50] have been added to the text with relevant pictures.

Author contributions

S.K.M. contributed to conceptualization; S.K.M. and A.Y. contributed to collection and investigation; S.K.M. contributed to writing—original draft preparation; S.K.M.

and A.Y. contributed to writing—review and editing; A.Y. contributed to visualization. All authors read and approved the final version of the manuscript.

Funding

This research is a part of independent research, and the findings of research investigations presented here were not part of any funded research project, nor any funding was received to conduct this research.

Conflict of interest

Authors have no potential conflict of interest pertaining to this submission whether financial or non-financial, professional, or Proceedings from a Conference.

Ethics committee approval

No procedures performed in studies involved human participants and the ethical standards of the institutional ethical committee and with the 1964 Helsinki declaration and its later amendments were followed.

Abbreviations

A	anus
AM	amphidial papilla
AS	alate spicule
B	buccal flange
BT	buccal teeth
C	cephalic papilla at margin of cephalic flange
CA & Ca	caudal alae
Cl	Cluster of papillae around margin of oral aperture
Cm	cephalic papilla in mid-circle
Cp	costiform papillae
CP	cephalic papillae
Cr and Cd	cephalic papilla first row adjacent to buccal flange
CSP	single cephalic papilla
D, D_1, and D_2	deirid
DV, E	encapsulated wall of anus
Eh	elevated hump
EP, Er	muscular elevation interrupting incompletely developed or feebly developed cuticular dentigerous lining inside oral aperture
Ex	excretory pore
FP	foliate papilla
FR, F	sclerotized connectives
GP	genital pore
I	denticles
IC	intestinal ceca

K	keychain head papilla
LA	Lateral alae
LL	lateral lobe
LP	linguiform papilla
Lvl	left ventro-lateral
M	mucron
ML	median lobe
O	oral aperture
OP	peripheral papillae around labial flange
P	phasmid
PS	sensory pit
R	dentigerous ridge
RP	rosette papillae
Rvl	right ventro-lateral
S	scattered sessile papillae
SF	sunflower papilla
SP	spicule
Sl	spicule
So	Sucker-organ like muscular papilla
Sp	button-shaped sessile cephalic papilla
T_1, T_2, T	tail
VA and Va	ventricular appendix
V	vulva
Vg	vagina

Author details

Sandeep K. Malhotra[1] and Anita Yadav[2*]

1 Parasitology Laboratory, Department of Zoology, University of Allahabad (a Central University), Allahabad, U.P., India

2 Department of Zoology, C.M.P. P.G. College (a Constituent College of the University of Allahabad), University of Allahabad (a Central University), Allahabad, U.P., India

*Address all correspondence to: anitaydv997@gmail.com

References

[1] Moravec F. Some aspects of the taxonomy, biology, possible evolution and biogeography of nematodes of the spirurine genus *Rhabdochona* Railliet, 1916 (Rhabdochonidae, Thelazioidea). Acta Parasitologica. 2010;**55**(2):144-160. DOI: 10.2478/s11686-010-0017

[2] Rautela AS, Malhotra Sandeep KA. Contribution to the study of taxa differentiation in nematode taxonomy in the Himalayan ecosystem. The Himalayan Journal of Science. 1982;**2**(1):23-37

[3] Yadav A, Kapoor N, Arif A, Malhotra SK. Energy dispersive X-ray microanalysis in conjunction with scanning electron micrography to establish nematodes as bioindicators in marine fish environment. Journal of Parasitic Diseases. 2022;**46**:664-671. DOI: 10.1007/s12639-022-01480-8

[4] National Institute of Health (NIH). (.gov) Nematode genome evolution – WormBook. USA: National Institute of Health; 2005. Available from: https://www.ncbi.nlm.nih.gov.books.NBK19768

[5] Mejia-Madrid HH, Choudhury A, Perez-Ponce de Leon G. Phylogeny and biogeography of Rhabdochona Railliet, 1916 (Nematoda: Rhabdochonidae) species from the Americas. Systematic Parasitology. 2007;**67**:1-18. DOI: 10.1007/s11230-006-9065-3

[6] Strahler AN, Strahler AH. Elements of Physical Geography. NY: John Wiley and Sons; 1989. p. 561

[7] Travassos L, Artigas P, Pereira C. Fauna helmintholojica dos peixes de agua doce de Brasil. Archivos do Instituto Biologico Sao Paulo. 1928;**1**:5-68

[8] Moravec F. Reconstruction of the nematode genus *Rhabdochona Railliet* 1916, with a review of the species parasitic in fishes of Europe and Asia. Studies CSAV. 1975;**8**(8):104

[9] Skrjabin KI, Moravec F. The development of Procamallanus laeviconchus (Wedl, 1862) (Nematoda: Camallanidae). Věstnik Československe Společnosti Zoologické. 1915;**39**(1):23-38

[10] Anderson RC. Nematode Parasites of Vertebrates. Their Development and Transmission. 2nd ed. Willingford: CABI Publishing; 2000. p. 550

[11] Gibbons LM. CIH Keys to the Nematode Parasites of Vertebrates: Suppl Vol Commonw Agric Bur. UK: Farnham Royal; 2000. p. 416

[12] Jaiswal N, Malhotra Sandeep K. Molecular characterization of host-specific Raphidascaridoid Worms from the Gangetic garfish (Teleostomi: Belonidae) in India. Intern. Journal of Molecular Biology. 2017;**4**(6): 00158. 16pp. DOI: 10.15406. IJMBOA.2017.02.00007

[13] Singh MK *Studies on the morphology and bio-ecology of nematode fauna of Rewa. D.Phil. Thesis, APS Univ, Rewa*. Chapter IV. Studies on the morphology and bio- cology of nematode fauna of Rewa. Ph.D. thesis submitted to A.P.S. Univ., Rewa under Dr. C.B. Singh. *Paracamallanus*%20 Species/*Procamallanus*%20*chauhanensis*. Shodhganga.pdf. Ph.D. Thesis. 1995: 44-54

[14] Neeshma J, Anshu M, Malhotra Sandeep K. Distribution and abundance relationship in infracommunities of proteocephalid tapeworms infesting

sharks of Arabian Sea at Goa. Proceedings of the Zoological Society of India. 2007;**6**(2):58-63.28

[15] Yadav A, Jaiswal N, Malhotra Sandeep K. Molecular, morphological and genetic characterization of *Tridentocamallanus indica* n.gen., n.sp. from Indian syncroaker of Aarabian Sea with revision of systematics of class chromadorea and a revised key to genera of Tridentocamallaninae n.subfam. Journal of Parasitic Diseases. 2025

[16] Railliet A. L'emploi des medicaments dans le traitement des maladies causees par des Nematodes. Recueil de Medecine Veterinaire Paris. 1915;**91**:490-513

[17] Hodda M. Phylum Nematoda: Trends in species descriptions, the documentation of diversity, systematics, and the species concept. Zootaxa. 2022;**5114**(1):290-317

[18] Railliet A, Henry A. Sur les nematodes du genre *Camallanus* Raill. and Henry, 1915 (*Cucullanus* auct., non Mueller, 1777). Bulletin de la Société de pathologie exotique. 1915;**8**(7):446-452

[19] Travassos L. Contribuicoes para o conhecimento da fauna helmintologica brasileira. Oxyascaridae n.fam. Arch Esc Sup Agric Med Vet. 1920;**4**(1):15

[20] On YLS. The reconstruction of the genus *Camallanus* Railliet et Henry, 1915. Journal of Helminthology. 1960;**34**:107-116

[21] Ali SM. Studies on the nematode parasites of fishes and birds found in Hyderabad state. Indian Journal of Helminthology. 1957;**8**:1-83

[22] Olsen LS. Some nematodes parasitic in marine fishes. Publications of the Institute of Marine Science. 1952;**2**:173-215

[23] Moravec F, Sey O. Nematodes of freshwater fishes from North Vietnam. Part 1. Camallanoidea and habronematoidea. Acta Societatis Zoologicae Bohemicae. 1988;**52**:12

[24] Moravec F, Scholz T. Observations on some nematodes parasitic in freshwater fishes in Laos. Folia Parasitologica. 1991;**38**:163-178

[25] Moravec F, Thatcher VE. *Procamallanus* (*Denticamallanus* subg.n.) *dentatus* n.sp. (Nematoda:Camallanidae) from the characid fish, *Bryconops alburnoides*, in the Brazilian Amazon. Parasite. 1997;**4**:239-243

[26] Petter A-J. Essai de classification de la sous-famille des Camallaninae (Nematoda, Camallanidae). Bulletin du Muséum national d'histoire naturelle. 1979;**4e sér., sect. A; 1**:991-1008

[27] Jothy AA, Fernando CH. A new camallanid nematode, *Malayocamallanus intermedius* gen. Et. sp. nov., from a Malayan freshwater fish, Fluta alba (Zuiew) with a key to the genera of the subfamily Procamallaninae. Helminthologia. 1970;**11**:87-91

[28] Bilqees FM, Akram M. Revision of the family Camallanidae Railliet and Henry, 1915 (Nematoda:Camallanoidea). Biologia. 1982;**28**:45-60

[29] Jackson JA, Tinsley RC. Representatives of *Batrachocamallanus* n.g. (Nematoda: Procamallaninae) from *Xenopus* Spp. (Anura:Pipidae): Geographical Distribution, Host Range and Evolutionary Relationships. Syst. Parasit. 1995;**31**:159-188

[30] Jaiswal N, Yadav A, Malhotra Sandeep K. Redescription of alien nematode, Rostellascaris spinicaudatum (Malhotra and Anas, 2001) of evolutionary significance with revised

key to the family Raphidascarididae Hartwich. Journal of Parasitic Diseases. 1954;**48**:460-473. DOI: 10.1007/s12639-024-01679-x

[31] Yadav A, Kapoor N, Malhotra SK. Faunal change over 3 decades to reveal *Rotundocollarette capoori* n.gen., n.sp., a unique anisakid from *Johnius dussumieri* from the central west coast of India at Goa. Journal of Parasitic Diseases. 2022;**46**(4):1110-1126. DOI: 10.1007/s12639-022-01533-y

[32] Jaiswal N. Spectral Signatures in Ichthyophthiriasis and co-Occurring Parasitic Infracommunity Variations in Freshwater and Marine Habitats. Unpublished Ph.D. Thesis. Prayagraj, U.P., India: University of Allahabad; 2006. 387 p

[33] Jaiswal N, Malhotra A, Malhotra SK, Gopal R. Roundworms of marine fishes from central west coast of India at Goa. I. *Paracamallanus tridenti* n.sp. from *Lutjanus malabaricus*. In: Proceedings of the International Conference of Zoology. Thiruvananthapuram: INCOZ; 2006. pp. 17-22

[34] Moravec F, Van As LL. Studies on some spirurids (Nematoda: Spirurida) from fishes of the Okavango River, Botswana. System Parasite. 2015;**91**:119-138. DOI: 10.1007/s11230-015-9565-0

[35] Pinheiro RHS, Melo FTV, Monks S, Santos JN, Giese EG. A new species of *Procamallanus* Baylis, 1923 (Nematoda, Camallanidae) from *Astronotus ocellatus* (Agassiz, 1831) (Perciformes, Cichlidae) in Brazil. ZooKeys. 2018;**790**:21-33. DOI: 10.3897/zookeys.790.24745

[36] Moravec F, Taraschewski H, Thairungroj Anantaphruti M, Maipanich W, Laoprasert T. *Procamallanus* (*Spirocamallanus*) *anguillae* sp. n. (Camallanidae) and some other nematodes from the Indonesian shortfin eel *Anguilla bicolor* in Thailand. Parasitology Research. 2006;**100**:69-75. DOI: 10.1007/s00436-006-0245-5

[37] Rodriguez H, De O, Pinto RM, Noronha D. Key to the species of Brazilian *Procamallanus* with general considerations (Nematoda, Camallanoidea). Memórias do Instituto Oswaldo Cruz, Rio de Jeneiro. 1991;**86**(1):107-113

[38] Khalifa RMA, Mohamadain HS, YFM K. Redescription and systematic studies on *Procamallanus* (*Procamallanus*) *elatensis* Fusco and Overstreet, 1979 from three Red Sea *Siganus* sp. fishes. Journal of the Egyptian Society of Parasitology. 2019;**49**(1):81-90

[39] Choudhury A, Nadler SA. Phylogenetic relationships of Cucullanidae (Nematoda) with observations on Seuratoidea and the monophyly of *Cucullanus*, *Dichelyne* and *Truttaedacnitis*. Journal of Parasitology. 2016;**102**:87-93

[40] Jaiswal N, Malhotra A, Malhotra Sandeep K. Bioinvasion: A paradigm shift from marine to inland ecosystem. Journal of Parasitic Diseases. 2014;**40**(2):348-358. DOI: 10.1007/s12639-014-0506-7

[41] Yadav A, Malhotra SK. Critical add-on SEM observations on oral armature and life cycle of raphidascaridoid worm, *Indospinezia multispinatum* Jaiswal and Malhotra (2017). International Journal of Molecular Biology: Open Access. 2023;**6**(1):59-62. DOI: 10.15406/ijmboa.2023.06.00153

[42] Akther M, Alam A, D'Silva J, Bhuiyan AI, Bristow GA, Berland BJ. *Goezia bangladeshi* n. sp. (Nematoda: Anisakidae) from an anadromous fish *Tenualosa ilisha* (Clupeidae). Journal of Helminthology. 2004;**78**(2):105-113. DOI: 10.1079/joh2003219

[43] Yadav A, Jaiswal N, Malhotra Sandeep K. A contribution on first report of morphogenetic characterization of *Anisakis typica* parasitizing Indian sand whiting, *Sillago sihama* from central west coast of India. Helminthologia. 2024;**61**(3):232-243. DOI: 10.2478/helm-2024-0027

[44] Koie M. On the histochemistry and ultrastructure of the tegument and associated structures of the cercaria of *Zoogonoides viviparus* in the first intermediate host. Ophelia. 1971;**9**:165-206

[45] Abollo E, Gestal C, Pascual S. *Anisakis* infestation in marine fish and cephalopods from Galician waters: An updated perspective. Parasitology Research. 2001;**87**:492-493

[46] Geetanjali MSK, Malhotra A, Ansari Z, Chatterjee A. Role of nematodes as bioindicators in marine and freshwater habitats. Current Science. 2002;**82**(5):505-507

[47] Jaiswal N, Malhotra A, Malhotra Sandeep K. Bioinvasion: A paradigm shift from marine to inland ecosystems. Journal of Parasitic Diseases. 2016;**40**(2):348-358. DOI: 10.1007/s12639-014-0506-7

[48] Yadav A. Studies on Helminth Parasites of Fresh and Marine Water Fishes. Unpublished Ph.D. Thesis. Prayagraj, U.P., India: University of Allahabad; 2023. 243 p

[49] Diesing F. Histoire naturelle des helminthes ou vers intestinaux. Librairie Encyclopedique de Roret. Paris.1845; xvi + 654 + 15 pp., pls. 1-12

Chapter 5

Amyloodiniosis in Semi-Intensive Aquaculture

Florbela Soares, Márcio Moreira, Rui Sousa and Cátia Lourenço-Marques

Abstract

Fish ectoparasites are one of the pathogen groups that are greatly concerned with the aquaculture industry. The dinoflagellate *Amyloodinium ocellatum* is responsible for amyloodiniosis, a parasitological disease with a strong economic impact in temperate and warm water aquaculture, mainly in earthen pond semi-intensive systems. Amyloodiniosis represents one of the most important bottlenecks for aquaculture, and with the predictable expansion of the area of influence of this parasite to higher latitudes due to global warming, it might also be a threat to other aquaculture species that are not yet parasitized by *A. ocellatum*. This book chapter aims to better understand the dynamics of amyloodiniosis in semi-intensive aquaculture production systems regarding the life cycle characterization, identification, diagnosis, parasite-host interactions, host physiological responses, prevention, and treatments.

Keywords: aquaculture, diseases, *Amyloodinium ocellatum*, detection, earthen ponds, prevention, treatments

1. Introduction

Most aquaculture production in the southern Mediterranean region is made by small producers in semi-intensive earthen pond production systems, at densities ranging from 1 to 5 kg/m^3 [1]. The main farmed species in these ponds are gilthead seabream (*Sparus aurata*), European bass (*Dicentrarchus labrax*), and meagre (*Argyrosomus regius*) and, at lower rates, Senegalese sole (*Solea senegalensis*) [1]. Due to the less intensive nature of these systems, the total number of fish produced is significantly lower than in intensive systems, such as offshore or recirculating aquaculture systems (RAS), being less representative of the total European production. Due to these conditions, semi-intensive production is perceived as a high-end niche market fish with high environmental standards [1]. These same fish production conditions, along with the presence of accessory species in the earthen ponds, create not only a complex ecosystem where energy and nutrients are cycled in a more diverse manner (multitrophic system) than in a monoculture (single-species) system but also unique pathological challenges, as disease dynamics can be more complex due to interactions between different species and differ from those typically encountered in more intensive production systems. Although amyloodiniosis is not an obligatory reported disease in the European Union (EU), according to Council Directive 2006/88/EC of 24 October 2006 on animal health requirements for aquaculture [2], it is important to recognize the significant impact of this disease on semi-intensive production systems—a key aquaculture production methods worldwide. This underscores the urgent need for continuous research and development efforts to better understand the disease dynamics, improve management strategies, and enhance the resilience of aquaculture operations. Amyloodiniosis outbreaks manifest as rapid, often asymptomatic outbreaks with high morbidity and mortality rates [3, 4], sometimes reaching 100% mortality in semi-intensive production systems within a very short period—often less than 48 hours—where conditions are frequently ideal for its growth, spread, and infection [5]. These phenomenon outbreaks are linked to the specific environmental characteristics of these production systems, including the occurrence of such microalgal blooms, potential anoxic conditions during early morning hours, and sedimentation that harbors various life stages of parasites [4].

Regarding the economic impact of this disease on producers, Shinn et al. [6] demonstrated that reported cases of amyloodiniosis in a milkfish (*Chanos chanos*) incubator in 2004 and Nile tilapia (*Oreochromis mossambicus*) in the Salton Sea caused total losses between US$20,000 and US$6–77 million, solely from fish mortality. Summing up the indirect cost of labor, fish retrieval and disposal, and treatments, it is enough to bring small-scale companies that operate in earthen ponds to bankruptcy. This is a non-obligatory report of disease in the EU, according to Council Directive 2006/88/EC of October 24, 2006 on animal health requirements for aquaculture [2] and non-listed disease in the Aquatic Animal Health Code [7], that leads to a subestimation of the real impact of this disease. Moreover, the expected increase in the infestation period of *A. ocellatum* due to global warming will likely increase both the impact of the disease and its associated economic burden [6, 8–10]. Thus, given the high mortality rates associated with this parasite in semi-intensive systems and the lack of effective treatments, this chapter aims to evaluate the current status of amyloodiniosis in semi-intensive aquaculture systems and provide strategies to help producers manage the disease.

2. Life cycle and physiological impact on the host

2.1 Parasite hosts, life cycle, and conditions for propagation

Taxonomically, *A. ocellatum* belongs to the Oodiniaceae family, the only member of the *Amyloodinium* genus [11]. Regarding the hosts, this parasite is one of the few that can infest both elasmobranchs and teleosts [11–16], affecting nearly all finfish within its ecological range, from flatfish to pelagic fish [12, 17–24]. This parasite also presents a high potential of co-infecting different fish species produced at the same location [25, 26], which is very common in semi-intensive production, where one or more fish species can coexist. Additionally, several commercially important shrimp species reported moderate to intense tissue inflammation [26]. There are also reports of co-infection of *A. ocellatum* with *Vibrio alginolyticus* in European seabass [27] and a more recent case of co-infection with *Chilodonella hexasticha* in farmed silver carp (*Hypophthalmichthys molitri*) [28]. Moreover, *Amyloodinium ocellatum* can also hyperparasite other fish parasites like *Neobenedenia melleni* [27].

A. ocellatum has a direct triphasic life cycle that comprises the following stages (**Figure 1**).

- *Trophont*: The parasitic stage of the parasite attaches firmly to the gill/skin/mouth epithelium of the host through rhizopod-like structures and feeds using a stomatopod. When it reaches 80–140 μm in width, or there is a sudden change in the physicochemical conditions in the water, the trophont detaches from the gill and encysts, transforming itself into a comment [28].

- *Tomont*: The reproductive encysted stage of the parasite is usually found on the gills, in the tank sediment, and, occasionally, in the intestinal tract of the hosts [29]. Under optimal physicochemical conditions, each moment can divide into limits and produce up to 256 dinospores within three days at 25°C [30], which are then released into the water column.

- *Dinospores*: Free-living, infestant stage of the parasite. These are small anteroposteriorly compressed, thinly armored peridinin-type dinoflagellates, measuring 6.1 ± 0.8 μm in length, 11.7 ± 0.5 μm in width, and 11.1 ± 1.2 μm in-depth [13, 28, 31, 32]. They have a life span of up to 10 days [33, 34] and can infest a potential host [34].

Regarding the outbreak conditions for amyloodiniosis, several environmental conditions that modulate *A. ocellatum* outbreaks are summarized in **Figure 2**.

Among them, some play a more important role in the modulation of *A. ocellatum* pathogenicity and life cycle speed, such as temperature and salinity [34–37]. *Amyloodinium ocellatum* can reproduce at temperatures ranging from 16 to 30°C, with optimal limits of production between 23 and 27°C. Nevertheless, amyloodiniosis sporadic outbreaks were reported at 36°C, where *A. ocellatum* trophonts are expected to arrest their development. Below 16°C, the division is charged, and mont mortality may occur at temperatures below 8°C [38]. Regarding salinity levels, *A.* ocellatum can tolerate salinities between 10 and 60 psu, with an optimum salinity range between

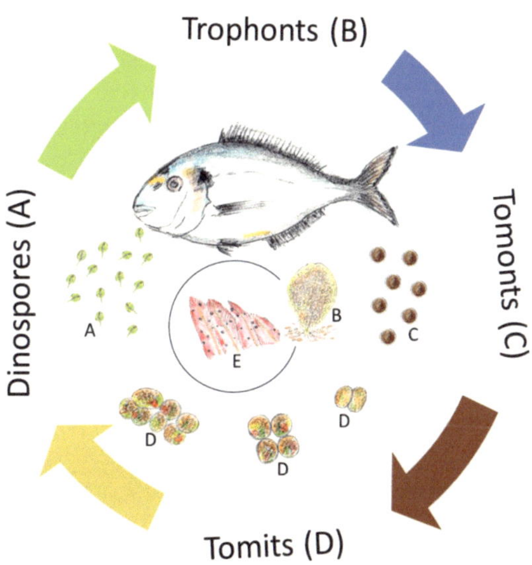

Figure 1.
Life cycle of the fish parasite Amyloodinium ocellatum. *A—dinospores, B—trophonts, C—tomonts, D—tomits, and E—parasitized gills.*

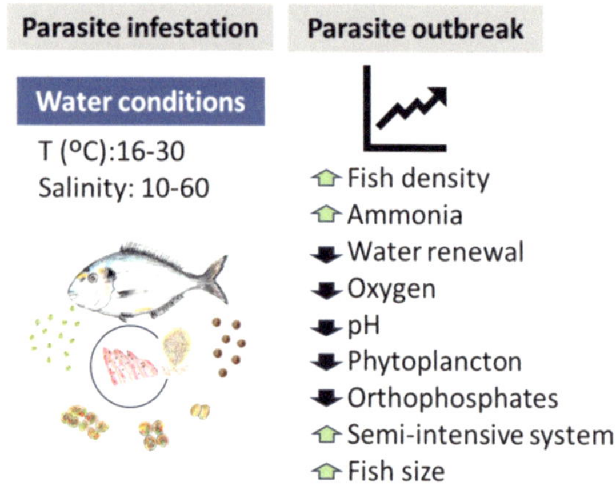

Figure 2.
Factors modulating amyloodiniosis outbreaks.

18 and 39 psu [34, 38–40]. However, sporadic cases have been reported at 46 psu and 7 psu, indicating that other factors also play an important role in amyloodiniosis outbreak modulation. Pereira et al. [35] reported that dissolved oxygen, water temperature, pH, and phytoplankton biomass significantly negatively correlate with *A. ocellatum* outbreaks in gilthead seabream. Seoud et al. [41] reported a strong, significant negative correlation between pH and water temperature levels, a strong, significant positive correlation with salinity, and a weak but significant positive correlation between ammonia levels and parasitic infestation in a European seabass infestation in Egypt. Tahraoui et al. [42] reported a high concentration of ammonia (10–10.4 mg/L) and low levels of orthophosphates (0.8–0.9 μg/L) during a natural outbreak of *A. ocellatum* on the Atlantic coast of Morocco. Moreover, other reports highlight the importance of water renewal rates [35], fish density [43], and fish size [9] as significant important factors in the modulation of amyloodiniosis outbreaks [4].

2.2 Symptomatology and host responses

Behaviorally, amyloodiniosis symptomatology is characterized by jerky or uncoordinated movements, slow swimming at the water surface, and decreased appetite (**Figure 3**) [4, 44]. Other disease signs include an increased respiratory rate with possible "piping" and gasping, pruritis (with flashing behavior or rubbing on tank walls, substrate, or other structures/fish), gathering near areas with higher dissolved oxygen concentrations or water current, and darkened skin and/or skin lesions in some fish species [11, 42, 45]. Since the infestation also affects the skin, fish may develop a "velvety" white or brown coloration and a cloudy appearance, most visible under indirect lighting, such as a flashlight [46].

Fish mortality is often linked to anoxia and gill damage [47] and can occur within 12–24 hours when parasite loads are high. However, sudden deaths can also happen at moderate parasite levels, indicating that other factors such as hypoxia, osmotic imbalance, secondary bacterial infections, and the possible presence of toxins [13, 48] may play a role. An *in vitro* study on gilthead seabream cell cultures found that certain compounds associated with the attachment phase of dinospores and the feeding phase of trophonts exhibit hemolytic properties, meaning they can destroy red blood cells [49]. This could trigger an array of physiological responses from the host.

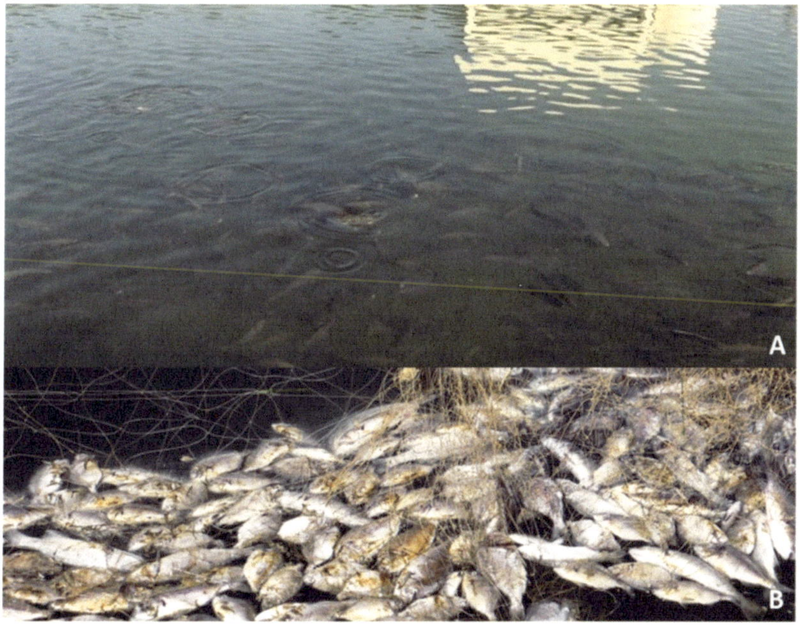

Figure 3.
(A) Fish presenting amyloodiniosis symptomatology at the surface of a semi-intensive pond. (B) Fish mortality associated with the same Amyloodinium ocellatum *outbreak.*

The information about these physiological responses from the host is nevertheless limited and very fragmented. Hematological indicators of response to an *A. ocellatum* reported an increase in red blood cell count, mean corpuscular hemoglobin concentration, and a decrease in mean corpuscular volume (MCV) in infested yellowtail amberjack (*Seriola lalandi*) in comparison with healthy, unparasitized individuals [50]. In white seabream (*Diplodus sargus*), Moreira et al. [51] reported a significant increase in the white blood cell count and MCV levels at 5 h post-infestation. Regarding the metabolic and stress indicators, higher levels of glucose and triglyceride concentrations and lower levels of total protein, albumin, and globulin were reported in infested California yellowtail (*Seriola dorsalis*) [52]. Another study with healthy, unparasitized individuals in infested white seabream reported a significant increase in cortisol and glucose levels at 5 h post-infestation [45]. Gilthead seabream also presents a substantial rise in cortisol and lactate levels at 18 h post-infestation [52]. These responses can indicate a primary and secondary response to stress caused by the parasite's attachment to the gills [52]. As for osmoregulatory indicators, there is a huge lack of information about the host responses to an *A. ocellatum* outbreak. The only work that has studied these parameters reported a significant decrease in the gill Na+, K+ ATPase levels in gilthead seabream with amyloodiniosis at 18 h post-infestation, which could be associated with anoxia and physiological impact caused by trophont-induced damage [52, 53]. The immune response can be divided into two major systems. The vertebrate innate immune system recognizes both pathogenic and non-pathogenic microorganisms via germline-encoded pathogen pattern recognition receptors (PRRs), which evolved to sense pathogen-associated molecular patterns (PAMPs), initiating a well-coordinated innate immune response [54]. The adaptive immune system, on the other hand, is mediated by antigen receptors, with some species-specific variations in fish [55]. In amyloodiniosis, available research highlights the role of PRRs in recognizing *A. ocellatum* PAMPS, with toll-like receptors (TLR) being key players in initiating this immune response. Interestingly, in infested European seabass, TLR1, TLR2, TLR4, and TLR9 were not activated in the gills. However, increased mRNA abundance for TLR9 was observed in the head kidney, suggesting parasitic DNA being recognized through TLR9 in this organ [56]. TLR22 has also been identified as an important immune gene involved in the antiparasitic immune response of yellowtail amberjack to *A. ocellatum*, which aligns with its role in the antiparasitic immune response in teleost fish [57, 58]. Other studies on fish immune responses to *A. ocellatum* have explored innate immunity and other branches of the immune system, depending on the affected tissue. *Amyloodinium ocellatum* causes tissue damage in the gill and skin due to epithelial shedding and rhizoid penetration, leading to inflammation, bleeding, and necrosis [59], which is expected to trigger a host immune response. This was observed in the gills of naturally infested European seabass, where increased transcripts of interleukin 8 (IL-8), chemokine CC1, and cyclo-oxygenase two transcripts were observed, all of which are usually associated with inflammatory responses [56]. Additionally, gilthead seabream presents a differential expression of apolipoprotein1 (ApoA1) and fibrinogen beta chain in response to epithelial damage in an amyloodiniosis outbreak [52]. In another study with *A. ocellatum* infection in yellowfin seabream (*Acanthopagrus latus*) both in individual fishes and cell lines, increased expression of apoptosis and inflammation-related genes was observed, including caspase 3 (Casp 3), interleukin 1 (IL-1), interleukin 10 (IL-10), and tumor necrosis factor-alpha (TNF-α) [59]. Furthermore, IL-1β and TNFα gene expression levels increased in the intestines of symptomatic European seabass [44]. Since the intestine is not an infested tissue by *A. ocellatum*, the elevated levels of these pro-inflammatory markers may simply reflect a response to metabolic changes associated with the disease [44]. This is supported by the increased mRNA expression levels of hepatic PPARα transcripts in the same study, suggesting the activation of metabolic pathways that promote lipids utilization to cope with the metabolic burden of the infestation and restore homeostasis. Proteome data obtained from gilthead seabream plasma also indicated a differential expression of hemopexin, ApoA1, and fibrinogen beta-chain proteins. These markers are usually associated with acute-phase and inflammatory responses [52]. Other humoral substances and cell secretions also contribute to the natural resistance of fish to pathogenic and infectious agents, such as complement, transferrin, anti-proteases, lytic enzymes, lectins, C-reactive protein, antimicrobial peptides (AMP), interferons, and enzyme inhibitors [60, 61]. In response to amyloodiniosis, a series of AMPs, including histone-like proteins, piscidin 2, ApoA1, and HbβP-1, have been shown to affect both the dinospores and trophont phase of *A. ocellatum* [52, 62, 63]. Hepcidin, an AMP also involved in iron metabolism, showed an increased mRNA expression level in the gills of European seabass naturally infected with *A. ocellatum* [56]. Interestingly, an increase in hemopexin expression was also observed in the liver of gilthead seabream infected with this ectoparasite, suggesting an important role of iron transport and metabolism during the development of the disease, most likely related to the appearance of hemorrhages [13, 64]. Another interesting response is the increase in plasma lysozyme in some fish species. However, since some studies do not report lysozyme activity, this may be a host-specific response to *A. ocellatum* [64–66]. Additionally, another cytokine production is expected in response to severe hyperplasia and inflammatory reactions [59], leading to the recruitment of neutrophils. However, this response has not been consistently observed across studies. In European seabass affected by spontaneous *A. ocellatum* outbreaks, an increased number of macrophages was detected, primarily in the secondary lamella epithelium, with macrophage numbers rising proportionally to the parasite burden [67]. Nevertheless, other studies have reported only limited infiltration of macrophages, lymphocytes, and eosinophil granular cell migration in the gills of juvenile fish infested with *A. ocellatum* [39]. Recently published time-course studies reported that meager (*Argyrosomus* regius) showed an increase in peripheral blood neutrophils 9 h after exposure to the parasite, alongside a decrease in the relative proportion of circulating lymphocytes [64].

More data regarding the adaptive response to amyloodiniosis needs to be available. The role of the adaptative immune response to *A. ocellatum* has been known for a long time because the antisera from fish intraperitoneally immunized with dinospores can agglutinate live dinospores at concentrations as low as 0.156–2.5% and immobilize infective dinospores at serum concentrations of 5% *in vitro* [68]. Antibodies against *A. ocellatum* were detected in the sera of experimentally immunized blue tilapia (*Oreochromis aureus*) and hybrid striped bass (*Morone saxatilis* ♀ × *Morone chrysops* ♂) that survived an amyloodiniosis outbreak [69], as well as in a cultured population of European seabass following an outbreak of the disease [53]. More recent studies reported a high expression of the immunoglobulin IgT in the gills and head-kidney of infected European seabass, even in the absence of gene expression for genes coding for molecules related to adaptive immunity (e.g., MHC I, MHC II, and IgM) [53]. Other studies reported the activation of components of gill-associated lymphoid tissue in European seabass [70]. These adaptative immune responses highlight the importance of research and the development of vaccines as a viable approach to prevent and reduce mortalities from amyloodiniosis.

3. *Amyloodinium ocellatum* incidence in semi-intensive systems

3.1 Semi-intensive production systems

The parasite *A. ocellatum* is widespread, affecting intensive and semi-intensive aquaculture systems. However, fish produced in earthen ponds, characteristic of the Mediterranean region, are particularly susceptible to this parasite [10]. This is due to the specific conditions of these production systems, which involve sediment bottom (mud) ponds that allow the parasite to remain "dormant" when conditions are unfavorable for its development, serving as a reservoir for new reinfections. Since these ponds usually exceed 0.5 ha, the bottom is not disturbed during the production cycle, which lasts over 14 months in the Mediterranean, for species like sea bream and sea bass [4]. As a result, the pond bottoms can only be treated at the end of the production cycle, after fish harvest.

Moreover, the water renewal rate is usually low, and primary production is higher in warm weather, leading to lower oxygen levels during the night. Taking advantage of this operational characteristic, the parasite remains in the sediment and opportunistically infests the fish population when favorable conditions arise. This makes this type of production system especially vulnerable to *A. ocellatum*. Although this production system does not account for the highest fish production in the Mediterranean, this problem is not given the importance it has [4].

Due to the characteristics of semi-intensive production systems, amyloodiniosis poses a major bottleneck for aquaculture production in Southern Europe because it affects most fish farms and causes extremely high mortalities. According to Soares et al. [4], it is a "quiet" disease because when the fish farmer notices the first symptoms and mortality, it is often too late, and the fish do not

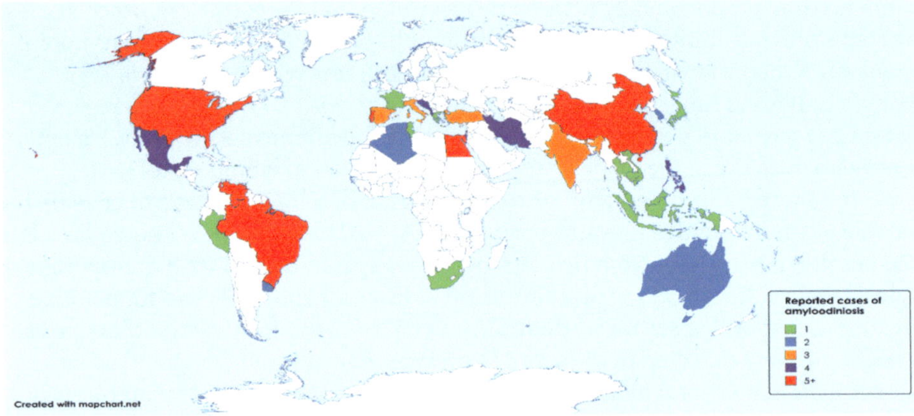

Figure 4.
Published cases of Amyloodinium ocellatum *worldwide, based on the data presented by Moreira et al. [9].*

respond to treatment. This situation occurs in Mediterranean countries between spring and autumn, when water temperatures range from 16 to 30°C, a range expected to increase due to global warming [13, 71, 72]. The increased stress can trigger disease outbreaks during the summer when the fish harvest is more frequent due to higher selling prices.

3.2 Amyloodiniosis incidence and reported cases

Amyloodiniosis distribution, based on reported cases in aquaculture experimental facilities or production sites worldwide, confirms that *A. ocellatum* has a wide geographical distribution [4, 12, 13, 73]. Its prevalence is higher in tropical and temperate regions or areas influenced by warm water currents, where conditions for completing the parasite cycle are fulfilled [13] (see **Figure 4**). Other factors contributing to the expansion of *A. ocellatum* include aquaculture development, production intensification, stock/larvae movement, and the widespread use of advanced detection techniques [14, 40].

Regarding incidence, A. *ocellatum* affects several fish species from different phylogenetic families, at various ages, and in almost all available production systems [13, 74–77]. However, there are more reports of outbreaks in semi-intensive systems compared to other production systems worldwide [10, 13]. Typically, there is an increase in affected aquaculture facilities following the first country detection. Several factors contribute to this pattern, including the open design of many aquaculture systems, which facilitates the spread of *A. ocellatum* to new areas within its ecological range where outbreaks can start [76, 77]; the transfer of infested fish between rearing facilities [78–80]; and higher awareness among aquaculture technicians and national veterinary bureaus regarding this issue [71, 79, 81].

4. Amyloodiniosis detection, prevention, and available treatments

4.1 Amyloodiniosis assessment and detection

Accurate and precise diagnostics are crucial for assessing infestation severity in fish parasitosis. In the case of amyloodiniosis, one of the critical factors is the selection of the individuals chosen for examination [13]. Fish should be alive or caught immediately after death. If the fish is already dead, it should be handled so that there is no contact with freshwater or ice to avoid parasite detachment. This detachment can result in inaccurate assessments of parasite load, leading to incorrect diagnoses of infestation levels and potentially increasing mortality due to the disease [30]. Another important aspect is the speed of diagnosis. *Amyloodinium ocellatum* is an opportunistic pathogen that can rapidly proliferate under favorable conditions. Therefore, rapid assessment and detection of amyloodiniosis are critical for minimizing its impact, even if the process is often challenging due to the infection's rapid progression and sometimes asymptomatic nature [11].

Additionally, the species produced in the same pond should be considered to better understand the situation and guide the sample. In polyculture systems, collecting representative samples from each reared species is essential to thoroughly evaluate the outbreak in the production tank [13]. It is important to recognize that a thorough diagnosis has significant implications for recommending effective measures to address infestations and manage mortality rates associated with the disease. In the case of amyloodiniosis, one of the critical factors is the selection of individuals for examination, as it may condition the diagnosis. Fish should be alive or examined immediately after death, as the parasite's trophonts often detach from the host shortly after death. This detachment can lead to inaccurate assessments of parasite load and potentially result in incorrect diagnoses (**Figure 5**) [4, 10, 13, 82].

Early detection of *A. ocellatum* infestations often rely on observing behavioral and physiological changes in fish. An infestation is then confirmed by assessing the presence of the parasite in the gills and the mucosa of the branchial cavity, where infestations primarily occur [25]. Parasites can also be found on the skin, fins, and eyes, especially in severe cases, with reports of 50–200 trophonts per gill filament [83]. Additionally, their presence has been documented on the skin of gilthead seabream during both larval and post-larval stages [84]. One diagnostic method involves microscopic observation, as the trophonts (parasitic stage) are easily visible at low magnification under a light microscope (**Figure 6**). Examining gill, skin, or mucus samples to identify the parasitic stages of *A. ocellatum* is a common procedure for diagnosing amyloodiniosis. Regular random fish sampling is recommended for early detection, especially in systems with recurring outbreaks. However, some diagnostic methods are invasive and may require the sacrifice of the animals, as accurate observation often necessitates cutting the gill arch [13].

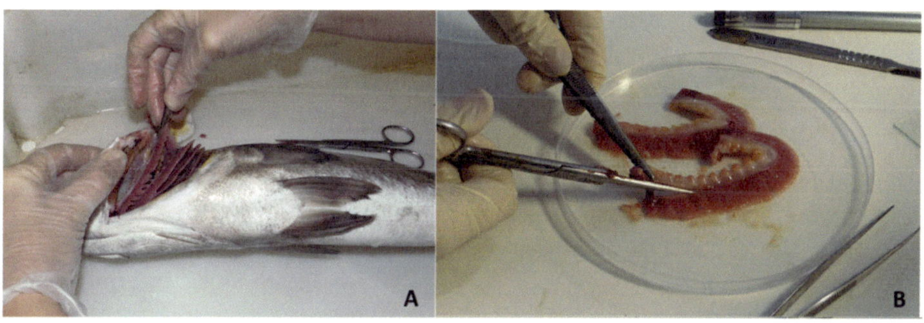

Figure 5.
Analysis of the fish gills to assess the presence of Amyloodinium ocellatum. *(A) Collection of fish gills for* A. ocellatum *fresh visualization. (B) Separation of gill filaments from the arch for better parasite observation.*

Microscopic identification of the parasite is necessary to accurately diagnose amyloodiniosis [30, 85]. Typically, this involves cutting the gill arch for observation. Detection is possible under a light microscope for larvae and post-larvae, as the infestation primarily affects the skin [13]. When dealing with fish that cannot be sacrificed, such as broodstock, trophonts can be collected by gently brushing or scraping the skin or gills for microscopic examination [46, 85–87]. Environmental conditions in aquaculture production are crucial for the proliferation of *A. ocellatum* [25]. Therefore, monitoring water parameters such as salinity, temperature, and dissolved oxygen levels is essential for implementing early warning systems and conducting risk assessments. This monitoring is particularly important during high-risk periods, as it can prevent amyloodiniosis outbreaks [88].

Risk-based surveillance strategies are increasingly being implemented to assess the prevalence of amyloodiniosis. This approach targets identifying systems or conditions at higher risk of infection, such as farms with a history of *A. ocellatum* outbreaks and areas where environmental conditions favor the parasite's growth. Producers can allocate resources more efficiently by concentrating monitoring efforts on high-risk zones, enabling earlier intervention and reducing the likelihood of widespread infection [89]. Fish mortality is often linked to anoxia and can occur within 12–24 hours when parasite loads are high. However, sudden deaths can also happen at moderate parasite levels, suggesting that other factors, such as hypoxia, osmotic imbalance, secondary bacterial infections, and the possible presence of toxins [49, 90], may contribute to mortality. An *in vitro* study on gilthead seabream cell cultures found that certain compounds associated with the attachment phase of dinospores and the feeding phase of trophonts exhibit hemolytic properties, meaning they can destroy red blood cells, which may trigger various physiological responses in the host [49].

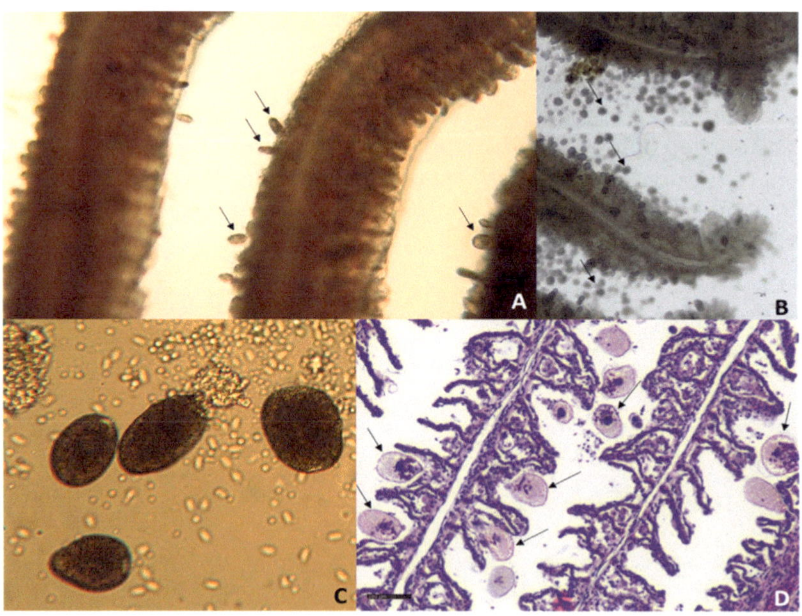

Figure 6.
Microscope observation of Amyloodinium ocellatum. *(A) Early trophonts in gill filaments (100×); (B) tomonts detaching from the gills (40×); (C)* A. ocellatum *comments expelling the dinospores (400×); (D) histological observation of* A. ocellatum *trophonts attached in a fish gill (100×), stained with hematoxylin-eosin.*

Early detection of *A. ocellatum* infection in fish is critical for effective and timely treatment. Along with monitoring fish behavior and conducting routine sampling of fish in production, detecting the free-swimming dinospore stage in tanks' water is particularly important [91]. Identifying the parasite at this early stage allows for rapid intervention, mitigating potential impacts on fish welfare and reducing mortality rates, thereby minimizing associated economic losses. A study by Masson et al. [91] used formaldehyde to immobilize dinospores in seawater for quantification, but this method is time-consuming and imprecise. The application of molecular techniques has greatly enhanced the early detection and management of *A. ocellatum* infections, providing a valuable tool for controlling and treating this parasitic disease. In this context, a rapid and sensitive method for *A. ocellatum* identification was developed by Levy et al. [92]. However, it is important to highlight a potential source of error: the reverse primer referenced in their study is presented in the 3′–5′ direction rather than the commonly accepted 5′–3′ orientation.

Loop-mediated isothermal amplification (LAMP) has also been developed to detect *A. ocellatum* in water [52, 93]. These highly sensitive techniques can detect the parasite at very low concentrations, such as 10 dinospores/mL of water [93]. These techniques allow precise pathogen load monitoring and early identification of infections, even before clinical signs become apparent [4, 44, 91, 93–95].

Recently, Zhuang et al. [29] have developed an efficient diagnostic method for *A. ocellatum* detection. This quantitative PCR (qPCR) technique offers a specific, sensitive, and quantitative diagnostic tool compared to conventional PCR and other diagnostic techniques. This novel qPCR method is suitable for assessing *A. ocellatum* population dynamics and predicting disease outbreaks in aquaculture systems. It can accurately detect as few as 8–10 dinospores in 300 L of seawater. However, although promising, this method has yet to be tested in a real farming scenario.

Given the importance of early and accurate detection of amyloodiniosis to minimize its impact on aquaculture, a combination of regular clinical observations, microscopic examination, environmental monitoring, and advanced molecular tools offers the most effective approach for managing this parasitic disease. Although significant efforts have been made, the rapid onset and high mortality associated with *A. ocellatum* outbreaks highlight the need for continuous research into effective prevention and control measures [13].

4.2 Prevention and treatment

Amyloodiniosis is an asymptomatic disease in the early stages of infestation, with clinical signs usually appearing only in the later stages. These delayed onset symptoms often result in high morbidity and mortality. Consequently, preventive measures are very important for effective disease prevention and mitigation.

Current and emergent strategies for preventing amyloodiniosis fall into five categories: zootechnical control, physical disinfection systems, functional feeds, vaccination, and mixed approaches [13]. Zootechnical measures, such as closely monitoring fish rearing (particularly during amyloodiniosis season), play a key role in managing outbreaks. Early detection of *A. ocellatum* in fish gills or water is essential to controlling the parasite effectively [13]. Maintaining good water quality within production ponds, ensuring appropriate stocking densities, and implementing a high-water renewal rate during the most critical months for amyloodiniosis outbreaks are important steps to reduce or even prevent *A. ocellatum* infestations [35]. When the parasite is detected early or infestation levels are low, frequent water changes might help to manage the infestation without treatment by diluting and washing out motile dinospores as they emerge from comments [96].

Nevertheless, this might not be enough to stop disease progression if amyloodiniosis reaches the mid-to-late stages of infestation [97]. Routine hygiene protocols, such as removing dead fish from tanks, must be performed to prevent the release of parasite loads and the degradation of water quality [13]. Another critical procedure is removing the sediment top layer during sanitary breaks, as comments typically settle on the bottom of a tank. This action significantly decreases parasite load for the next fish grow-out cycle, lowering the chances of more severe outbreaks caused by high infestation levels. For earthen ponds, this can be done by scraping the sediment surface, complementing sterilization procedures, such as exposure to sunlight and desiccation of the tank bottom for some time, or sterilizing with sodium hydroxide. In the case of cement or fiberglass tanks, the tank surface should be scrubbed with an acid solution [97]. All these measures should be incorporated into risk management plans to effectively address this disease. Such plans can be complemented with informatic tools specifically designed for this purpose. A new software and a mobile app designed to help predict amyloodiniosis outbreaks based on environmental parameters and fish behavioral factors communicated by the producers, are currently in the final phases of implementation. This system has been statistically validated to help early detect *A. ocellatum* outbreaks in sea bream and sea bass rearing ponds [98].

Physical disinfection systems, such as ultraviolet (UV) light, ozone, and chlorine, can be implemented before the water enters the tank, and quarantine periods for newcoming fish can also limit the introduction of parasites in aquaculture systems [28, 94]. However, these methods have limited applicability in open systems with tanks ranging from 0.4 to 1 ha. Another interesting approach involves using functional ingredients [62, 83, 99–101], which have shown interesting results. For example, a diet supplemented with the live yeast *Debaryomyces hansenii* stimulated the immune system of juvenile leopard grouper (*Mycteroperca rosacea*), leading to enhanced resistance against *A. ocellatum* [102]. Similar results have been reported with several prebiotics supplemented in the diet [103]. Vaccination represents the most appropriate method for pathogen control currently available to the aquaculture sector, and a protective vaccine against *A. ocellatum* could be a viable future development. Early studies have investigated the use of inactivated parasites as vaccine agents. Byadgi et al. [103] evaluated the protective effects of fragmented dinospores administered intracoelomatically in European seabass. This study presented some preliminary, promising results in immune system modulation [104]. The Portuguese Institute for the Ocean and Atmosphere, Aquaculture Research Station (EPPO-IPMA) pathology research group focused on possible vaccine development for European seabass, using hydrophilic extracts from *A. ocellatum* tomonts [103]. However, the need for a standardized method to produce *A. ocellatum* dinospores or trophonts severely hampers the scale-up in this research [13].

The available amyloodiniosis treatments must be highly effective, as *A. ocellatum* outbreaks must be treated swiftly to avoid catastrophic consequences [10]. As shown in **Table 1**, the free-living stage (dinospores) is the primary target for treatment development, as they are more susceptible to chemotherapy. In contrast, the parasitic and encapsulated states of trophonts and tomonts are more difficult to eradicate or treat, hampering the efforts to manage infestations over time [4].

Controlling environmental factors in production settings is rarely feasible [105]. An alternative is short freshwater baths that dislodge most trophonts in most fish species [28, 106]. For example, a treatment regimen tested on six-finger threadfin

Treatment	Doses/time	Effectivity	Feasibility in semi-intensive systems
Abiotic parameters			
Freshwater baths	5 minutes	High trophont gill release. Noneffective in tomont stage	Nonapplicable
Lower salinity	NA	Low delays parasite cycle	Not applicable
Lower temperature	15°C	Arrest parasite cycle	Not applicable
Biological			
Artemia salina nauplii	1 nauplii for 2500 dinospores or 1 nauplii for every 1250 dinospores	Dinospores were eliminated after 20 h and 8 h, respectively	Not applied yet
Chemical			
Copper sulfate	0.15–0.2 mg/L for 10–14 days	Effective in dinospore removal. High trophont gill release. Noneffective in tomont stage	Effective in earthen ponds.
Hydrogen peroxide	25 ppm for 30 min to 200 ppm for 1 h	Effective in dinospore removal. High trophont gill release. Noneffective in tomont stage	Less effective in earthen ponds.
Formalin	100–200 ppm for 6–9 h; 51 ppm for 1 h; 4 ppm for 7 h.	Effective in dinospore removal. High trophont gill release. Noneffective in tomont stage	Less effective in earthen ponds.
Sodium hypochlorite (NaOCl)	Chlorine ≥250 ppm for 1 h	Inactivation of tomonts (100%)	NA
Virkon S	1000 ppm for 1 h	Inactivation of tomonts (66%). No release of dinospores	NA
Ox-Virin (5% peracetic acid solution)	500 ppm for 48 h	Inactivation of tomonts (100%)	NA
Chloroquine diphosphate	10 mg/L water baths	Effective in dinospore removal. Noneffective in tomont stage	Not applicable
3, N-methylglucamine lasalocid	0.001 to 1 ppm	Inhibition of dinospore motility. Trophont inactivation and removal at higher doses. Reduces comment division rate	Not applicable
Tomatine	50–6.25 μg/ml for 1 hour	Inhibition of dinospore motility	NA
2′,4′-Dihydroxychalcone	50 and 25 μg/ml for 1 hour	Inhibition of dinospore motility	NA

NA—non-available data.

Table 1.
Treatments available for amyloodiniosis.

(*Polydactylus sexfilis*) involved a 5-minute freshwater bath followed by transfer to a clean tank, repeated three times every 3 days. This approach is more effective since it removes the dinospore and most of the trophont load while reducing the moment population through tank transfers [94, 107]. Biological treatments have also been explored; nauplii of brine shrimp (*Artemia salina*) were tested as a biological resource to reduce dinospores, achieving a reduction of 65% in trophont gill load in the red drum and a reduction in dinospore load in the water *in vitro* [108].

Nevertheless, the applicability of this method on an industrial scale has yet to be demonstrated. Regarding chemical treatments for amyloodiniosis, several products have achieved mixed results. The most common treatment for controlling and eliminating this parasite is copper sulfate, a chemical widely used in agriculture and as an algicide. Its ease of use and effectiveness against dinospores and for trophont gill release make it suitable for almost all the production systems available [109]. During copper sulfate treatments, the active component is the copper ion, which must remain in the water at a concentration of 0.15–0.2 mg/L for 10–14 days to effectively control the epidemic since comments are resistant to the treatment [106]. High concentrations of copper should be avoided as they are toxic to fish, invertebrates, and algae.

Additionally, free copper is unstable in water, so its levels should be closely monitored to maintain a desirable and safe concentration [4, 109]. It should be noted that at high water temperatures (25–30°C), amyloodiniosis outbreaks and treatments with copper sulfate may last for over a month, leading to increased costs for the producers [13]. There are several combinations to optimize the use of this product as a treatment. For example, a combined influx of freshwater to reduce salinity to 10 ppt alongside a lower dose of copper sulfate (0.1 ppm) showed positive results in trials with European seabass [110]. Another option is to mix 5-hydrate copper sulfate with citric acid monohydrate to yield 0.15 ppm copper ion concentration in the water [110]. Formalin (37% formaldehyde) is another product used to control ectoparasites in fish culture [71, 111]. Treatment with 100–200 ppm of formalin for 6–9 h causes trophonts of *A. ocellatum* to detach from gills. However, comments can resume division after removing the chemical, as formalin does not inactivate the moment stage [112]. Hydrogen peroxide (H_2O_2) is an ecofriendly therapeutic for amyloodiniosis. It effectively targets both dinospores and trophont life phases, with minor impact on tomonts at therapeutic dosages [106, 111]. However, it must be used within the therapeutic limits, as it can be lethal to the fish [113]. Several hydrogen peroxide treatment configurations were effective in the amyloodiniosis outbreak. In flathead gray mullet (*Mugil cephalus*), fry mortality lowered within 3 days following treatment with 25 ppm of hydrogen peroxide for 30 min [114]. In six-finger threadfin, treatments with hydrogen peroxide at 75–150 ppm for 30 min eliminated trophonts without affecting fish survival [113]. In milkfish (*Chanos chanos*) or gray snapper (*Lutjanus griseus*), a combined treatment of 1 h of freshwater immersion and 1 h immersion in 200 ppm of hydrogen peroxide before passing the fish to clean seawater effectively removed 100% of the trophonts [115]. European sea bass, treated with 100 and 200 ppm of hydrogen peroxide for 30 min, significantly decreased the number of trophonts in their gills [41]. There are also new treatments being tested against amyloodiniosis. Sodium hypochlorite (NaOCl) can be used for treatment or pond disinfection since it significantly impairs tomont division after 48 h at concentrations as low as 10 ppm and completely arrests it after 24 h at 250 ppm, also impairing dinospores' movement [111]. Virkon S (Dupont) and Ox-Virin (Grupo OX; TLH Lda) (5% peracetic acid solution) can also be used for tomont inactivation and dinospore impairment [111]. The administration of the antimalarial chloroquine diphosphate was effective against *A. ocellatum* dinospores in 10 mg/L water baths, being ineffective against the comment phase [116, 117]. The water-soluble ionophore 3, N-methylglucamine lasalocid, effectively reduced the moment division rate, inhibiting dinospore eclosion at concentrations greater than 0.001 ppm. In *in vitro* and *in vivo* studies with red drum (*Sciaenops ocellatus*) fry, trophont infection rates decreased by up to 80% at 0.1 ppm [118].

New treatments are still in the early testing phase, including tomatine, a glycoalkaloid derived from the tomato (*Solanum lycopersicum*), and 20,40-Dihydroxychalone, isolated from the plant *Zuccagnia punctate*; both showed promising results in inactivating the dinospores *in vitro*, being ineffective against the comment stage [116]. Over the last year, some innovative approaches to amyloodiniosis treatment have been published, with interesting results for amyloodiniosis treatment. Recent innovative techniques to treat amyloodiniosis involve inserting galvanized material into fish tanks to prevent and control *A. ocellatum* infestations. This method has shown good results in inhibiting dinospore infectivity and reducing trophont levels in fish gills, although it does not affect the tomont hatching rate and eclosion time [118]. However, most of the treatments described above are difficult to implement in open, semi-intensive production systems due to the extension of the tanks and the costs associated with treatment.

5. Conclusions

The fish parasite *Amyloodinium ocellatum* is the etiological agent of amyloodiniosis, a disease easily diagnosed in fish produced in aquaculture. However, it remains a significant issue due to its economic and environmental impacts. The inexistence of established effective preventive measures for its occurrence in earthen ponds combined with the inapplicability of most of the treatments in these systems—due to factors such as tank size and environmental impact—as well as the lack of recognition by the relevant authorities of the applicable ones creates a huge bottleneck for such production systems. While several articles have focused mainly on parasite diagnosis and its relationship with the host through physiological parameters analysis such as immune response, hematology, stress response, and proteomics, few studies are addressing the environmental impact of the treatments used or the economic losses associated with the occurrence of this parasite. Therefore, despite numerous scientific studies providing results that could serve as potential foundations for regulation, treatment licensing, or the development of prevention protocols, practical concerns regarding animal welfare, environmental impact, and consumer safety often arise. Addressing these aspects is crucial for providing clarity and support for production in semi-intensive systems in the Mediterranean region.

Acknowledgements

This work was financially supported by SAÚDE&AQUA II (MAR-021.1.3-FEAMPA-00018) and "Pacto da Bioeconomia azul" (Project No. C644915664-00000026) within the WP5 Algae Vertical, funded by Next Generation EU European Fund, the Portuguese Recovery and Resilience Plan (PRR), under the scope of the incentive line "Agendas for Business Innovation" through the funding scheme C5-Capitalization and Business Innovation, and with the support of Portuguese Blue Biobank project (Blue Economy Pact, operation code C644915664-00000026), funded by Plano de Recuperação e Resiliência (PRR).

Author details

Florbela Soares[1,2*], Márcio Moreira[2], Rui Sousa[2] and Cátia Lourenço-Marques[1,2]

1 IPMA—Portuguese Institute for the Ocean and Atmosphere, EPPO—Aquaculture Research Station, Olhão, Portugal

2 S2AQUA—Collaborative Laboratory, Association for a Sustainable and Smart Aquaculture, Olhão, Portugal

*Address all correspondence to: fsoares@ipma.pt

References

[1] EUMOFA. The EU Fish Market - Edition 2016. 2016th ed. Brussels: European Commission, Directorate-General for Maritime Affairs and Fisheries, Director-General; 2016. pp. 1-94

[2] Parliament E. Regulation (EU) 2016/429 of the European Parliament and of the Council of 9 March 2016 on transmissible animal diseases and amending and repealing certain acts in the area of animal health (Animal Health Law) (Text with EEA relevance) Text with EEA relevance: European Union. 2021. Available from: https://eur-lex.europa.eu/eli/reg/2016/429/2021-04-21

[3] Paperna I, Robin M. Parasites and diseases of mullets (Mugilidae). In: Oren OH, editor. Aquaculture of Grey Mullets. International Biological Programme. Great Britain: Cambridge University Press; 1981. p. 517

[4] Soares F, Quental Ferreira H, Cunha E, Pousão-Ferreira P. Occurrence of *Amyloodinium ocellatum* in aquaculture fish production: A serious problem in semi-intensive earthen ponds. Aquaculture Europe. 2011;**36**(4):13-16

[5] Francis-Floyd R, Floyd MR. *Amyloodinium Ocellatum*, an Important Parasite of Cultured Marine Fish. Southern Regional Aquaculture Center; 2011

[6] Shinn AP, Pratoomyot J, Bron JE, Paladini G, Brooker EE, Brooker AJ. Economic costs of protistan and metazoan parasites to global mariculture. Parasitology. 2015;**142**:196-270

[7] Health WOfA. Aquatic Animal Health Code 2024. Available from: https://www.woah.org/en/what-we-do/standards/codes-and-manuals/aquatic-code-online-access/?id=169&L=1&htmfile=index.htm

[8] Rowley AF, Baker-Austin C, Boerlage AS, Caillon C, Davies CE, Duperret L, et al. Diseases of marine fish and shellfish in an age of rapid climate change. iScience. 2024;**27**(9):110838

[9] Moreira M, Costas B, Rodrigues PM, Lourenço-Marques C, Sousa R, Schrama D, et al. Amyloodiniosis in aquaculture: A review. Reviews in Aquaculture. 2024;**16**(3):1042-1068

[10] Oidtmann BC, Mladineo I, Cook A, Beraldo P, Palenzuela O, Christofilogiannis P, et al. Main parasitic infections in gilthead seabream and European seabass aquaculture: Risk factors from stakeholders' perspective. Aquaculture International. 2024;**32**(4):4275-4302

[11] World Register of Marine Species (WoRMS) [Internet]. WoRMS Editorial Board. 2023. Available from: https://www.marinespecies.org

[12] Lawler AR. Studies on *Amyloodinium ocellatum* (Dinoflagellata) in Mississippi sound - natural and experimental hosts. Gulf Research Reports. 1980;**6**(4):403-413

[13] Boylan S, Skoy J, Ellis H, editors. Who needs the foul-line when you have the "trifecta" of bonnethead (*Sphyrna tiburo*) infectious diseases in captivity: Erpocotyle monogeneans, *Fusarium solani*, and *Amyloodinium*. In: Proceedings of the Eastern Fish Health Workshop Conference; Shepherdstown, WV, USA. Cornvallis, Oregon, USA: AFS Fish Health Section; 2014

[14] Smith M, Warmolts D, Thoney D, Hueter R, Murray M, Ezcurra J. The

Elasmobranch Husbandry Manual II: Recent Advances in the Care of Sharks, Rays and their Relatives. Columbus, Ohio: Special Publication of the Ohio Biological Survey; 2017

[15] Goertz CE. Protozoal diseases of elasmobranchs. In: The Elasmobranch Husbandry Manual: Captive Care of Sharks, Rays and their Relatives. Vol. 589. Columbus: Special Publication of the Ohio Biological Survey; 2004. pp. 417-426

[16] Nigrelli RF. The Morphology, Cytology and Life-History of *Oodinium Ocellatum* Brown: A Dinoflagellate Parasitic on Marine Fishes. New York, USA: New York University; 1936

[17] Brown EM, Hovasse R. *Amyloodinium ocellatum* (Brown), a Peridinian parasitic on marine fishes. A complementary study. Proceedings of the Zoological Society of London. 1946;**116**(1):33-46

[18] Nigrelli RF. Mortality statistics for specimens in the New York Aquarium, 1939. Zoologica. 1940;**25**(4):525-552

[19] Kingsford E. Treatment of Exotic Marine Fish Diseases. New York, USA: Palmetto Publishing Company; 1975

[20] Brown EM. On *Oodinium ocellatum* Brown, a parasitic Dinoflagellate causing epidemic disease in marine fish. Proceedings of the Zoological Society of London. 1934;**104**(3):583-607

[21] Simkatis H. Salt-Water Fishes for the Home Aquarium. USA: Lippincott, Cornell University; 1958

[22] Inagaki KY. Dieta e parasitas do peixe-porco *Stephanolepis hispidus* (Linnaeus, 1766) em duas localidades da costa brasileira: Universidade Federal de Santa Catarina, Brasil. 2017

[23] Bahri S. Protozoan and myxozoan infections in wild gilthead seabream (*Sparus aurata* L.) from North Lake of Tunis, Tunisia. Acta Parasitologica. 2012;**57**(2):114-121

[24] Sanchez-Garcia N, Raga JA, Montero FE. Risk assessment for parasites in *Diplodus puntazzo* (Sparidae) cultures in the Western Mediterranean: Prospects of cross infection with *Sparus aurata*. Veterinary Parasitology. 2014;**204**(3-4):120-133

[25] Soares F, Quental-Ferreira H, Moreira M, Cunha E, Ribeiro L, Pousao-Ferreira P. First report of *Amyloodinium ocellatum* in farmed meager (*Argyrosomus regius*). Bulletin of the European Association of Fish Pathologists. 2012;**32**(1):30-33

[26] Aravindan NCKAS. Protozoan parasites in commercially important shrimp species from northeast coast of Andhra Pradesh, India. Journal of Experimental Zoology, India. 2007;**10**(1):9-20

[27] Beraldo P, Massimo M. Chapter 38 - Amyloodiniosis. In: FSB K, Baldisserotto B, Chong RS-M, editors. Aquaculture Pathophysiology. London, United Kingdom: Academic Press; 2022. pp. 475-483

[28] Lawler AR. Dinoflagellate (Amyloodinium) Infestation of Pompano. Amsterdam: Elsevier Scientific Publishing Company; 1977. pp. 257-264

[29] Zhuang J, Li Z, Cao J, Luo Z, Wang B, Han Q, et al. A quantitative real-time PCR assay for rapid detection and quantification of *Amyloodinium ocellatum* parasites in seawater samples. Aquaculture. 2025;**595**:741651

[30] Landsberg JH, Steidinger KA, Blakesley BA, Zondervan RL. Scanning

Electron-microscope study of Dinospores of *Amyloodinium Cf ocellatum*, a pathogenic Dinoflagellate parasite of marine fish, and comments on its relationship to the Peridiniales. Diseases of Aquatic Organisms. 1994;**20**(1):23-32

[31] Ragab RH, Elgendy MY, Sabry NM, Sharaf MS, Attia MM, Korany RMS, et al. Mass kills in hatchery-reared European seabass (*Dicentrarchus labrax*) triggered by concomitant infections of *Amyloodinium ocellatum* and *Vibrio alginolyticus*. International Journal of Veterinary Science and Medicine. 2022;**10**(1):33-45

[32] Yang S-M, Zhou W-T, Bu X-L, Hu G-R, Zou H, Li W-X, et al. Y Co-Infection of *Amyloodinium ocellatum* and *Chilodonella hexasticha* in Farmed Silver Carp, *Hypophthalmichthys molitri*: A Case Report. Rochester, NY, USA: SSRN - Elsevier. DOI: 10.2139/ssrn.4947326

[33] Cheung PJ, Nigrelli RF, Ruggieri GD. Development of *Oodinium ocellatum* (Dinoflagellida): A scanning electron microscopic study. Transactions of the American Microscopical Society. 1981;**100**(4):415-420

[34] Kuperman BI, Matey VE. Massive infestation by *Amyloodinium ocellatum* (Dinoflagellida) of fish in a highly saline lake, Salton Sea, California, USA. Diseases of Aquatic Organisms. 1999;**39**(1):65-73

[35] Pereira JC, Abrantes I, Martins I, Barata J, Frias P, Pereira I. Ecological and morphological features of *Amyloodinium ocellatum* occurrences in cultivated gilthead seabream *Sparus aurata L.*: A case study. Aquaculture. 2011;**310**(3-4):289-297

[36] Saraiva A, Jeronimo D, Cruz C. *Amyloodinium ocellatum* (Chromalveolata: Dinoflagellata) in farmed turbot. Aquaculture. 2011;**320**(1-2):34-36

[37] Beraldo P, Byadgi O, Massimo M, Bulfon C, Volpatti D, Galeotti M, editors. Grave episodio di amyloodiniosi in giovanili di branzino (*Dicentrarchus labrax*): Analisi dei determinanti di malattia e rilievi anatomopatologici. In: Conference Proceedings of the XXIII Convegno Nazionale Società Italiana di Patologia Ittica, Lecce. Legnaro, Italy: Istituto Zooprofilattico Sperimentale delle Venezie; 2017

[38] Paperna I. Reproduction cycle and tolerance to temperature and salinity of *Amyloodinium ocellatum* (Brown, 1931) (Dinoflagellida). Annales de Parasitologie Humaine et Comparée. 1984;**59**(1):7-30

[39] Paperna I. *Amyloodinium ocellatum* (Brown, 1931) (Dinoflagellida) infestations in cultured marine fish at Eilat, Red-Sea - Epizootiology and pathology. Journal of Fish Diseases. 1980;**3**(5):363-372

[40] Vidya R, Raja RA, Avunje S, Bhuvaneswari T, Kumar TS, Aravind R, et al. A report on outbreak of *Amyloodinium ocellatum* infestation in broodstock of Java rabbitfish, *Siganus javus* (Linnaeus, 1766). Journal of Parasitic Diseases. 2024;**48**(1):1-12

[41] Seoud SSM, Zaki VH, Ahmed GE, El-Khalek NKA. Studies on Amyloodinium infestation in European Seabass (*Dicentrarchus labrax*.) fishes with special reference for treatment. International Journal of Marine Science. 2017;7(24)

[42] Tahraoui S, Ennaffah B, Belattmania Z, Reani A, Sabour B. First report on the occurrence and dynamics of the Ectoparasitic Dinoflagellate *Amyloodinium ocellatum* in the Moroccan

Atlantic Coast. Research Journal of Environmental Sciences. 2018;**12**:153-159

[43] Alves-Ferreira M, da Silva ECC, Ferreira-Pereira A, Scofano HM. Regulatory differences between Ca2+-ATPase in plasma membranes from chicken (nucleated) and pig (anucleated) erythrocytes. Comparative Biochemistry and Physiology Part C: Toxicology & Pharmacology. 2002;**131**(4):405-415

[44] Buchmann K. Impact and control of protozoan parasites in mariculture fishes. Parasitology. 2015;**142**(1):168-177

[45] Picón-Camacho SM, Thompson WP, Blaylock RB, Lotz JM. Development of a rapid assay to detect the dinoflagellate *Amyloodinium ocellatum* using loop-mediated isothermal amplification (LAMP). Veterinary Parasitology. 2013;**196**(3-4):265-271

[46] Levy MG, Litaker RW, Goldstein RJ, Dykstra MJ, Vandersea MW, Noga EJ. Piscinoodinium, a fish-ectoparasitic dinoflagellate, is a member of the class Dinophyceae, subclass Gymnodiniphycidae: Convergent evolution with Amyloodinium. The Journal of Parasitology. 2007;**93**(5):1006-1015

[47] Li Z, Zhuang J, Wang H, Cao J, Han Q, Luo Z, et al. Gill lesions are the main cause of death in yellowfin seabream (*Acanthopagrus latus*) following infection with Amyloodinium ocellatum. Microbial Pathogenesis. 2024;**194**:106845

[48] Noga E, Levy M. Dinoflagellate parasites of fish. In: Fish Diseases I: Protozoan and Metazoan Infections. Vol. 1. Oxfordshire, Wallington, United Kingdom: CAB International; 1995. pp. 1-25

[49] Moreira M, Soliño L, Marques CL, Laizé V, Pousão-Ferreira P, Costa PR, et al. Cytotoxic and hemolytic activities of extracts of the fish parasite dinoflagellate amyloodinium ocellatum. Toxins. 2022;**14**(7):467

[50] Vivanco-Aranda M, Del Río-Zaragoza OB, Lechuga-Sandoval CE, Viana MT, Rombenso AN. Health response in yellowtail Seriola dorsalis exposed to an *Amyloodinium ocellatum* outbreak. Ciencias Marinas. 2018;**44**(4):267-277

[51] Moreira M, Cordeiro-Silva A, Barata M, Pousão-Ferreira P, Soares F. Influence of age on stress responses of white seabream to amyloodiniosis. Fishes. 2019;**4**(2):26

[52] Moreira M, Schrama D, Soares F, Wulff T, Pousão-Ferreira P, Rodrigues P. Physiological responses of reared sea bream (*Sparus aurata* Linnaeus, 1758) to an *Amyloodinium ocellatum* outbreak. Journal of Fish Diseases. 2017;**40**:1545-1560

[53] Moreira M, Herrera M, Pousão-Ferreira P, Navas Triano JI, Soares F. Stress effects of amyloodiniosis in gilthead sea bream *Sparus aurata*. Diseases of Aquatic Organisms. 2018;**127**(3):201-211

[54] Alvarez-Pellitero P. Fish immunity and parasite infections: From innate immunity to immunoprophylactic prospects. Veterinary Immunology and Immunopathology. 2008;**126**(3-4):171-198

[55] Byadgi O, Beraldo P, Volpatti D, Massimo M, Bulfon C, Galeotti M. Expression of infection-related immune response in European sea bass (*Dicentrarchus labrax*) during a natural outbreak from a unique dinoflagellate *Amyloodinium ocellatum*. Fish & Shellfish Immunology. 2019;**84**:62-72

[56] Panda RP, Chakrapani V, Patra SK, Saha JN, Jayasankar P, Kar B, et al. First evidence of comparative responses of Toll-like receptor 22 (TLR22) to relatively resistant and susceptible Indian farmed carps to *Argulus siamensis* infection. Developmental & Comparative Immunology. 2014;**47**(1):25-35

[57] Reyes-Becerril M, Ascencio-Valle F, Alamillo E, Hirono I, Kondo H, Jirapongpairoj W, et al. Molecular cloning and comparative responses of Toll-like receptor 22 following ligands stimulation and parasitic infection in yellowtail (*Seriola lalandi*). Fish & Shellfish Immunology. 2015;**46**(2):323-333

[58] Ellis A. Innate host defense mechanisms of fish against viruses and bacteria. Developmental & Comparative Immunology. 2001;**25**(8-9):827-839

[59] Nozzi V, Strofaldi S, Piquer IF, Di Crescenzo D, Olivotto I, Carnevali O. *Amyloodinum ocellatum* in *Dicentrarchus labrax*: Study of infection in saltwater and freshwater aquaponics. Fish & Shellfish Immunology. 2016;**57**:179-185

[60] Li Z, Zhong Z, Zhuang J, Luo Z, Han Q, Cao J, et al. An experimental animal model of yellowfin seabream (*Acanthopagrus latus*) for *Amyloodinium ocellatum* infection. Aquaculture. 2023;**574**:739641

[61] Noga EJ, Fan Z, Silphaduang U. Histone-like proteins from fish are lethal to the parasitic dinoflagellate *Amyloodinium ocellatum*. Parasitology. 2001;**123**(Pt 1):57-65

[62] Colorni A, Ullal A, Heinisch G, Noga EJ. Activity of the antimicrobial polypeptide piscidin 2 against fish ectoparasites. Journal Fish Diseases. 2008;**31**(6):423-432

[63] Ullal AJ, Noga EJ. Antiparasitic activity of the antimicrobial peptide HbβP-1, a member of the β-haemoglobin peptide family. Journal of Fish Diseases. 2010;**33**(8):657-664

[64] Nogueira AFV. Impacto fisiológico do parasita dinoflagelado Amyloodinium ocellatum (Brown, 1931) em corvina-legítima (*Argyrosomus regius,* Asso, 1801) produzida em aquacultura [master thesis]. Faro, Portugal: University of Algarve; 2015

[65] Henry M, Nikoloudaki C, Tsigenopoulos C, Rigos G. Strong effect of long-term *Sparicotyle chrysophrii* infection on the cellular and innate immune responses of gilthead sea bream, *Sparus aurata*. Developmental & Comparative Immunology. 2015;**51**(1):185-193

[66] Mutoloki S, Jørgensen JB, Evensen Ø. The adaptive immune response in fish. Fish Vaccination. 2014;**9**:104-115

[67] Colorni A. Diseases of Mediterranean fish species: Problems, research, and prospects. Bulletin of the European Association of Fish Pathologists. 2004;**24**(1):22-32

[68] Cecchini S, Saroglia M, Terova G, Albanesi F. Detection of antibody response against *Amyloodinium ocellatum* (Brown, 1931) in serum of naturally infected European sea bass by an enzyme-linked immunosorbent assay (ELISA). Bulletin of the European Association of Fish Pathologists. 2001;**21**(3):104-108

[69] Smith SA, Levy MG, Noga EJ. Detection of anti-amyloodinium ocellatum antibody from cultured hybrid striped bass (*Morone saxatilis* × *M. chrysops*) during an epizootic of Amyloodiniosis. Journal of Aquatic Animal Health. 1994;**6**(1):79-81

[70] Massimo M, Volpatti D, Galeotti M, Bron JE, Beraldo P. News insights into the host-parasite interactions of amyloodiniosis in European Sea bass: A multi-modal approach. Pathogens (Basel, Switzerland). 2022;**11**(1):62

[71] Cascarano MC, Stavrakidis-Zachou O, Mladineo I, Thompson KD, Papandroulakis N, Katharios P. Mediterranean aquaculture in a changing climate: Temperature effects on pathogens and diseases of three farmed fish species. Pathogens (Basel, Switzerland). 2021;**10**(9):1205

[72] Macnab V, Barber I. Some (worms) like it hot: Fish parasites grow faster in warmer water and alter host thermal preferences. Global Change Biology. 2012;**18**(5):1540-1548

[73] Becker CD. Flagellate parasites of fish. Parasitic Protozoa. 1977;**1**:357-416

[74] Paperna I, Colorni A, Ross B, Colorni B. Diseases of Marine Fish Cultured in Eilat Mariculture Project Based at the Gulf of Aqaba, Red Sea. Rome (Italy): FAO; 1980. Report No.: 92-5-000964-X Contract No.: 57

[75] Rigos G, Troisi G. Antibacterial agents in Mediterranean finfish farming: A synopsis of drug pharmacokinetics in important euryhaline fish species and possible environmental implications. Review in Fish Biology and Fisheries. 2005;**15**(1-2):53-73

[76] Mladineo I. Check list of the parasitofauna in Adriatic Sea cage-reared fish. Acta Veterinaria. 2006;**56**(2-3):285-292

[77] Pérez-Sánchez T, Mora-Sánchez B, Balcázar JL. Biological approaches for disease control in aquaculture: Advantages, limitations, and challenges. Trends in Microbiology. 2018;**26**(11):896-903

[78] Brugere C, Onuigbo DM, Morgan KL. People matter in animal disease surveillance: Challenges and opportunities for the aquaculture sector. Aquaculture. 2017;**467**:158-169

[79] Chintagari S, Hazard N, Edwards G, Jadeja R, Janes M. Risks associated with fish and seafood. In: Thakur, S Kniel, KE editors. Preharvest Food Safety. Washington, DC, USA: ASM Press; 2018. pp. 123-142

[80] Sitjà-Bobadilla A, Oidtmann B. Chapter 5 - integrated pathogen management strategies in fish farming. In: Jeney G, editor. London, UK: Fish Diseases: Academic Press; 2017. pp. 119-144

[81] Paladini G, Longshaw M, Gustinelli A, Shinn AP. Parasitic diseases in aquaculture: Their biology, diagnosis and control. In: Austin BA, Newaj-Fyzul A, editors. Diagnosis and Control of Diseases of Fish and Shellfish. West Sussex, UK: John Wiley & Sons Ltd; 2017. pp. 37-107

[82] Noga EJ, Borron PJ, Hinshaw J, Gordon WC, Gordon LJ, Seo JK. Identification of histones as endogenous antibiotics in fish and quantification in rainbow trout (*Oncorhynchus mykiss*) skin and gill. Fish Physiology and Biochemistry. 2011;**37**(1):135-152

[83] Alvarez-Pellitero P, Adilla ASB, Franco-Sierra A, Palenzuela O. Protozoan parasites of gilthead sea bream, *Sparus aurata* L., from different culture systems in Spain. Journal of Fish Diseases. 1995;**18**(2):105-115

[84] Gonzales R. Sensitivity of a LAMP assay for detection of the dinoflagellate *Amyloodinium ocellatum* in simulated field conditions and freeze tolerance of the parasite [master's theses]. Hattiesburg, Missisípi, USA: The University of Southern Mississippi; 2022

[85] Noga EJ. Fish Disease: Diagnosis and Treatment. Iowa, USA: John Wiley & Sons; 2010

[86] Masson I, Blaylock RB, Lotz JM. Susceptibility and tolerance of spotted seatrout, cynoscion nebulosus, and red snapper, *Lutjanus campechanus*, to experimental infections with *Amyloodinium ocellatum*. Journal of Parasitology. 2011;**97**(4):577-585

[87] Sabo-Attwood T, Apul OG, Bisesi JH Jr, Kane AS, Saleh NB. Nano-scale applications in aquaculture: Opportunities for improved production and disease control. Journal of Fish Diseases. 2021;**44**(4):359-370

[88] Arthur R, Bondad-Reantaso MG, Campbell ML, Hewitt C, Phillips M, Subasinghe RP. Understanding and Applying Risk Analysis in Aquaculture: A Manual for Decision-Makers. Rome, Italy: Food and Agriculture Organization of the United Nations; 2009

[89] Noga EJ, Levy MG. Phylum Dinoflagellata. In: Fish Diseases and Disorders, Protozoan and Metazoan Infections. Vol. 1. Switzerland: CABI Publishing; 2006. pp. 16-45

[90] Marques CL, Medeiros A, Moreira M, Quental-Ferreira H, Mendes AC, Pousão-Ferreira P, et al. Report and genetic identification of *Amyloodinium ocellatum* in a sea bass (*Dicentrarchus labrax*) broodstock in Portugal. Aquaculture Reports. 2019;**14**:100191

[91] Masson I, Lotz JM, Blaylock RB. Population model for *Amyloodinium ocellatum* infecting the spotted seatrout *Cynoscion nebulosus* and the red snapper *Lutjanus campechanus*. Diseases of Aquatic Organisms. 2013;**106**(2):139-148

[92] Levy MG, Poore MF, Colorni A, Noga EJ, Vandersea MW, Litaker RW. A highly specific PCR assay for detecting the fish ectoparasite *Amyloodinium ocellatum*. Diseases of Aquatic Organisms. 2007;**73**(3):219-226

[93] Louzao MC, Espiña B, Cagide E, Ares IR, Alfonso A, Vieytes MR, et al. Cytotoxic effect of palytoxin on mussel. Toxicon. 2010;**56**(5):842-847

[94] Noga EJ. Amyloodinium ocellatum. In: Woo PTK, Buchmann K, editors. Fish Parasites: Pathobiology and Protection. Preston, UK: CABI Publishers; 2012. pp. 19-29

[95] Noga EJ, Silphaduang U, Park NG, Seo JK, Stephenson J, Kozlowicz S. Piscidin 4, a novel member of the piscidin family of antimicrobial peptides. Comparative Biochemistry and Physiology Part B, Biochemistry & Molecular Biology. 2009;**152**(4):299-305

[96] Abreu PC, Robaldo RB, Sampaio LA, Bianchini A, Odebrecht C. Recurrent Amyloodiniosis on Broodstock of the Brazilian flounder *Paralichthys orbignyanus*: Dinospore monitoring and prophylactic measures. Journal World Aquaculture Society. 2005;**36**(1):42-50

[97] Kabata Z. Parasites and Diseases of Fish Cultured in the Tropics. Berkeley, USA: Taylor & Francis Ltd.; 1985

[98] Buentello JA, Neill WH, Gatlin DM. Effects of dietary prebiotics on the growth, feed efficiency, and non-specific immunity of juvenile red drum *Sciaenops ocellatus* fed soybean-based diets. Aquaculture Research. 2010;**41**(3):411-418

[99] Smith SA, Schwarz MH. Getting Acquainted with Amyloodinium Ocellatum. Petersburg, USA: Virginia Seafood Agricultural Research and Extension Center, Virginia Tech: Virginia State University; 2019. p. 2

[100] Byadgi O, Beraldo P, Massimo M, Bulfon C, Galeotti M, Volpatti D. The first pilot study on amyloodiniosis vaccine efficacy trial in European seabass (*Dicentrarchus labrax*). In: Atti del XXIV Convegno Nazionale SIPI (Società Italiana di Patologia Ittica); 11-13 Ottobre 2018; Torino (Italia). Legnaro, Italy: SIPI, Istituto Zooprofilattico Sperimentale delle Venezie; 2018. p. 58

[101] Reyes-Becerril M, Tovar-Ramirez D, Ascencio-Valle F, Civera-Cerecedo R, Gracia-Lopez V, Barbosa-Solomieu V. Effects of dietary live yeast *Debaryomyces hansenii* on the immune and antioxidant system in juvenile leopard grouper *Mycteroperca rosacea* exposed to stress. Aquaculture. 2008;**280**(1-4):39-44

[102] Ribeiro APFJM. Utilizing hydrophilic extracts of *Amyloodinium ocellatum* (Brown, 1931) in the development of new marine fish therapies [master thesis]. University of Algarve; 2022

[103] Byadgi O, Massimo M, Dirks RP, Pallavicini A, Bron JE, Ireland JH, et al. Innate immune-gene expression during experimental amyloodiniosis in European seabass (*Dicentrarchus labrax*). Veterinary Immunology and Immunopathology. 2021;**234**:110217

[104] Barbaro A, Francescon A. Parassitosi da *Amyloodinium ocellatum* (Dinophyceae) su larve di *Sparus aurata* allevate in un impianto di riproduzione artificiale. Oebalia. 1985;**11**:745-752

[105] Rigos G, Padrós F, Golomazou E, Zarza C. Antiparasitic approaches and strategies in European aquaculture, with emphasis on Mediterranean marine finfish farming: Present scenarios and future visions. Reviews in Aquaculture. 2024;**16**(2):622-643

[106] Paperna I. Chemical control of *Amyloodinium ocellatum* (Brown 1931) (Dinoflagellida) infections: In vitro tests and treatment trials with infected fishes. Aquaculture. 1984;**38**(1):1-18

[107] Fajer-Avila EJ, Abdo-de la Parra I, Aguilar-Zarate G, Contreras-Arce R, Zaldivar-Ramirez J, Betancourt-Lozano M. Toxicity of formalin to bullseye puffer fish (*Sphoeroides annulatus* Jenyns, 1843) and its effectiveness to control ectoparasites. Aquaculture. 2003;**223**(1-4):41-50

[108] Pathinathan P, Kumar DK, Sirisha H, Pravalika P. Prevalent Diseases and Effective Management Strategies in Asian Seabass (*Lates calcarifer)* Vigyan Varta an International E-Magazine for Science Enthusiasts. 2024;**5**(8):17-21

[109] Bessat M, Fadel A. Amyloodiniosis in cultured *Dicentrarchus labrax*: Parasitological and molecular diagnosis, and an improved treatment protocol. Diseases of Aquatic Organisms. 2018;**129**(1):41-51

[110] Sousa R, Laizé V, Lourenço-Marques C, Barata M, Pousão-Ferreira P, Soares F. Inactivation in vitro of the marine parasite *Amyloodinium ocellatum*. Diseases of Aquatic Organisms. 2024;**159**:183-197

[111] Oestmann DJ, Lewis DH. Improved cell culture propagation of *Amyloodinium ocellatum*. Diseases of Aquatic Organisms. 1996;**24**(3):173-178

[112] Montgomery-Brock D, Sato VT, Brock JA, Tamaru CS. The application of hydrogen peroxide as a treatment for the ectoparasite *Amyloodinium ocellatum* (Brown 1931) on the Pacific threadfin *Polydactylus sexfilis*. Journal of the World Aquaculture Society. 2001;**32**(2):250-254

[113] El-Deen A, Eissa I, Osman H, Zaid A, Darwish O. Studies on prevailing parasitic fish diseases in pre-mature

cultured Sea bass, *Dicentrarchus labrax*, Sea bream and *Mugil cephalus* at Ismailia, province with special references to control. International Journal of Veterinary Science. 2020;**9**(4):558-562

[114] Cruz-Lacierda ER, Maeno Y, Pineda AJT, Matey VE. Mass mortality of hatchery-reared milkfish (*Chanos chanos*) and mangrove red snapper (*Lutjanus argentimaculatus*) caused by *Amyloodinium ocellatum* (Dinoflagellida). Aquaculture. 2004;**236**(1-4):85-94

[115] Tedesco P, Beraldo P, Massimo M, Fioravanti ML, Volpatti D, Dirks R, et al. Comparative therapeutic effects of natural compounds against *Saprolegnia* spp. (Oomycota) and *Amyloodinium ocellatum* (Dinophyceae). Frontiers in veterinary. Science. 2020;7:83. DOI: 10.3389/fvets.2020.00083

[116] Ramesh Kumar P, Nazar AA, Jayakumar R, Tamilmani G, Sakthivel M, Kalidas C, et al. *Amyloodinium ocellatum* infestation in the broodstock of silver pompano *Trachinotus blochii* (Lacepede, 1801) and its therapeutic control. Indian Journal Fish. 2015;**62**(1):131-134

[117] Oestmann DJ, Lewis DH. Effects of 3, N-methylglucamine lasalocid on *Amyloodinium ocellatum*. Diseases of Aquatic Organisms. 1996;**24**(3):179-184

[118] Luo Z, Zhong Z, Li Z, Zhuang J, Li H, Wang B, et al. Galvanized material is a promising approach to control *Amyloodinium ocellatum* infection in fishes. Aquaculture. 2024;**578**:740045

Chapter 6

Mass Production and Field Application of Some Parasitoids in Egypt

Ahmed Amin Ahmed Saleh and Ahmed Shamkhi Jabbar

Abstract

In the Arab Republic of Egypt, work was done to study some aphid species, Nezara viridula whitefly, and *Sesamia cretica* infestation-associated parasitoids with aphid species. Diaeretiella rapae emerged as a major parasitoid of aphid species. All parasitoids that emerged from collected egg masses of Nezara viridula were identified as *Trissolcus megalocephalus*. The general means of parasitism were 21.84 and 29.61% in the 2021 and 2022 seasons, respectively. Incidentally, both *Encarsia formosa* and *Eretmocerus mundus* were the most effective biocontrol agents of *B. tabaci*, respectively. The comparable findings were the same *Bracon brevicornis* as a native primary gregarious ectoparasitoid that targets *Sesamia cretica*, *Ostrinia nubilalis*, *Chilo agamemnon*, *Helicoerpa armigera*, and *Pectinophora gossypiella* were detailed. Not only was longevity affected by temperature and food, but also, the female bias in offspring production was affected, not the host species. Further to illustrate the repeatability of this behavioral response of the parasitoid at different host densities these parasitoids were also chlorinated. A higher host density led to shorter host-searching and initial sting durations, but a higher number of stings and mummies were obtained according to both results obtained from the study held. This study pinpointed the role of some parasitoids as a pest control method in greenhouses and open fields. Moreover, this aphid parasitoid is not always efficient pest control when aphids are at higher population densities. Therefore, it is concluded that where these parasitoids are used as biological control agents, they should be used in environments with low host densities.

Keywords: parasitoids, mass production, release, Egypt, ecology, biology

1. Introduction

Different kinds of parasitic relationships (parasitoids may or may not kill their host; e.g., mistletoe is a parasitic plant that needs a living host plant to survive) [1–4]. Micro-parasites, for example, bacteria and viruses, can infect a host as a disease (e.g., tulip-break or mosaic virus, which produces dramatic color streaks in flowers) [5–7]. Most of the plants, like powdery mildews, leaf spots, rusts, are parasitic types deleterious to the host plant's chance of survival [8, 9]. One example of a parasite that does not always kill its host is mistletoe, which is a parasitic plant that depends on a living host plant to survive [1–4]. There are various kinds of parasitic relationships. Bacteria and viruses are examples of microparasites that parasitize host plants and cause disease (such as mosaic virus or tulip-break virus, which causes striking color streaks in the flowers) [5–7]. Powdery mildews, leaf spots, rusts, and other common plant diseases are detrimental to plants and lower their chances of survival [8, 9]. Biological control, which includes the use of biotic agents like parasites, predators, and pathogens, is one of the most crucial technologies for control measures to lessen environmental pollution caused by pesticides [10–12]. Under the Integrated Pest Management (IPM) Program, biological control is an effective tactic. Applying parasitoids to control insect pests falls under the category of actions that contribute to keeping the pest population at a low level [12]. Aphid parasitism has been demonstrated to be density-dependent [11, 13]. Species that attack oothecae and feed on multiple embryos (considered predators), species where one individual can dominate the nest of a social insect (known as "nest parasitoids"), and cases where the host is only castrated by the "parasitoid" [13–15] will not be considered. For the sake of clarity, we refer to a parasite's action as "parasitism" rather than "parasitoids" [16, 17]. The larval stage of parasitoids develops on or inside one host and eventually kills the host, while the adult stage is usually free-living, making them ideal for biological control [18]. There are two kinds of endoparasitoids that grow from an egg laid inside the host and ectoparasitoids that live and attack from outside the host [19, 20]. The parasitoids *Eretmocerus eremicus* and *Encarsia formosa* serve as the hosts for whitefly larvae [21]. Their effectiveness as biological control agents is further enhanced by the fact that many adult parasitoid wasps are also predators—they kill and feed as predators, frequently killing one or more insects every day [22–25]. Koinobionts are usually endoparasitoids; parasitism symptoms do not appear until the host has grown enough, and the emerging larva starts feeding on and destroying it. Before beginning development, the parasitoid koinobiont leaf miner *Dacnusa sibirica* must pupate; the majority of koinobionts target the early stages of exposed hosts [26, 27]. The aphid parasitoid *Aphidius* spp. undergoes pupariation concurrently with the parasite [19, 20]. Numerous caterpillar parasitic wasps are gregarious parasites; multiple individuals may emerge from a single host's body as a single brood. From a single caterpillar host, *Cotesia glomerata* can occasionally produce 20–40 larvae [1]. The parasitoid leaf miner *Diglyphus isaea* exhibits this as well; as it can produce two or even three adults from a single host in the field, this wasp excels. However, hyperparasites kill the first layer during its maturation stage by parasitizing another layer, usually the primary host's larval stage, to later mature as a second layer [21, 28].

The host-modifying behavior of insect parasitoids is something animals can observe without magnifying lenses, like traditional animal husbandry before the discovery of lenses [29–31]. Parasitic concepts were slower to be understood as a result [19]. Since many parasitoids are internal feeders, it was hard to provide visual evidence, and determining the presence of parasitoids required rearing or dissection of insects [2, 29]. The English doctor Martin Lister was the first to write down the correct understanding of how insects can be parasitic, and in 1685, he described the ichneumon wasps he examined as a different species of insect, one that hatched from eggs inserted into caterpillars [14, 16]. It is hard to count the number of insects that are parasitoid [30]. There are also planned larvae in many species that do the aggressive invasion and incorporation of host body tissues, which changes the behavior of the parasitoid [1, 31].

The following aspects are the focus of the study:

1. Aphids (*Brevicoryne brassicae*, *Aphis gossypii*, *Aphis craccivora*, *Aphis nerii*, *Rhopalosiphum padi*, *R. maids*, and *Hyalopterus pruni*) are surveyed for seasonal abundance, and the percentages of parasitism on the aphid species' and parasitoids population sizes over two seasons are estimated.

2. Seasonal abundance of *Bemisia tabaci* and *Nezara viridula* parasitoids are estimated.

3. Calculating how temperature and relative humidity, two weather variables, affect the number of aphid parasitoids and its aphid hosts.

4. Researching the host suitability and biological characteristics of *D. rapae* and the most common parasitoid on specific aphid species.

5. Assessing how well the parasitoid *D. rapae* controls the cauliflower and cabbage aphid in the field.

6. The biology and effectiveness of *Bracon brevicornis* on *Sesamia cretica* in the laboratory and the parasitoid D. rapae on particular *B. brassicae*.

7. Producing large quantities and calculating the contribution of the parasitoid *D. rapae* to the management of the cowpea aphid, *Aphis craccivora* (Koch), *A. gossypii* Glover, and the cabbage and cauliflower aphid, *Brevicoryne brassicae* (L.), in greenhouses and the field.

2. Aphid parasitoids

2.1 Ecological studies

Aphids infesting cabbage and cauliflowers were known as *Brevicoryne brassicae*. Only one species of parasitoid, *Diaeretiella rapae,* was found emerging from the mummified aphids of *B. brassicae* [18, 20]. *D. rapae* was the main parasitoid that emerged from the mummified aphid. One of the major aphid species that infest faba bean crops is *Aphis craccivora* [21–24]. Three parasitoids emerged from the mummified aphids. *D. rapae*, *Ephedrus persica,* and *Trioxys* sp. [31, 32]. *Aphidius colemani* and *Diaeretiella rapae* are recognized as two important parasitoid species that target the aphid *Hyalopterus pruni*. In the case of Dafla plants, specifically *Nerium oleander*, *Aphis nerii* was the predominant aphid species causing infestations [33]. Research has shown that three parasitoids—*D. rapae, Aphidius matricariae*, and a species of *Aphelinus*—emerged from mummified aphids (see **Table 1**). A study conducted in Greece revealed that the most frequently encountered parasitoids attacking the oleander aphid *A. nerii* included *A. colemani, Binodoxys angelicae, D. rapae,* and *P. volumetri*. When it comes to *A. nerii*, five primary parasitoids were identified: *D. rapae* and various *Aphidius* species, alongside hyperparasitoids like *Pachyneuron* sp., *Alloxysta* sp., and *Aphidencyrtus* sp. *Aphis gossypii*, on the other hand, was the primary aphid species infesting cucumber crops. From the mummified aphids of this species, primary parasitoids such as *Lysiphlebus*

Host plant	Host insect	Parasitoids	Status
Sweet basil	*Nezara viridula*	*Trissolcus megalocephalus*	Primary
Cucumber	*B. tabaci*	1. *Encarsia Formosa*	1.Primary
		2. *Eretmocerus mundus*	2. Primary
Corn	*Sesamia cretica*	*Bracon brevicornis*	Primary
Navel orange trees	1.*Aphis gossypii* Glover	1. *Aphidius matricariae Haliday*	Primary
	2. *Aphis citricola (van der Goot)*	2. *Trioxys sp*	Primary
	3. *Myzus persicae (Sulzer)*	3. *Praon sp*	Primary
	4. *Aphis craccivora Koch*	4. *Alloxysta (Charips) sp.*	Secondary
Cabbage and Cauliflower	*Brevicoryne brassicae* (L.)	*Diaeretiella rapae (M'Intosh)*	Primary
		Pachyneuron sp.	Secondary
		Alloxysta sp. (Cynipidae)	
Faba bean	*Aphis craccivora* (Koch)	*Diaeretiella rapae* (M'Intosh)	Primary
		Ephedrus persicae Froggatt	
		Trioxys sp. (Aphidiidae)	
		Pteromalidae	Hyper
Dafla (Oleander plants)	*Aphis nerii* (Boyer)	*Diaeretiella rapae* (M'Intosh)	Primary
		Aphidius matricariae Haliday (Aphidiidae)	
		Aphelinus sp.(Nees) (*Aphelinidae*)	
		Pteromalidae	Hyper
Hagna (Reed plants)	*Hyalopterus pruni* (Geoffroy)	*Diaeretiella rapae* (M'Intosh)	Primary
		Aphidius *Colemani viereck*	
		Aphelinus sp.(Nees)	
Cucumber plants	*Aphis gossypii* Glover	*Lysiphlebus fabarum* Marshall	Primary
		Diaeretiella rapae (M'Intosh)	
		Binodoxys angelica (Haliday)	
		Pachyneuron sp.	Hyper
Cowpea	*Aphis craccivora* (Koch)	*Lysiphlebus fabarum*	Primary
		Marshall *Diaeretiella rapae* (M'Intosh)	
		Trioxys sp.	
		Aphidencyrtus sp.	Hyper
Corn	*Rhopalosiphum maidis*	*Diaeretiella rapae* (M'Intosh)	Primary
	Rhopalosiphum padi	*Paron* sp.	Primary
	Linnaeus		

***Table 1** is the modified version of table taken from Ref. [33].*

Table 1.
Parasitoids surveyed from pest species on different host plants in Egypt.

fabarum, D. rapae, and *Binodoxys angelicae* emerged. Additionally, a secondary parasitoid, *Pachyneuron* sp., was also found (see **Table 1**).

In the case of *A. gossypii* on cucumber, other parasitoids like *Ephedrus cerasicola*, *Lysiphlebus testaceipes,* and *A. colemani* were recorded from mummified specimens [32, 33]. For the cowpea aphid, *A. craccivora*, the study documented both primary and hyperparasitoid species [29, 33]. The primary parasitoids observed included *Lysiphlebus fabarum, D. rapae*, and *Trioxys* sp., while the hyperparasitoids consisted of *Aphidencyrtus* sp. Furthermore, *Trioxys angelicae* (Hal.) was noted as a parasitoid of *A. craccivora* [34]. Four hymenopterous parasitoid species were recorded during the study, three of them were primary parasitoids, *A. matricariae*, *Trioxys* sp., and *Praon* sp., and one was a secondary parasitoid, *Alloxysta* (*Charips*) sp. The most prevalent aphid (*A. gossypii, A. craccivora*, *Aphis spirocola* Putch, and *Myzus persicae* (Sulzer)) species on navel orange trees (see **Table 1**).

2.2 Seasonal abundance of green bug *Nezara viridula* parasitoids

2.2.1 Background

Trissolcus basalis is a Scelionidae of the Hymenoptera order [35]. Native to Mediterranean Europe, it is common in Spain (**Figure 1**) but is a cosmopolitan species. Parasitizes eggs of *Nezara viridula* (L.) but not monophagous has been shown to parasitize other pentatomid species [36, 37]. The wasp lays an egg inside the host egg. After hatching, the young parasite goes through three larval stages, a pre-pupal and a pupal stage (taking around 12–15 days, **Figure 1**), before emerging as an adult [38].

However, all emerged parasitoids from egg masses of *Nezara viridula* were identified as *Trissolcus megalocephalus* (Ashmead) (Hymenoptera: Scelionidae). The parasitism was first noticed at a level of 8.16% in the fourth week of June, with a progressive increase until it reached 42.39% in the third week of July in the first season of the study. During the first season of the study, the parasitism was initially detected at 8.16% in the fourth week of June and increased gradually until it reached 42.39% in the third week of July. The parasitic rate was 21.84% in 2021 and 29.61% in 2022 seasons, respectively. Maximum adult emergence of *Trissolcus megalocephalus* was 92.31% during the third week of July, while the minimum was 71.43% during the first week of July during the season of 2021 (**Table 2**). In the 2022 season, the maximum emergence percentage of the parasitoid's adults was observed in the third week of July by 92.45% and the minimum percentage was 60.00% in the fourth week of June (**Table 2**). The highest sex ratio (as females), 2 females: 1 male, was achieved

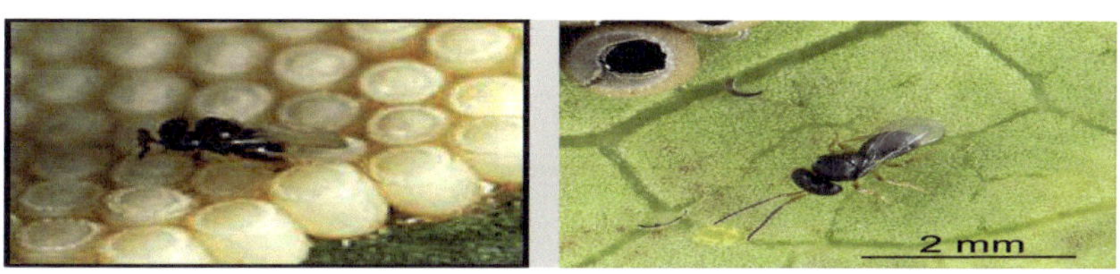

Figure 1.
Shows Trissolcus basalis *parasitizing Southern green stink bug eggs and egg parasitoid,* Trissolcus basalis *Platygasteridae after emergence. Photographer J. K. Clark, University of California Statewide IPM Program.*

Sampling date	No. of examined host egg masses		Total host eggs/masse		Parasitism%		Parasitoid adult emergence %		Parasitoid sex ratio % (as female)	
	2021	2022	2021	2022	2021	2022	2021	2022	2021	2022
June 3rd	00	2	00	89	00	3.37	00	66.67	00	50.00
4th	1	2	49	98	8.16	5.10	75.00	60.00	66.67	66.67
July 1st	1	3	57	158	12.28	21.52	71.43	76.47	60.00	53.85
2nd	2	2	123	114	20.33	51.75	84.00	86.44	57.14	54.90
3rd	3	2	184	119	42.39	44.54	92.31	92.45	54.17	55.10
4th	2	1	119	47	26.05	42.55	90.32	90.0	57.14	61.11
Aug. 1st	00	1	00	39	00	38.46	00	86.67	00	61.54
Total	9	13	532	664	00	00	00	00	00	00
Mean ± SE	1.8 ± 0.37	1.86 ± 0.26	106.4 ± 24.68	94.86 ± 15.72	21.84 ± 6.00	29.61 ± 7.42	82.61 ± 4.11	79.81 ± 4.70	59.02 ± 2.12	57.60 ± 2.15

Table 2.
Parasitism percentage of egg-parasitoid Trissolcus megalocephalus *on* N. viridula *eggs on sweet basil plants during 2021 and 2022 seasons.*

in the fourth week of June in both studied seasons. The mean sex ratio was 1.47♀:1♂ in the 2021 season and 1.40♀:1 ♂in the 2022 season (**Table 2**).

2.3 Whitefly, *Bemisia tabaci*, *Bemisia argentifolii*, and parasitoids

2.3.1 Background

Many researches were performed to find powerful natural enemies of whiteflies so as to establish organic manipulation because of useless and high-priced chemical control [39–42]. Thus, as biological control appears to be the most promising technique of dealing with whiteflies, I recognition on it in this thesis. Biological controls, whether or not herbal or delivered, are the handiest long-term answers for controlling whitefly populations. Biological control retailers like *Encarsia formosa*, *Encarsia luteola*, and *Eretmocerus* californicus have been a success in greenhouses (**Figure 2**). Insect pathogenic fungi (*Verticillium lecanii*, *Paecilomyces fumosoroseus*, and *Beauveria bassiana*) can successfully control whiteflies in greenhouse and area vegetation (**Figure 2**). Whitefly predators encompass beetles (Coccinellidae), authentic insects (Miridae, Anthocoridae), lacewings (Chrysopidae, Coniopterygidae), mites (Phytoseiidae), and spiders (Araneae) [41]. Many studies have been carried out to find effective herbal enemies of whiteflies with a purpose to establish organic control as a result of ineffective and steeply priced chemical control [39–43]. Reducing the use of pesticides to govern whiteflies and defensive agricultural merchandise at a lower price is a desire of organic management [42]. In greenhouses, biological management agents such as *Eretmocerus californicus, Encarsia luteola,* and *Encarsia formosa* had demonstrated success [41–43]. Whiteflies in greenhouses and subject crops can be effectively managed by insect pathogenic fungi (*Verticillium lecanii, Paecilomyces fumosoroseus,* and *Beauveria bassiana*) [44]. Beetles (Coccinellidae), spiders (Araneae), mites (Phytoseiidae), lacewings (Chrysopidae, Coniopterygidae), and real bugs (Miridae, Anthocoridae) are among the predators of whiteflies [41].

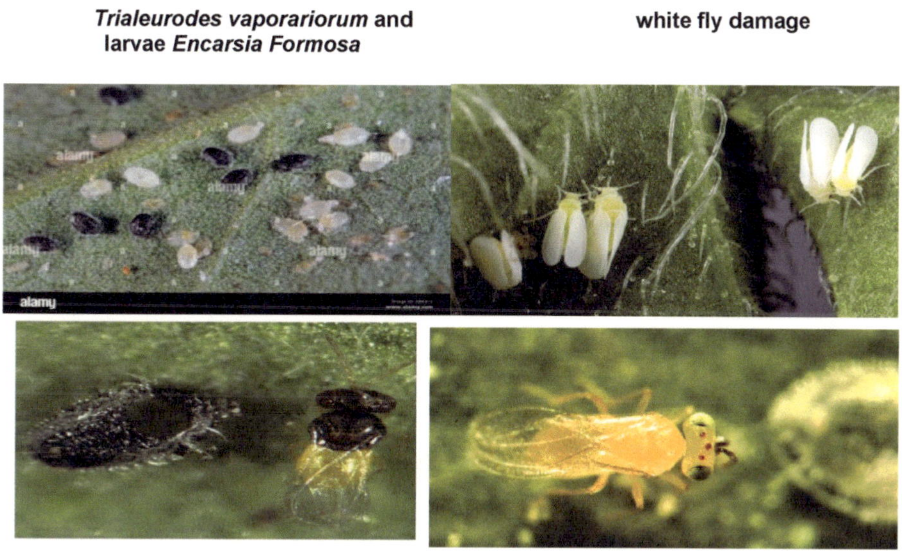

Figure 2.
Whitefly and its parasitoids Encarsia formosa *and* Eretmocerus eremicus.

3. Biological studies

3.1 Host selection and preference for hosts parasitized

Natural enemies are becoming a more viable option, and biological management is the cornerstone of the Integrated Pest Management (IPM) paradigm [6, 45]. Using both short-range and long-range cues is the foundation of parasitoids' host selection strategy [44]. In order to find and comprehend their hosts, parasitoids respond to every semiochemical and physiological stimulus [33]. These responses are both because of aphid sex pheromones appearing as kairomones or due to aphid-brought-about plant volatiles, performing as synomones. Various interactions, like genetic, studying, and conditioning elements, which play a crucial position in the host selection behavior of foraging parasitoids, were mentioned with the aid of Saleh [33].

3.2 *Diaeretiella rapae* life cycle when raised on *B. brassicae* at 18 ± 1°C and 60 ± 5% relative humidity

In the lab at 23 ± 1°C, different *D. rapae* lifestyle ranges were examined on *Myzus persicae*. After oviposition, parasitized aphids continued to feed and cling to the host plant's leaves. Larva: After 72 ± 1 hours, creamy white larvae were found in the aphid's stomach, feeding on smooth tissue.

The mummified aphid changed into golden yellow (**Figure 3B** and **C**). Our observations were associated with Hafeez [46]. After 96 ± 2 h., dissections confirmed that creamy white larvae changed into yellow coloration [20, 38]. They changed into a brown eye spot gift on the pointed give-up (anterior location) (**Figure 3D**).

On the fifth day, the color of the larvae changed into nevertheless yellow, but it became absolutely modified from the fourth-day larvae; there was truly differentiation among the head, thorax, and abdomen [35, 47, 48]. Antennae, legs, and wings commenced to increase; however, they were obviously in shade (**Figure 4E**). There were four larval instars completed inside the mummified aphid. The abdomen was wiped clean out, and then the thorax and head [48]. Larvae on the sixth day, initiation

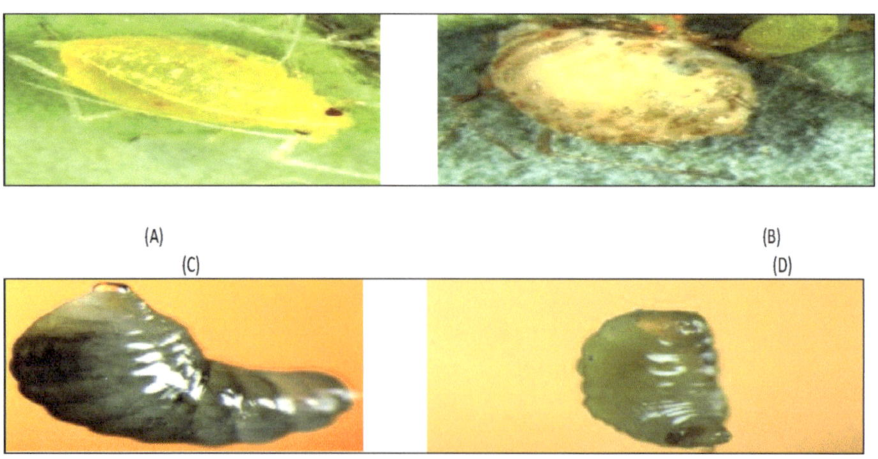

Figure 3.
Life cycle of D. rapae *on* M. persicae. *Development of* D. rapae *larvae; parasitized aphid (A), mummified aphid (B), newly hatched larvae (C), and 4 days old larva (D).*

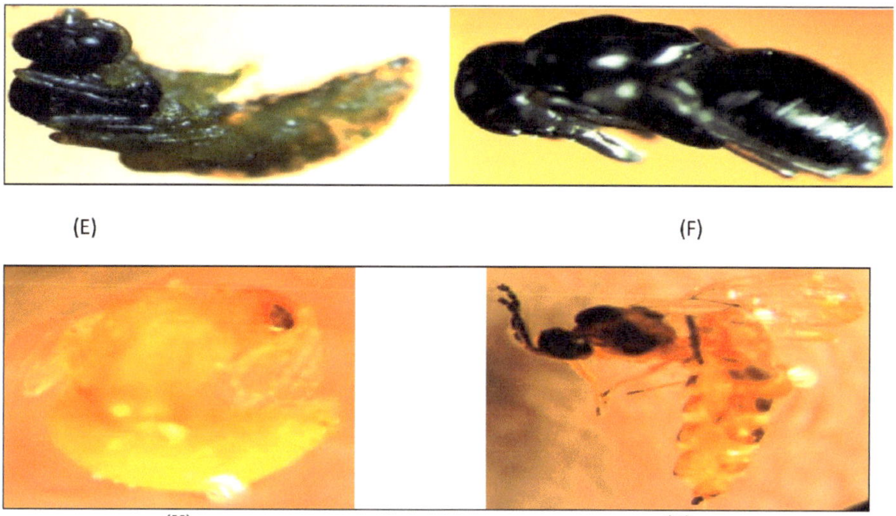

Figure 4.
Development of D. rapae *larva to pupa; 5 days old larvae (E), 6 days old larvae (F), 7 days old larvae (G), and on the 9th larvae changed into pupae (H).*

segmentations, the head, and thorax changed to black color; antennae and wings had not been absolutely developed at that point (**Figure 4F**). On the seventh day, no considerable change occurred within the larvae (**Figure 4G**). Pupae and adult: On the ninth day, larvae completely modified and changed into pupae, which have been black (**Figure 4H**). Pupal period lasts for about 2 days, and it is modified into a grown-up on the 11th day (**Figure 5I**) [38]. On the same day, grownups emerged by making a hollow within the abdomen of their host (**Figure 5J**). After the emergence of *D. rapae*, a lifeless host is called a mummy (**Figure 5K**) [38]. The total life cycle of *D. rapae* in the host (*M. persicae*) from oviposition to emergence becomes finished in 11.5 days [49]. An internal parasitoid called *Diaeretiella rapae attacks* aphids and lays its eggs inside the host's body; the larva goes through four instars. According to the results in **Table 3**, the range of egg level duration was 2–4 days, with a mean of 4.01 ± 0.35 days. The median duration of the larval stage was 6.23 days, with a range of 4–7 days. The median pupal duration was 7.19 ± 0.24 days, with a range of 5–8 days. With a mean of 17.43 ± 0.91 days, the average existence cycle from egg to person's emergence varied between 12 and 19 days (**Table 3**).

3.3 Biological aspects of *Bracon brevicornis* reared on *Sesamia cretica*

Sesamia cretica Led. is taken into consideration as one of the most negative agricultural pests, which causes severe financial harm and reduces the crop yield. This pest species is hard to be controlled by using touch insecticides because the larvae bore into plant tissues shortly after hatching. In addition, pesticide residues in food are becoming increasingly unacceptable to purchasers [50]. The parasitoid, *Bracon brevicornis* Wesm., is an indigenous, primary gregarious ectoparasitoid on Sesamia cretica, *Ostrinia nubilalis* Hb.; *Chilo agamemnon* Bles.; and *Helicoerpa armigera* (Hubner) and *Pectinophora gossypiella* (Saunders) [50, 51]. The parasitoid is extensively allotted over decrease and top Egypt and has 24 generations within the laboratory in line with 12 months [50].

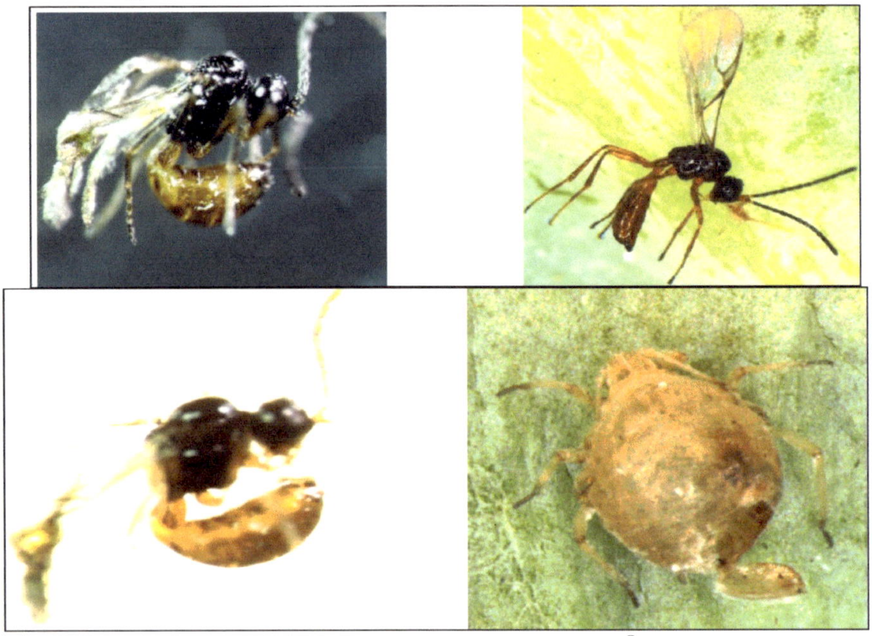

Figure 5.
Development of D. rapae *larva; pupae changed into an adult at 11 days (I), on the same day emerged from host (J, K, and L).*

Host aphid	Egg (days)	Larval (days)	Pupal (days)	Life cycle (days)
Brevicoryne brassicae	4.01 ± 0.35[a] (2–4)	6.23 ± 0.51[b] (4–7)	7.19 ± 0.24[c] (5–8)	17.43 ± 0.91[d] (12–19)
LSD 0.05	0.49947	0.79915	0.9989	1.9978

Means with different letters in the same row indicate a significant difference ($p \leq 0.05$).

Table 3.
Brevicoryne brassicae *and* Diaeretiella rapae *life cycle at 18.00 ± 1 °C and 65 ± 5 RH%.*

3.3.1 Biology Bracon brevicornis

Data in **Table 4** showed the biological elements of the parasitoid *Bracon brevicornis* beneath the laboratory conditions of 25 ± 2°C and 60 ± 4 RH. The incubation duration of eggs lasted for 2 to 3 days, with a mean of two, 2.72 ± 0.11 days. The percentage of hatchability became 95.97%. Larval level lasted a mean of 5.35 ± 0.47 days with a range of 4–7 days. The mortality percentage is 3.17% (**Table 4**). The pupal length ranged from 7 to 9 days, with a mean of 7.98 ± 0.73 days (**Table 4**). The overall developmental duration (egg–Adult) lasted 14–18 days, with a mean of 16.05 ± 1.44 days. The mean percentage of adult emergence changed to 95.74%. The sex ratio changed to 1 male:0.54 lady (**Table 4**). The pre-ovipositional length of grown-up females, furnished with *Sesamia cretica* full-grown larvae, becomes 1.67 ± 0.33 days, with

Stage		Duration in days	
		Range	Mean ± SE
Egg	Incubation period	2–3	2.72 ± 0.11
	Hatchability %	90–100%	95.97%
Larva	Duration	4–7	5.035 ± 0.47
	Mortality	—	3.17%
Pupal period		7–9	7.98 ± 0.73
Total developmental period (egg-adult)		14–18	16.05 ± 1.44
Adult emergence %		—	95.74%
Sex ratio (Male: Female)		—	1:0.54
Adult female	Pre-ovipositional period	1–2	1.67 ± 0.33
	Ovipositional period	13–25	21.17 ± 1.78
	Post-ovipositional period	2–4	2.67 ± 0.74
	Female longevity	16–29	25.51 ± 2.20
Male longevity		9–15	12.67 ± 0.84
No. of eggs/female		121–339	209.08 ± 4.1
No. of eggs/larva		2–21	8.19 ± 0.901

Table 4.
Biological aspects of the parasitoid Bracon brevicornis *on* S. cretica *at 25 ± 2 °C and 60 ± 4% RH.*

a variety of 1–2 days. The ovipositional period becomes 21.17 ± 1.78 days, with quite a number of 13–25 days (**Table 4**). Post-ovipositional duration turned into 2.67 ± 0.74 days, with a variety of 2–4 days. The mean female longevity changed to 25.51 ± 2.20 with more than a few 16–29 days. The suggested male toughness became 12.67 ± 0.84 with more than a few 9–15 days (**Table 4**). The mean range of deposited eggs for *Bracon brevicornis* became 209.08 eggs/female, with a range of 121–339 eggs. The mean quantity of eggs/host larva became 8.19 eggs (**Table 4**), while the parasitoid reared on *S. cretica* complete-grown larvae (**Table 4**).

4. Aphid parasitoid mass production and field application

4.1 Effect of parasitoid densities on parasitization rate

Data presented in illustrated **Table 5** show that the parasitoid density had an impact on the parasitism percentage; for *D. rapae*, which was maintained at a rate of 15 parasitoid females per cage, the maximum percentage was 87.75% and the minimum was 48.60% at three parasitoids per cage. There were significant differences in the total numbers of parasitized aphid and the total percentage of parasitism at all densities. The maximum number of parasitized aphids by *D. rapae* (175.5) was recorded at 15 parasitoids per cage and a minimum of 97.2 was recorded at three parasitoids per cage. The highest percentage of adult's emergence was 82.41% for *D. rapae* at three parasitoids per cage. These findings agree with those of Refs. [33, 52–54].

Parasitoid density	Mean ± SD				
	No. of emerged adults	No. of non emerged adults	No. of parasitized aphid (Mummies)	Percentage of parasitism	Percentages of adult emergence
3♀	80.1E ± 4.89	17.1D ± 2.12	97.2E ± 6.25	48.6E ± 2.96	82.41A ± 3.11
6♀	95D ± 3.96	28.5C ± 1.27	123.5D ± 5.21	61.75D ± 2.53	80.13B ± 2.39
9♀	112C ± 2.71	32.5C ± 1.41	144.5C ± 4.03	72.25C ± 2.25	76.18C ± 2.02
12♀	120B ± 5.21	39.0B ± 3.22	159B ± 7.01	79.5B ± 3.03	73.35E ± 1.68
15♀	132.1A ± 8.71	43.4A ± 6.31	175.5A ± 5.09	87.75A ± 2.60	75.27D ± 4.09
LSD 0.05	1.68407	4.125106	5.179249	0.729223	0.0197474

Table 5.
Effect of parasitoid density on percentage of parasitism and percentage of adult emergence in the field under 19 ± 10 C and 74 ± 3% R.H [23].

4.2 *Diaeretiella rapae* inundative release in greenhouses

4.2.1 In greenhouses D. Rapae inundative release

Table 6 shows the results from 2010/2011 concerning the release of *D. rapae* at various ratios of parasitoids to hosts on cauliflower plants to manage *B. brassicae*. After 8 days, the lowest total parasitism rates were 32.37, 19.91, 11.80, and 9.18% for ratios of 1:4, 1:8, 1:12, and 1:16, respectively. Over the next 28 days, these rates increased to 100, 78.70, 73.57, and 36.62% for the same ratios. The average parasitism rates in greenhouses were 73.94, 60.74, 54.29, and 39.98% for the ratios 1:4, 1:8, 1:12, and 1:16.

Table 7 details another study in 2011–2012 that observed the release of *D. rapae* at ratios of 1:8 and 1:12 in the field on cauliflower plants against *B. brassicae*. The lowest total parasitism rates were 13.32 and 9.69% for the 1:8 and 1:12 ratios, while a farmer's observation noted a rate of 8.44% after 4 days. However, the total parasitism rates later rose to 98.57 and 84.73% for those same ratios.

The average parasitism rates in the field were recorded at 58.39, 50.01, and 32.49% when the ratios of parasitoids to hosts were 1:8 and 1:12, respectively. The parasitoid *D. rapae* can effectively control *B. brassicae* in cauliflower farms both in greenhouses and in open fields at these same ratios [55].

In the studies on *B. brassicae*, various parasitoids to host ratios of 1:4, 1:8, 1:12, and 1:16 were used. **Table 8** presents data showing how temperature and humidity relate to the population density of *B. brassicae* over two growing seasons. In the first season, lower temperatures had a significant negative effect, while higher temperatures had a positive impact [46, 56]. During the second season, higher humidity was positively correlated at a 1:4 ratio. At a 1:8 ratio, both low and high humidity showed positive correlations, and high temperatures also had a positive correlation at a 1:12 ratio during the first season. In 2011, low humidity showed a positive correlation in the second season, as noted by Saleh [23, 33] in **Table 8**.

The study examined how temperature and humidity affect the population of the aphid *B. brassicae* and its parasitoid *D. rapae* in greenhouses, considering different ratios of parasitoids to hosts. **Table 9** shows the population density of *B. brassicae* over 2 years. Temperature variations explained 25.8 to 22.1%, 69.2 to 2.3%, 0.1 to 24.1%, and 27.3 to 23.3% of the population density during the first season. In the second

Sampling dates	Dates after release	Parasitoid: host ratio				
		1:4	**1:8**	**1:12**	**1:16**	**Control**
16-12-10	4	0	0	0	0	0
20-12	8	32.37	19.91	11.89	9.18	8.81
24-12	12	49.67	25.71	18.19	12.29	10.13
28-12	16	68.09	36.62	23.79	15.90	14.44
1-1-2011	20	73.48	48.2	41.58	20.13	16.0
5-1	24	89.74	65.74	54.49	28.75	18.7
9-1	28	100	78.70	73.57	36.62	16.22
13-1	32	100	93.28	81.75	58.25	20.67
17-1	36	100	100	92.03	78.93	25.12
21-1	40	100	100	100	86.6	32.74
25-1	44	100	100	100	93.08	35.17
Average		73.94 ± 10.19	60.74 ± 11.01	54.29 ± 11.17	39.98 ± 10.11	18.59 ± 2.80

Table 6.
Percentages of parasitism on B. brassicae *after release of* D. rapae *at different parasitoid: host ratios under green houses on cauliflower plants during 2010/2011 [23].*

Sampling dates	Dates after release	Parasitoid: host ratio		In the farmer
		1:8	1:12	
15-12-11	4	13.32	9.69	8.44
19-12	8	17.67	14.22	10.81
32-12	12	20.62	16.67	14.13
27-12	16	33.88	21.68	16.44
31-12	20	41.89	32.47	22.00
4-1-2012	24	51.47	40.61	27.7
8-1	28	62.68	53.07	39.22
12-1	32	74.25	62.75	48.67
16-1	36	86.28	70.98	45.12
20-1	40	98.57	84.73	52.47
24-1	44	100	93.92	48.17
28-1	48	100	100	56.46
Average		58.39	50.01	32.49

Table 7.
Percentages of parasitism on B. brassicae *after release of* D. rapae *at different parasitoid: host ratios in the field on cauliflower plants during 2011/2012 [23].*

Weather factors	Correlation coefficient (R)			
	2010–2011			
	1:4	1:8	1:12	1:16
Min. temp.	−0.508*	−0.226	0.316	−0.258
Max. temp	0.470*	−0.276	0.419*	0.483
Min. R.H.	−0.366	0.600*	0.106	−.0567*
Max. R.H.	0.077	0.522*	−0.104	0.074
	2011–2012			
Min. temp.	−0.162	0.227	−0.020	0.061
Max. temp	−0.344	−0.217	0.073	0. 179
Min. R.H.	−0.238	−0.381	−0.421	0.545
Max. R.H.	0.681*	0.095	0.304	0.088

* *Significant*

Table 8.
Simple correlation coefficient between temperature, relative humidity, and the total numbers of B. brassicae *at different parasitoid: host ratios under green houses on cauliflower plants during the two season 2010/2011 and 2011/ [23].*

season, the explained variance ranged from 1.0 to 29.2%, 34.2 to 33.7%, 5.6 to 4.0%, and 2.9 to 14.4%. Relative humidity also varied significantly, with minimums and maximums ranging from 5.0 to 10.3%, 18.9 to 0.2%, 24.1 to 7.0%, and 1.0 to 2.0% in 2010. In 2011, these ranges were 3.1 to 46.3%, 14.5 to 8.7%, 17.7 to 10.7%, and 1.8 to 12.6%. The overall impact of both factors averaged 82.1, 94.5, 41.3, and 38.2% in the 2011 season across the four ratios of 1:4, 1:8, 1:12, and 1:16.

Weather A: Simple	Regression equation (*B. brassicae*)							
	1:4		1:8		1:12		1:16	
	2010–2011 R2	2011–2012 R2	2010–2011 R2	2011–2012 R2	2010–2011 R2	2011–2012 R2	2010–2011 R2	2011–2012 R2
Min. temp.	0.258	0.001	0.692*	0.342	0.010	0.056	0.273	0.029
Max. temp	0.221	0.292	0.023	0.337	0.241	0.040	0.233	0.144
Min. R.H.	0.005	0.031	0.189	0.145	0.001	0.177	0.001	0.018
Max. R.H.	0.103	0.463*	0.020	0.087	0.070	0.107	0.020	0.126
B: Multiple	0.821*	0.945*	0.945*	0.786*	0.413	0.645*	0.382	0.345

** Significant*

Table 9.
Numerical relation between temperature, relative humidity, and the total numbers of B. brassicae *during the two season 2010/2011 and 2011/2012 [23].*

4.3 On *D. Rapae* in cauliflower at parasitoid/host ratios 1:4,1:8,1:12, and1:16

The data in **Table 10** revealed the correlation between temperature, humidity, and the population density of *D. rapae* over the 2-year study period. During the first year, the minimum temperature showed a strong negative correlation, while the minimum relative humidity also displayed a significant negative correlation at a parasitoid/host ratio of 1:4. In contrast, the maximum temperature revealed a strong negative correlation at a ratio of 1:8 and a significant negative correlation at a ratio of 1:16 in the same period. In the second year, temperature and relative humidity influenced the correlations, which varied from slight negative to positive across different parasitoid/host ratios, as shown in **Table 10**.

Table 11 shows the relationship between temperature, humidity, and the population density of *D. rapae* over two study seasons. The variance explained by temperature, both

Weather factors	correlation coefficient (R)			
	2010–2011			
	1:4	1:8	1:12	1:16
	−0728**	−0.334	−0.018	−0.413
Max. temp	−0.049	−0.782**	−0.363	−0.580*
Min. R.H.	−0.574*	0.160	−0.422	−0.265
Max. R.H.	−0.196	0.264	−0.431	−0.076
	2011–2012			
Min. temp.	−0.069	0.184	−0.012	0.029
Max. temp	−0.425	−0.319	0.032	0.379
Min. R.H.	0.339	−0.296	0.396	0.065
Max. R.H.	0.323	0.184	0.167	−0.136

** Significant*
*** Highly significant*

Table 10.
Simple correlation coefficient between temperature, relative humidity, and the total numbers of D. rapae *during the two season 2010/2011 and 2011/2012 [23].*

Weather factors	Regression equation (B. brassicae)							
	1:4		1:8		1:12		1:16	
seasons	2010–11 R2	2011–12 R2	2010–11 R2	2011–12 R2	2010–11 R2	2011–12 R2	2010–11 R2	2011–12 R2
A:Simple Min. temp.	0.530	0.153	0.026	0.231	0.106	0.100	0.174	0.178
Max. temp	0.132	0.181	0.612	0.102	0.222	0.168	0.336	0.049
Min. R.H.	0.330	0.140	0.135	0.150	0.140	0.053	0.029	0.297
Max. R.H.	0.030	0.102	0.025	0.135	0.185	0.005	0.011	0.134
B: Multiple	0.906	0.684	0.977	0.881	0.623	0.671	0.711	0.816

Table 11.
Numerical relation between temperature, relative humidity, and the total numbers of D. rapae *during the two season 2010/11 and 2011/2012 [23].*

minimum and maximum, influenced *D. rapae* density with effects ranging from 13.2 to 61.2% in the first season and from 10.2 to 18.1% in the second season. The relative humidity levels ranged from 3.0 to 33.0% in 2010. The combined impact of temperature and humidity averaged between 62.3 and 97.7% in the first season and between 67.1 and 88.1% in the second season at various parasitoid-to-host ratios of 1:4, 1:8, 1:12, and 1:16.

4.4 On *B. brassicae* and *D. rapae* in cauliflower at parasitoid/host ratios 1:8 and 1:12 in field

Table 12 presents the correlation coefficients for temperature, relative humidity, and the population densities of *B. brassicae* and *D. rapae* during the 2011–2012 season. Temperature had a varied impact, showing correlations that ranged from slightly positive to negative for *D. rapae*. High relative humidity resulted in a significant negative correlation for *B. brassicae* at a parasitoid/host ratio of 1:4 and a slightly negative

Weather factors	Correlation coefficient (R)	
	B. brassicae	
	1:8	1:12
Min. temp.	0.315	−0.326
Max. temp	−0.054	−0.259
Min. R.H.	0.272	−0.362
Max. R.H.	−0.678**	0.113
	D. rapae	
Min. temp.	0.402	0.005
Max. temp	0.186	0.422
Min. R.H.	−0.262	−0.524*
Max. R.H.	−0.386	−0.137

Table 12.
Simple correlation coefficient between temperature relative humidity and the total numbers of B. brassicae *and* D. rapae *during the season 2011 at parasitoid: host ratios1:4 and1:8 in field [23].*

Weather	Correlation coefficient (R)			
A:Simple	*B. brassicae*		*D. rapae*	
	1:4	1:8	1:4	1:8
Min. temp.	0.020	0.098	0.0340	0.161
Max. temp	0.010	0.028	0.049	0.037
Min. R.H.	0.131	0.001	0.275	0.143
Max. R.H.	0.151	0.460	0.262	0.149
B: Multiple	0.558	0.524	0.568	0.520

Table 13.
Numerical relation between temperature, relative humidity, and the total numbers of B. Brassicae *and* D. rapae *during the season 2011 at parasitoid: host ratios1:8 and1:12 in field [23].*

correlation for *D. rapae* at a ratio of 1:8. In **Table 13**, the numerical relationships among temperature, relative humidity, and the population densities of these species for the 2011 season are shown. The explained variance for temperature (both minimum and maximum) concerning the population densities ranged from 2.0% to 1.0% for *B. brassicae* and from 3.4 to 4.9% for *D. rapae*, with extremes of 9.9 to 2.8% and 16.1 to 3.7%, respectively, at ratios of 1:4 and 1:8. Minimum and maximum relative humidity values varied from 13.1 to 15.1% and 27.5 to 26.2% for *B. brassicae*, and from 1.0–46% and 14.3 to 14.9% for *D. rapae* at the same ratios. The combined effect of temperature and humidity averaged 55.8, 56.8, 52.4, and 52.0% for *B. brassicae* and *D. rapae* at the respective ratios, as noted by Saleh [23, 33].

5. Conclusions

Under a comprehensive pest management system, biological control is an excellent program. The parasitoids' organic manipulation of the pest is the behavior that keeps the population of the pest at a lower level. *D. rapae* is a significant species that has the ability to parasitize a remarkable range of aphid species. It is generally accepted to be a highly effective organic aphid management agent, particularly for the cabbage aphid in Egypt's cauliflower and cabbage fields. Conversely, the observer suggested participating in Egypt's Integrated Pest Management Programs, which aim to influence *B. brassicae* initiatives. Based on the information provided, it was determined that *D. rapae* infested all *B. brassicae* ranges; however, the most successful adults of the Agricola were hatched from the third and fourth larvae. However, subsequent studies demonstrated that, after being taken advantage of in their parasitoid-host relationship, *L. fabarum* and *D. rapae* effectively control cowpeas, faba beans, cabbage, *A. craccivora,* and *B. brassicae*. In particular, when there are few *D. rapae* in the field, the pest should be released into the population. Coexisting with the pest population allows *D. rapae* to maintain a proactive biological control strategy. Furthermore, this experiment demonstrated that the parasitoid may offer ecosystem services by controlling the pest in specific settings, such as fields or greenhouses. Based on the results of the experiment, this aphid parasitoid performed better in an area where there were more aphids. We therefore draw the conclusion that if parasitoids are to be used for biological control, they ought to be discharged into fields where host densities are lower. All of the parasitoids that surfaced from the egg masses taken to be *Trissolcus megalocephalus*. The parasitism rates in two consecutive seasons are 21.84 and 29.61%, respectively. According to the results, *B. tabaci* was effectively controlled by the biological control agents *Eretmocerus mundus* and *Encarsia formosa*. Furthermore, *Eretmocerus mundus* and *Encarsia formosa* had the greatest effects on *B. tabaci*. Furthermore, it has been confirmed that the wasp *Bracon brevicornis*, a new gregarious ectoparasitoid of *Sesamia cretica, Ostrinia nubilalis*, *Chilo agamdemon*, or *Helicoverpa armigera*, and *Pectinophora gossypiella*, is established in Egypt. Thus, some of the pests listed under the Egyptian growing conditions may be biologically controlled by the results of these experiments with the parasitoids *L. fabarum*, *D. rapae, Encarsia formosa, Eretmocerus mundus,* and *Bracon brevicornis*. Therefore, it is strongly advised that in order to minimize the environmental dispersion of insecticides, the integrated pest management strategy that is advised for many of the pest management practices under Egyptian field conditions should include a recommendation to monitor the release timing of this parasitoid in the fields.

Author details

Ahmed Amin Ahmed Saleh[1] and Ahmed Shamkhi Jabbar[2*]

1 A.R.C., Plant Protection Research Institute, Giza, Egypt

2 Department of Plant Protection, College of Agricultural, University of Al-Qadisiyah, Al-Qadisiyah, Iraq

*Address all correspondence to: ahmed.shamkhi@qu.edu.iq

References

[1] Habashy AZN, Abd-Elsamed AA, Saleh AAA. Biological aspects of the parasitoid *Bracon brevicornis* Wesm (hymenoptera: Braconidae), reared on *Sesamia cretica* led. Under laboratory condition. Journal of Plant Protection and Pathology. 2012;**10**:1023-1032

[2] Saleh AAA, Amer SAM, Abd-Elsamed AA, Zawrah MFM. Performance of certain predators in controling *Aphis craccivora* koch and *Myzus persicae* (Sluzer). On broad bean plants. Journal of Plant Protection and Pathology. 2022;**13**(12):277-282

[3] Saleh AAA, El-Nagar H, Khalifa AA, Zawrah MFM. The role of *Chrysoperla carnea* (Steph.) and *Beauveria bassina* for controlling cabbage aphid, *Brevicoryne brassicae* L. on cabbage plants. Arab Journal of Plant Protection. 2023;**41**(3):321-326. DOI: 10.22268/AJPP-041.3.321326

[4] Saleh AAA, Sh Ali AM, Mohamed NE. Natural enemies attacking the mealy aphid *Hyalopterus pruni* (Geoffroy) in peach orchard at Ismailia governorate. Egyptian Journal of Agricultural Research. 2013;**91**(1):75-93

[5] Lokma N, Saleh AAA, Amer SAM, Zawrah MFM. Efficacy of some predators and *Lecanicillium lecanii* fungus in controlling of *Aphis gossypii* (glover) and *Myzus persicae* (Sulzer) in potato crop. Arab Journal of Plant Protection. 2023;**41**(2):152-160. DOI: 10.22268/AJPP-041.2.152160

[6] Sh Ali AM, Saleh AAA, Saleh FM. Bio efficacy of plants extracts and entomopathogenic fungi (*Trichoderma album*) in controling *Myzus persicae* and *Bemisia tabaci*. Plant Archives. 2020;**20**(Suppl 1):1450-1459

[7] Akram AM, Jamal HK, Zahid NAK. Selection of highly virulent entomopathogenic fungal isolates to control the greenhouse aphid species in Iraq. Egyptian Journal of Biological Pest Control. 2018;**28**:71. DOI: 10.1186/s41938-018-0079-3

[8] Kidd NAC, Jervis MA. Host-feeding and oviposition strategies of parasitoids in relation to host stage. Researches on Population Ecology. 1991;**33**:13-28

[9] Gamal MA, Lashin AAAS, Ali AM. Efficacy of entomopathogenic fungus *Isaria fumosorsea* (wize) and the parasitoid *Diaeretiella rapae* (M'Intosh) against cabbage aphid *Brevicoryne brassicae* L. (Hemiptera: Aphididae). In: The Eleventh International Environmental Conference. Egypt: Faculty of Science-Zagazig University, Bulletin of the Faculty of Science-Zagazig University; 2016. pp. 485-497

[10] Sarhan AA. Studies on the biological control of cotton white fly *Bemisia tabaci* (Genn.) in Egypt [thesis]. Egypt: Faculty of Agriculture, Cairo University; 1976. 164 p

[11] Saleh AAA, Ismail HA, Arafa EMF, Zawrah MFM. Ecological and biological aspects of aphid parasitoids on navel orange trees in Egypt. Journal of Plant Protection and Pathology. 2023;**14**(5):115

[12] Ismail HA, Saleh AAA, Abdel Hafez MM, El-Gendy RM. Estimating seasonal abundance of piercing-sucking insects and their natural enemies on sweet basil plants. Egyptian Academic Journal of Biological Sciences. 2024;**16**(1):65-75

[13] Walker GP, Nault LR, Simonet DE. Natural mortality factors acting on

potato aphid (*Macrosiphum euphorbiae*) populations in processing tomato field in Ohio. Environmental Entomology. 1984;**13**:724-732

[14] Al-Hadary SSNA, Saleh AAA. Knowledge needs of cotton farmers for using the *Trichogramma* parasitoid to control bollworms in certain villages in IN Sharqia governorate. Zagazig Journal of Agricultural Research. 2024;**51**(4):885-900

[15] Saleh AAA, Ismail HA, Eltahawe HS, Selem GS. Evaluating potential impact of certain natural enemies on key piercing-sucking insects infesting sweet basil plants. Egyptian Academic Journal of Biological Sciences. 2024;**17**(1):131-140

[16] Eggleton P, Belshaw R. Insect parasitoids: An evolutionary overview. Philosophical Transactions of the Royal Society of London (Series B). 1992;**337**:1-20

[17] Zawrah MFM, El Masry AT, Noha L, Saleh AAA. Efficacy of certain insecticides against whitefly *Bemisia tabaci* (genn) infesting tomato plants and their associated predators. Plant Archives. 2020;**20**(Suppl 2):2221-2228

[18] Saleh AAA. Storage of *Diaeretiella rapae* (M'Intosh) (hymenoptera: Aphidiidae) mummies in three aphid species; *Brevicoryne brassicae* (L.), *Aphis nerii* Boyer de fonscolombe and *Aphis gossypii* (Glov.) (Homoptera: Aphididae). Egyptian Journal of Biological Pest Control. 2008;**18**(1):39-42

[19] Saleh AAA, Ali SAM, Abd-Elsamed AA, Elsayed AAA. Development of the parasitoid *Diaeretiella rapae* (M'Intosh) reared on certain aphid species in relation to heat unit requirement. Journal of Entomology. 2014;**11**(3):127-141

[20] Saleh AAA. Ecological and biological studies of *Diaeretiella rapae* (M'Intosh) (hymenoptera: Aphidiidae), the parasitoid of some aphid species in Egypt. Egyptian Journal of Biological Pest Control. 2008;**18**(1):33-38

[21] Mahr DL, Ridgway NM. Biological control of insects and mites: An introduction to beneficial natural enemies and their use in pest management. North Central Regional Extension Publication. 1993;**481**:91

[22] Saleh AAA, Desuky WMH, Mohamed NE. Studies on some parasitoids of the cowpea aphid *Aphis craccvora* Koch (Homoptera: Aphididae) in Egypt. Egyptian Journal of Biological Control. 2009;**19**(1):11-16

[23] Saleh AAA. Evaluation of release of *Diaeretiella rapae* (M'Intosh) for controlling the cruciferous aphid, *Brevicoryne brassicae* L. on cauliflower plants at Sharkia governorate, Egypt. Plant Protection and Pathology. 2012;**3**(3):307-318

[24] Saleh AAA. Efficacy of the aphid parasitoid *Diaeretiella rapae* (M'Intosh) to control *Brevicoryne brassicae* L., *Aphis craccivora* (Koch) and *Aphis nerii* Boyer at Sharkia governorate. Egyptian Journal of Agricultural Research. 2012;**91**(1):21-31

[25] Abd-Elkareim AI, Jabbar AS, Marouf AE. Effects of feeding floral resource on potential of *Bemisia tabaci* parasitoids. Indian Journal of Ecology. 2019;**46**(3):636-639

[26] Watson AK, editor. Biological Control of Weeds Handbook. Champaign, IL: Weed Science Society of America; 1993. 202 p

[27] Saleh AAA, Hashem MS, Abd-Elsamed AA. *Aphidius colemani* iereck and *Diaeretiella rapae* (M'Intosh)

as parasitoids on the common reed aphid, *Hyalopterus pruni* (Geoffroy) in Egypt. Egyptian Journal of Biological Pest Control. 2006;**16**(2):93-97

[28] Saleh AAA, Ali SAM, El-Nagar H. Development of the parasitoid *Aphidius colemani* vierek on the mealy aphid, *Hyalopterus pruni* (Geoffroy) in relation to heat unit requirement. Egyptian Journal of Biological Pest Control. 2014;**24**(1):17-21

[29] Vázquez BSLL, Marucci RC. Natural Enemies of Insect Pests in Neotropical Agroecosystems. Biological Control and Functional Biodiversity. Switzerland: Springer Nature; 2019. DOI: 10.1007/978-3-030-24733-1

[30] Hanson PE, Gauld ID. Hymenoptera de la región neotropical. Memoirs of the American Entomological Institute. 2006;**77**:994

[31] Saleh AAA, Khedr MMA. Performance of the aphid parasitoid, *Diaeretiella rapae* (M'Intosh) towards certain aphid species in Egypt. Journal of Entomology. 2014;**11**(3):127-141

[32] Gullan PJ, Cranston OS. Insets - fundamentos da Entomologia – 5a Ed. Brasilla: Guanabara Koogan; 2017. 460 p

[33] Saleh AAA. Propagation, Manipulation, Releasing and Evaluation of Aphid Parasitoids in Egypt. Vol. 3. Springer Nature Switzerland AG: AAA. Propagation; 2020. pp. 73-132. DOI: 10.1007/978-3-030-33161-0_3

[34] Gauld I, Bolton B. The Hymenoptera. London: Oxford University Press, Oxford and the Natural History Museum; 1988. p. 332

[35] Jervis M, Kidd N. Insect Natural Enemies, Practical Approaches to their Study and Evaluation. London: Chapman & Hall; 1996. p. 491

[36] Abrahamian PE, Abou-Jawdah Y. Whitefly-transmitted criniviruses of cucurbits: Current status and future prospects. Virus Disease. 2014;**25**(1):26-38

[37] Colazza S, Bin F. Efficiency of *Trissolcus basalis* (hymenoptera: Scelionidae) as an egg parasitoid of *Nezara viridula* (Heteroptera: Pentatomidae) in Central Italy. Environmental Entomology. 1995;**24**(6):1703-1707

[38] El-Husseini MM, Draz KAA, El-Aw MAM, Askar SIS. Some biological and morphological aspects of *Trissolcus basalis* Wollaston (Hymenoptera: Scelionidae) an egg parasitoid of *Nezara viridula* (L.) (Heteroptera: Pentatomidae). Egyptian Journal of Biological Pest Control. 2006;**16**(2):111-114

[39] Gerling D, Mayer RT. *Bemisia*: Taxonomy, Biology, Damage, Control and Management. Andover, Hants, UK: Intercept LTD; 1996. 702 p

[40] Gerling D. Natural enemies of whiteflies: Predators and parasitoids. In: Gerling D, editor. Whiteflies: Their Bionomics. Pest Status and Management. Andover UK: Intercept Ltd; 1990. pp. 147-185

[41] Gerling D, Alomar O, Arno J. Biological control of *Bemisia tabaci* using predators and parasitoids. Crop Protection. 2001;**20**:779-799

[42] Hoddle MS. 1st International Symposium on Biological Control of Arthropods. USA: The Bugwood Network; 2003. pp. 3-16

[43] Cranshaw WS. Green House Whitefly. 2014. Available from: http://www.ext.colostate.edu/pubs/insect/05587.html

[44] Faria M, Wraight SP. Biological control of *Bemisia tabaci* with fungi. Crop Protection. 2001;**20**:767-778

[45] Ali SAM, Saleh AAA, Saleh FM. Biocontrol of certain piercing sucking pests infesting cucumber plants in Egypt. Plant Archives. 2020;**20**(1):3347-3357

[46] Thakur JN, Rawat US, Pawar AD, Sidhu S. Natural enemy complex of the cabbage aphid, *Brevicoryne brassicae* L. (Homoptera: Aphidiidae) in Kull Valley, Himachal Pradesh. Journal of Biological Control. 1989;**3**(1):69

[47] Hafeez M. Seasonal fluctuations of population density of the cabbage aphid *Brevicoryne brassicae* (L.) in the Netherlands and the role of its parasite *Aphidius* (*Diaeretiella*) *rapae* (Curtis). Tijschrift Over Planteziekten, Rehman and Powell. 1961;**309**(67):445-548

[48] Imran B. Biosystematics of Aphid Parasitoids from Punjab Province of Pakistan. Vol. 6. Rawalpindi, Pakistan: Faculty of Crop and Food Sciences Pir Mehr Ali Shah Arid Agriculture University; 2010. p. 206

[49] Dhiman SC. *Diaeretiella rapae* (M'Intosh) (Hymenoptera: Aphidiidae) a potential biocontrol agent of mustard aphid, *Lipaphis erysimi* (Kalt.). Advances in Indian Entomology: Productivity and Health. 2006;**11**:101-109

[50] Hegab Ola IM. Studies on certain insect vectors of plant pathogenic agents [thesis]. Egypt: Faculty of Agriculture, Zagazig University; 2001. 214 p

[51] Kares EA, Ebaid GH, El-Sappagh IA. Biological studies on the larval parasitoid species, *Bracon brevicornis* Wesm. (Hymenoptera: Braconidae), reared on different insect hosts. Egyptian Journal of Biological Pest Control. 2009;**19**(2):165-168

[52] Megahed HEA. Studies on aphids [thesis]. Egypt: Faculty of Agriculture, Zagazig University; 2000. 206 p

[53] Nematollahi MR, Fathipour Y, Talebi AA, Karimzadeh J, Zalucki MP. Parasitoid and hyperparasitoid-mediated seasonal dynamics of the cabbage aphid (Hemiptera: Aphididae). Environmental Entomology. 2014;**43**:1542-1551

[54] Sinha TB, Singh R. Studies on the bionomics of *Trioxys indicus* (Hymenoptera: Aphidiidae): Effect of population densities on sex ratio. Entomophaga 1979. 1979;**24**(3):289-294

[55] Sinha TB, Singh R. Studies on the bionomics of *Trioxys indicus* Subba Rao and Sharma (Hymenoptera: Aphidiidae): A parasitoid of *Aphis craccivora* Koch (Homoptera: Aphidiidae) the area of discovery of parasitoid. Zetschrift fur Angewandte Entomologie. 1980;**89**(2):173-178

[56] Le Ralec A, Ribulé A, Barragan A, Outreman Y. Qutraman host range limitation caused by incomplete host regulation in an aphid parasitoid. Journal of Insect Physiology. 2011;**57**(3):363-371

Chapter 7

From Helminths to *Blastocystis*: Intestinal Parasite Prevalence among Children of Northeast Texas

William Sorensen, Rebecca Swindall, Valerie Smith and Cheryl Cooper

Abstract

Parasitic infections in human populations vary depending on geographical region. Periodic epidemiological study of intestinal parasites informs on shifting infection rates. Soil transmitted helminths (STH) are global parasites that thrive in soil lacking proper sanitation, including contamination by human or animal feces. Prevalence studies of STH in children in East Texas have not been conducted for over 90 years. The goal of this study was to determine current prevalence rates of parasitic infection among children of East Texas. This was a Texas state government funded infectious disease surveillance study. Recruitment included completion of a short questionnaire and distribution of a stool sample kit to caregivers of children, with instructions to return for testing. Recruitment involved a convenience sampling method at health clinics in Cherokee, Gregg, and Smith counties. Of the 481 caregivers recruited, 221 (46%) provided their child's stool sample for testing of parasites. No STH parasites were found. However, we identified 20 children with parasitic protozoa and 1 with a multi-cellular intestinal worms (9.5% overall prevalence). Of the protozoa infections, nearly half (4.1%, n = 9) were infected with *Blastocystis hominis*. *B. hominis* infection was associated with the age of the child infected and the number of children in the household. STH in East Texas has declined over the decades, likely due to sanitation standards and cultural shifts towards sustained sanitation efforts. *B. hominis* may be emerging to fill this gap.

Keywords: intestinal parasites, children, Northeast Texas, screening and surveillance, stool ova, parasite testing

1. Introduction

Intestinal parasites have been in coexistence with human populations since the emergence of humanity. Parasites thrive in the presence of specific host behaviors and environmental conditions, have co-evolved with humans [1, 2], and continue to play a role in shaping the human genome [3]. Recent studies suggest that human traits, behaviors, and even cultural diversity have been linked to our parasitic alliance [2]. The human gut microbiome, a complex ecosystem, affects the entire host organism [4, 5]. Research has shown that homeostasis between the gut microbiota and the rest of the body is crucial for health [4]. For instance, helminths and protozoa have been observed to secrete molecules which may cause alteration in the ecology of gut microbiota influencing biochemical interactions and immune response [4].

1.1 Soil transmitted helminths (STH) prevalence study

STH are common global parasites found in soil that has been contaminated with infected animal and human feces, or at the very least, soil that is not considered "sanitary". Three STHs are often monitored together and are the launching point for this chapter: *Ascaris lumbricoides* (ascaris), *Trichuris trichiura* (whip worm) and either *Necator americanus* or *Ancylostoma duodenale* (hookworm). These three STHs are strictly human parasites and do not thrive in other animal hosts. However, there are many other STHs that share other mammalian hosts; for example, *Strongyloides stercoralis* is gaining prominence in epidemiological studies but will not be a pertinent subject for this chapter [6].

Heavy infestations with the three STHs of interest can result in serious health problems, especially in children. Among these problems are bowel obstruction, resulting from a large bolus of worms (*Ascaris*); nutritional deficiencies, such as iron deficiency anemia resulting in delayed physical and mental development or acute pulmonary reaction (hookworm); severe diarrhea, rectal prolapse, and/or growth retardation (*Trichuris*) [7]. There is also an increased risk of poor health associated with polyparasitism, when more than one species infects a child. For example, Sorensen, et al. [8] found significantly lower hemoglobin levels in Guatemalan children infected with more than one parasite, than those infected with just one parasite, regardless of egg intensity levels.

STHs have been characterized regularly throughout the twentieth century as "tropical diseases" [9], a dangerous precedent and relic from the colonial past since the term "tropical" casts an unconscious bias onto groups of people [10]. STHs have been more recently reperceived and relabeled as "neglected diseases of poverty" (NDP), most likely to reflect the fact that they are reappearing in the United States (U.S.); or they have never left but were never at the forefront of U.S. attention. These types of nuisance diseases were largely ignored while a high-tech "biomedical" approach was, by contrast, forefront in American perception [10].

However, pockets of poverty have always persisted in the U.S. Perhaps the attention was averted until the public health labels of "Social Determinants of Health" or "Disparities" came into wide use in the latter 20th and early 21st centuries, about the same time that the label NDP arose.

Along with this lack of attention to STHs for several decades, a parallel lack of research or surveillance concerning STHs ensued [11]. In Lynn and colleagues' review about this subject they claim that medical attention in the U.S. declined for about 40 years in spite of occasional case reports of STH infection from, the 1980s to the present. On the other hand, Starr et al. [12] reviewed studies from 1940 through 2010 and found sources indicating sporadic STH infection, "...throughout the southern United States and Appalachia as recently as 1982 (p. 680)." During this era, in these regions, hookworm prevalence ranged from 0% to 19.6%; *Trichuris trichiura* ranged from 0.5% to 55.2%; *Ascaris lumbricoides* ranged from 2.3% to 49.4%.

Persons living in poverty in temperate/tropical regions where there is poor sanitation or lack of waste treatment systems, who do not consistently wear shoes, and hands and food such as fruits and vegetables are not frequently washed are most vulnerable to STH infection [7]. Transmission of *Ascaris* and *Trichuris* is fecal-oral. Children are particularly vulnerable to ingesting the parasite eggs from unwashed hands after having contact with the soil. The parasites eventually migrate to the intestine. Unlike *Ascaris* and *Trichuris*, hookworm larvae usually penetrate the skin of the human foot, migrate to the bloodstream, then to the lungs and eventually to the small intestine. Once in the intestine, the adult female will produce many thousands of ova which will then be passed to the soil during host defecation, to continue the transmission cycle.

Hotez [13] describes poverty in the U.S. as unevenly distributed. The northeast Texas region is situated between two of Hotez' poverty hotspots, the border area with Mexico and the Mississippi Delta. He estimates that there are currently about four million cases of ascariasis in Appalachia and the "American South". He describes the Delta region as one with high poverty rates, inadequate housing, and poor health. Hotez cites earlier publications from the 1970's and 80's that indicate Louisiana having some of the highest rates of ascariasis in the U.S. Our study was managed within five northeast Texas counties, a mere three counties, or 120 kilometers from Louisiana. In addition, Hotez notes that STH have been recently detected in Mexican-born migrant workers living in the U.S. Two of the counties involved in our study, Cherokee and Smith, have high rates of migrant workers [14]. Cooper cites *colonia*-like conditions in many migrant farmer households in Cherokee County; that is sub-standard sanitary conditions [14].

Hotez et al. [15] remind us that poverty rates in Texas are greater than in the rest of the U.S. Furthermore, these authors make the argument that due to proximity with Mexico NDP in Texas are likely to be more common than in other parts of the country. They reported that STH are the most common NDPs in Mexico, led by trichuriasis (18 million cases), followed by ascariasis (9 million cases) and hookworm (1 million cases). In 2015, the incidence of ascariasis in Mexico was reported at 39.8 per 100,000 inhabitants [16].

The literature indicates that STH are native to the eastern Texas region and that infections may yet occasionally occur. For historical perspective, in 1932–1933, a researcher from Nacogdoches, Texas conducted a study to identify hookworm ova in the stool of school children in five northeast or central east Texas counties (Angelina, Nacogdoches, Panola, Sabine, and San Augustine). Nearly 1900 children (34%) were found to be infected with hookworm [17]. His report, completed nearly 90 years ago in the pre-antibiotic and pre-childhood-vaccine era, gives some indication of early twentieth century endemic environments.

Recently, we have seen renewed attention to this subject, perhaps brought on by the issues of: 1. Proximity to Mexico or the influx of migrants (globalization), 2. Climate change, 3. Social and Cultural change, and 4. New testing technology. Traditional low-tech diagnosis of STH is made through macroscopic observation of the worms or by microscopic observation of ova in the stool [7]. This is referred to as an ova and parasite (O&P) test.

The 2015 Texas Department of State Health Services (DSHS) data for Health Region 4 of Texas (consisting of 23 counties in the northeast corner of Texas) showed that, of the inhabitants, 15.8% were Hispanic, 65.7% non-Hispanic white and 15.2% non-Hispanic black. This region had a 2015 population of 1,149,721 persons of whom 19.6% were children. Furthermore, 17.4% of people in this region lived in poverty compared to 15.9% of people in Texas lived in poverty and 10.7% of the children in this region had no health insurance compared to 9.5% of children in Texas had no health insurance [18].

This study sought to identify the presence of the three common, multicellular intestinal parasites in the stool samples of northeast Texas children. The research questions were: 1. Is there any indication of STH infection (*Ascaris*, hookworm, or *Trichuris*) in northeast Texas children as evidenced by the presence of microscopic identification of ova or parasites in fecal samples? 2. If there is detection, what are the relative intensities of parasitic infection in these children? 3. If there is evidence of infection, do prevalence rates and intensities differ among demographic groups? 4. If there is evidence of infection, is there evidence of poly-infection (more than one parasite) in individuals?

1.2 *Blastocystis* subsequent analysis

How did *Blastocystis* begin to emerge as interesting for the researchers? Quite simply, we saw *Blastocystis* jump out ahead of other organisms in positive laboratory test counts.

Some studies have identified emerging species of intestinal protozoa, such as *Dientamoeba fragilis* and *B. hominis* as becoming increasingly relevant to global public health efforts and suggest that they may emerge as important gastrointestinal pathogens in the coming years [19].

Blastocystis currently classified as a genus of single-celled, anaerobic, intestinal protists, is defined with distinct structures between mammals and bird organisms compared to all others (ST1-ST17), ST1-ST9 in humans [20]. The most common subtype in humans is ST3, suggesting that this may be transmitted person-to-person (oral-fecal route), whereas the other eight subtypes are suspected of being zoonotic [21]. Prevalence of co-infection with more than one subtype can be as high as 14% and that is likely an underestimate [21].

There are four morphological forms: Vacuolar, granular, amoeboid, and cyst. The cyst is the one manifestation suspected of being the most infectious, when the cyst is found in the colon and ready for expulsion in the feces. *Blastocystis* is often confused with other microorganisms and when it is identified it is mostly in the cyst form [21].

For decades *B. hominis* has been considered a pathogenic human parasite [22, 23]. The Centers for Disease Control and Prevention (CDC) mention on their website that it is up for debate whether it is or it is not a parasite [23]. The debate includes recent studies citing evidence that it is not harmful, but rather a benign part of human micro-fauna [21, 24–26]. Indeed, some articles claim that *Blastocystis* is beneficial to health [27, 28]. Lukes et al. suggest labeling the collection of gut protists "eukaryomes" instead of "parasites", much like the natural collection of gut viruses are called "the virome" and the natural zoo of bacteria, "the microbiome" [27]. This study further sought to assess associations among types of infection and demographic variables.

2. Methods

During the summer of 2017, caregivers of children younger than 18 years of age were recruited, mostly at clinics that cater to the under-insured and underserved populations, in Cherokee, Gregg, Smith, and Upshur Counties, to have their child give a stool sample for testing of parasites. Two of the three clinics specifically served children as clients. The caregivers also filled out a short questionnaire about their children. The laboratory selected to test the stool specimens was a local healthcare laboratory that conducted a standard O&P test. Transportation of specimens from recruiting site to laboratory was organized by the investigators. An element of flexibility was built into the procedure as the study progressed; the possibility to reach out to other collaborators was reserved if needed. If the laboratory revealed a positive test, then doctors and caregivers of infected children were notified of the infection for follow-up treatment purposes. The DSHS funded this study. Institutional Review Board approval was received by a south-central public university (IRB #S2017-66).

Recruiters were crucial to this study. All were trained in public health methods of how to engage caregivers of small children in conversation about risks of intestinal parasites. Then, if the caregiver was interested, recruiters led the caregivers through the informed consent process and completion of the questionnaire. Next, recruiters educated them on how to collect a stool sample and informed them when to return the sample for laboratory delivery. If caregivers did not return the specimen within 24 hours, recruiters reached out to offer assistance or answer any questions. Further, a team of recruiters were selected to design their own nested study to recruit caregivers and stool specimens in rural areas and then transport to the laboratory. In order to transport the specimens the recruiters obtained a separate State-of-Texas training.

Study managers and recruiters were encouraged to text each other on their password-protected smart phones from the onset of the study. The research team texted each other to ask and respond to borrowing supplies if one site was low on an item to temporarily transport and restock supplies. In addition, recruiters texted summaries of their workday to management at the end of every day. Further, group texts were sent every evening to all recruiters with a summary of how many total stool kits were distributed, at what site, and how many stool specimens were noted as transported to the laboratory for testing.

The backbone of the research team were the recruiters with a State-of-Texas Certified Health Worker (CHW) credential. These CHWs understood the health issues involved and ensured the study was of high quality. In general, the CHW recruiters were assigned times to work in clinics, but also were given permission to conduct recruitment in the rural sites, at their own convenience. Other recruiters were university graduate students in the healthcare or public health field.

All recruiters were trained in motivational interviewing and informed consent techniques. They had to complete a university-required online ethics training course in order to proceed in the study. Ten different recruiters cycled through this study.

The program's field activities began 8 May 2017, and were completed in little over three months. The last day of collection activities was 14 August 2017. Activities were concentrated in clinics, then as the study progressed it expanded into non-clinical settings. The clinics were in Gregg and Smith counties; the rural sites included Cherokee, Rusk, and Upshur Counties. The total expected stool testing count was 440.

Next, laboratory and questionnaire data from the original STH prevalence study was reanalyzed with *B. hominis* classified separately from other organisms to enable a more detailed investigation for associations among specific demographic, health, and environmental variables. Statistical methods, including Kruskal-Wallis and Fisher's exact tests, were applied to identify significant differences among groups. While we report on significant findings or findings that trend towards significance, they should be interpreted with caution due to limited sample size. Analysis was performed with Stata v. 16.1 (College Station, Texas).

3. Results

Table 1 shows the breakdown by week and site of the actual number of stool kits distributed to recruited caregivers. That number is also the number of questionnaires completed and returned. The pattern from **Table 1** shows progression moving from one site to another. The pattern helps explain decisions made regarding personnel and sites. The last column, "Non-clinic", shows progression involving add-on sites. As the study progressed it expanded into non-clinical settings, however, only 71 of 481 (14.8%) were non-clinical sites.

Based on questionnaires completed and lab results matched to them, caregivers of 481 children were recruited through this study. This exceeded expectations by 9.3% (481 vs. 440). Stool testing was a different matter. Early in the study it was recognized that actual stool tests would fall short of recruitment efforts. Yet it is difficult to pin down a "standard" return rate for stool testing. One study done in adult refugees with O&P testing mention a return rate of 89.5% [29]. On the other hand, a stool test for fecal blood (cancer screening) revealed a response rate of 43.4% [30]. A recent study done in Texas showed only a 10.6% stool return rate [31].

These data showed that 221 stool specimens (46%) were returned for laboratory testing, with 165 laboratory results performed and received (34.3%), see **Table 2**. This "low-to-moderate" testing rate is due to various reasons: 1. At clinic Z only 1 of the 45 samples submitted for testing had the test performed; 2. Not all specimens were tested due to improper labeling; 3. Some specimens were thrown away due to time

	Clinic X	Clinic Y	Clinic Z	Non-clinic	Total
Week 1	28	0	0	0	28
Week 2	19	0	0	0	19
Week 3	38	4	0	0	42
Week 4	22	0	0	5	27
Week 5	20	4	0	2	26
Week 6	28	13	0	10	51
Week 7	33	11	0	2	46
Week 8	21	8	0	0	29
Week 9	0	4	0	0	4
Week 10	0	12	0	18	30
Week 11	0	2	8	8	18
Week 12	0	5	30	15	50
Week 13	0	10	39	4	53
Week 14	0	12	27	7	46
Week 15	0	12	0	0	12
Total	209	97	104	71	481

Clinic X: Smith County, non-profit private.
Clinic Y: Gregg County, public.
Clinic Z: Gregg County, non-profit private.

Table 1.
Tallies of stool kits distributed by facilities or sites, by week.

N (%)	All	Clinic X	Clinic Y	Clinic Z	Non-clinic
Collected (N-481)					
No	260 (54.1)	119 (45.8)	55 (21.2)	59 (22.7)	27 (10.4)
Yes	221 (46)	90 (40.7)	42 (19)	45 (20.4)	44 (19.9)
Tested (N-481)					
No	260 (54.1)	119 (45.8)	55 (21.2)	59 (22.7)	27 (10.4)
Yes	165(34.3)	85 (51.5)	40 (24.2)	1 (0.6)	39 (23.6)
Not tested	56 (11.6)	5 (8.9)	2 (3.6)	44 (78.6)	5 (8.9)
Pathogenic result (N-165)					
Negative	149 (90.3)	74 (49.6)	38 (26.4)	0 (0)	35 (89.7)
Positive	16 (9.7)	11 (68.8)	1 (6.3)	1 (6.3)	3 (18.8)
Infection type (N-16)					
Blastocystis hominis	9 (56.3)	6	0	0	3
Dientamoeba fragilis	5 (31.3)	4	1	0	0
Giardia lamblia	1 (6.3)	0	0	1	0
Enterobius vermicularis	1 (6.3)	1	0	0	0
Parasite Load					
None	460 (96.6)	195 (42.4)	95 (20.7)	103 (22.4)	67 (14.6)
Rare	6 (1.3)	5 (83.3))	0 (0)	1 (16.7)	0 (0)
Few	10 (2.1)	7 (70)	2 (20)	0 (0)	1 (1.4)
Moderate	4 (0.8)	2 (50)	0 (0)	0 (0)	2 (50)
Abundant	1 (0.2)	0 (0)	0 (0)	0 (0)	1 (1.4)
Poly-infection	1 (0.2)	1 (100)	0 (0)	0 (0)	0 (0)

Table 2.
Results of stool sample results by site specimen received.

expiration; 4. Nine laboratory results were received that did not match up with any questionnaire information (these 9 are not included in further data description or analysis). In terms of stool testing, this study fell short of expectations by about 50%. Interestingly, there was a higher proportion of stool samples returned among study participants contacted outside clinics compared to those contacted through a clinic, 62% vs. an average of 43% per clinic (Fishers Exact: p = 0.03).

Table 2 further details the 165 stool specimens tested, where 21 (12.7%) were positive, and 16 were pathogenic parasites (9.7%). Clinic X carried the bulk of positive pathogenic stool samples (68.8%, n = 11), non-Clinic with 18.8% (n = 3), and Clinic Y and Clinic Z both with 6.3% (n = 1). No STHs were detected; the identified parasites were mostly microorganisms: 9 with *Blastocystis* (56.3%), 5 with *Dientamoeba fragilis* (31.3%), 1 with *Giardia lamblia* (6.3%), and 1 with a common helminth *Enterobius vermicularis* (6.3%). All children testing positive for these parasites were referred for medical evaluation. **Figure 1** shows these counts graphically. There was no difference found in viral load between clinics or type of infection and only one poly infection was identified: *Endolimax* cysts and *Entamoeba coli* cysts.

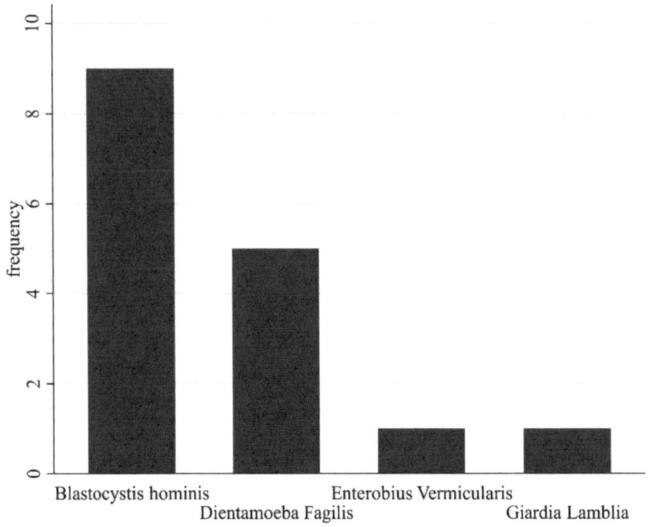

Figure 1.
Counts of intestinal pathogens discovered by the study.

Table 3 presents survey results among all caregivers surveyed and reports results of bivariate analysis comparing children with a positive or negative stool specimen. The median age of all children surveyed was 5 years (range 1–16). Of note, over half of the children were Hispanic, which corresponded with a higher proportion of caregivers reporting Spanish as their predominant language. No significant differences were observed between children with positive versus negative stool specimens. However, among racial/ethnic groups, a higher proportion of Asian children tested positive for parasites, 6.3% compared to 1.4%. Additionally, caregiver-reported assessments of child health, ranging from excellent to poor, as well as the number of days per week their child spends outdoors both, showed a trend towards statistical significance ($p = 0.08$ for each variable).

Anecdotal information from Clinic X's medical director included the observation that of the children infected, most do not show symptoms. In addition, the study uncovered evidence that the response rate (stool testing since initial enrollment) increased in more rural, community-based non-clinic sites. The rate of sampling return was about double in rural settings than urban clinic settings. Overall, the response rate improved, month to month. As to effectiveness of laboratory testing, we found that the rate of parasite detection is almost 3X greater in urban clinics than in rural settings.

Analysis of the 165 children who had stool results demonstrated significant differences in household size, child's age, and racial distribution across three stool sample result groups (negative/non-pathogenic, *B. hominis*, and other pathogenic). Children in households with *B. hominis* lived in households with a median of 4 children (range 2–5), compared to a median of 3 (range 0–7) for those children with a negative or non-pathogenic result and 3 (range 2–3) for children with other pathogenic infection ($p = 0.04$; **Table 4**). **Figure 2** demonstrates household size distribution by infection status, where the largest households are more likely to yield *B. hominis* infection. Additionally, children with *B. hominis* were younger (median age 3 years, range 1 to 8) compared to those in the negative/non-pathogenic and other pathogenic infection groups (6 years [1 to 15]

	All N = 481	Negative N = 149	Positive N = 16	p-value
Number of children in house[a]	3 (2–3)	3 (0–7)	3 (2–5)	0.12
Age of child in years[a]	5 (1–16)	6 (1–15)	5 (1–10)	0.29
Race/Ethnicity[b]				0.42
White-non Hispanic	117 (24.8)	46 (31.2)	3 (18.8)	
Hispanic	245 (51.9)	66 (44.6)	8(50)	
Black-non Hispanic	93 (19.7)	29 (19.6)	4 (25)	
Asian	5 (1.1)	2 (1.4)	1 (6.3)	
Multi-racial	12 (2.5)	5 (3.4)	0 (0)	
Language spoken at home[b]				0.28
English	264 (55.7)	89 (61.8)	8 (50)	
Spanish	121 (25.5)	33 (22.9)	6 (37.5)	
Both English and Spanish	83 (17.5)	19 (13.2)	1 (6.3)	
Other	6 (1.3)	2 (2.1)	1 (6.3)	
Child's health, over past year[b]				0.08
Excellent	188 (39.4)	65 (43.6)	5 (31.3)	
Good	235 (49.3)	68 (45.6)	7 (43.8)	
Fair	52 (10.9)	16 (10.7)	3 (18.8)	
Poor	2 (0.4)	0 (0)	1 (6.3)	
Days since last illness	142 (52–269)	154 (52–365)	141 (23–249)	0.53
Ever worms in child's poop[b]	11 (2.3)	4 (2.7)	0 (0)	
Attend daycare[c]	76 (18.5)	19 (15.5)	2 (16.7)	0.59
Days child outside, per week[c]	5 (3–7)	6 (4–7)	5 (3–6)	0.08
Child wears shoes outside[b]				0.95
Yes, always	229 (48.2)	73 (49.3)	9 (56.3)	
Yes, usually	124 (26.1)	29 (19.6)	3 (18.8)	
Yes, half-the-time	111 (23.4)	44 (29.7)	4 (25.0)	
No-usually not	11 (2.3)	2 (1.4)	0 (0)	
Handles animals[b]	319 (71.1)	100 (73)	9 (69.2)	0.50
Pets or animals child handles				
Dog[b]	266 (59.2)	78 (56.9)	8 (61.5)	0.49
Cat[b]	120 (26.7)	47 (34.3)	3 (23.1)	0.31
Horse[b]	22 (4.9)	7 (5.1)	0 (0)	0.52
Rabbit[b]	9 (2)	4 (2.9)	1 (7.7)	0.37
Chicken[b]	4 (0.9)	4 (2.9)	0 (0)	0.69
Water source[b]				1.00
City water – piped in	397 (87.6)	129 (90.9)	14 (93.3)	
Private – well/pump	18 (3.97)	3 (2.1)	0 (0)	

	All N = 481	Negative N = 149	Positive N = 16	p-value
Stream/River/Lake	5 (1.1)	2 (1.4)	0 (0)	
Filtered/Bottled	33 (7.3)	8 (5.6)	1 (6.7)	
Toilet source[b]				0.90
Inside flush toilet	438 (98.7)	136 (99.3)	14 (100)	
Inside no flush toilet	4 (0.9)	1 (0.7)	0 (0)	
Outside toilet	2 (0.5)	0 (0)	0 (0)	
Septic tank[b]				0.27
Yes	167 (37.4)	57 (40.4)	4 (26.7)	
No	268 (60.1)	81 (57.5)	10 (66.7)	
No-not connected	11 (2.4)	3 (2.0)	1 (6.7)	

[a]*Median (Range)/Kruskal Wallis.*
[b]*Number (%)/Fishers Exact.*
[c]*Median (Inter Quartile Range)/Kruskal Wallis.*

Table 3.
Questionnaire results among 481 participants surveyed, and bivariate analysis among 165 children with negative or positive stool specimens.

	Negative/ Non-pathogenic N = 151	*Blastocystis hominis* N = 9	Other pathogenic N = 5	p-value
Children in house[a]	3 (0–7)	4 (2–5)	3 (2–5)	0.04
Age of child in years[a]	6 (1–15)	3 (1–8)	8 (4–10)	0.04
Race/Ethnicity[b]				0.05
White-non Hispanic	47 (31.3)	2 (22.2)	0 (0)	
Hispanic	69 (46)	3 (33.3)	2 (40)	
Black-non Hispanic	28 (18.7)	3 (33.3)	1 (20)	
Asian	1 (0.7)	1 (11.1)	1 (20)	
Multi-racial	5 (3.3)	0 (0)	0 (0)	
Health, over past year[b]				0.39
Excellent	65 (43.1)	3 (33.3)	2 (40)	
Good	69 (45.7)	3 (33.3)	3 (60)	
Fair	16 (10.6)	3 (33.3)	0 (0)	
Poor	1 (0.7)	0 (0)	0 (0)	
Report of illness	104 (68.9)	7 (77.8)	1 (20)	0.07
Handles animals[b]	104 (74.3)	4 (66.7)	1 (25)	0.09

[a]*Median (Range)/Kruskal Wallis.*
[b]*Number (%)/Fishers Exact.*

Table 4.
Comparison among 165 children by stool sample result negative/non-pathogenic, Blastocystis hominis, *or other pathogenic infection.*

DOI: http://dx.doi.org/10.5772/intechopen.1008962

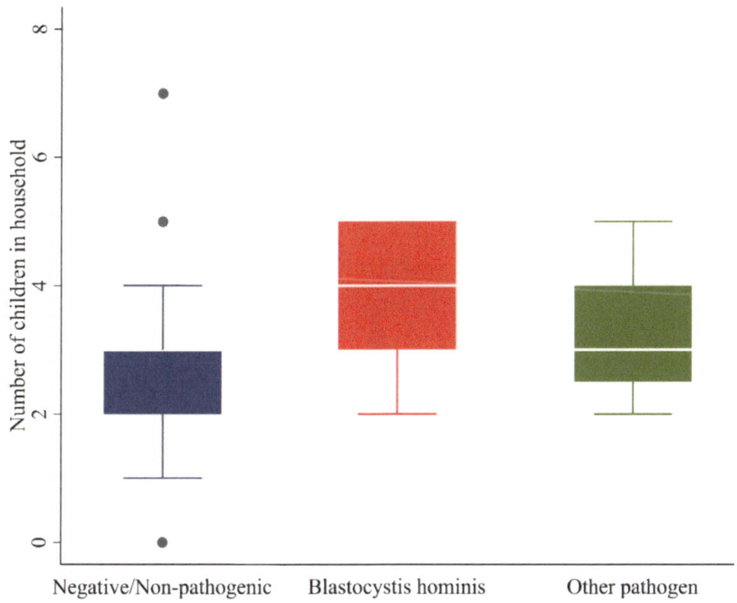

Figure 2.
Infection status by number of children in household.

and 8 years [4 to 10], respectively; p = 0.04). The oldest children were more likely to be infected with another pathogen. **Figure 3** demonstrates median age by infection status.

B. hominis was most prevalent among Black non-Hispanic (33.3%) and Hispanic children (33.3%). Comparing each infection group, Hispanics also had the most negative/non-pathogenic children (46%) and other pathogenic positive samples (40%), undoubtably due to the high proportion of Hispanic study participants. **Figure 4**

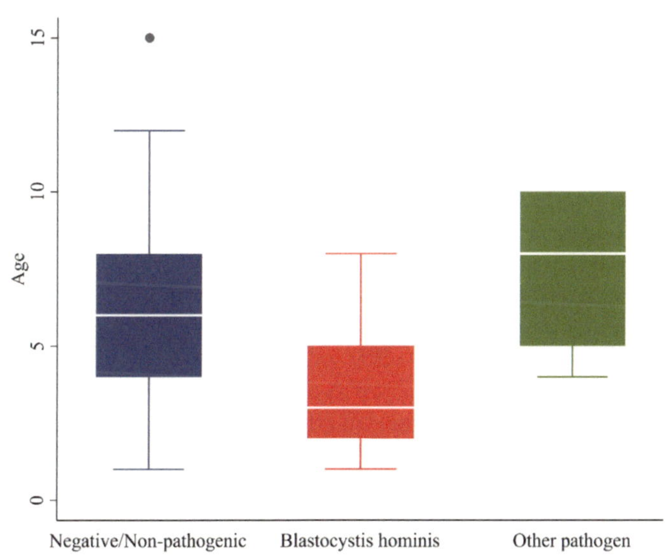

Figure 3.
Infection status by age.

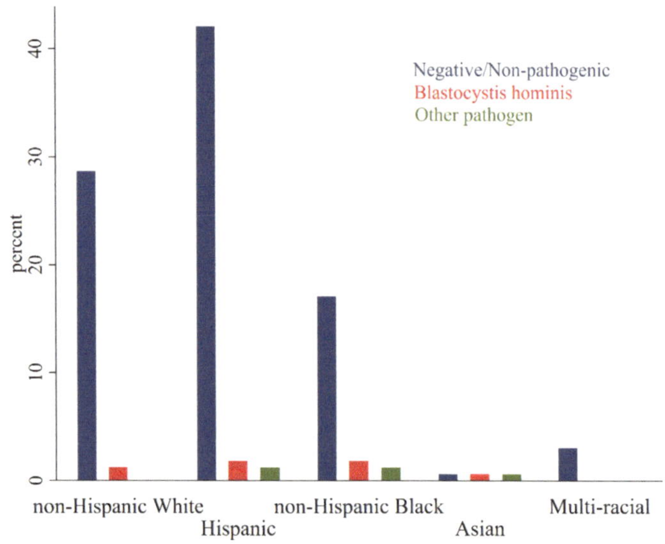

Figure 4.
Infection status by race/ethnicity.

shows the different proportions of infection status by racial/ethnic groups. Caregiver report of child's health over the past year did not differ between infection status groups (**Table 4**). However, a caregiver report of illness in the past year was more frequent in the *B. hominis* group (77.8%) compared to the negative/non-pathogenic group (68.9%) and the other pathogenic group (20%). Animal handling was less common among children in the other pathogenic group (25%) compared to the *B. hominis* group (66.7%) and negative/non-pathogenic group. However, illness report and animal handling did not reach statistical significance, $p = 0.07$ and $p = 0.09$, respectively. See **Table 4**.

4. Discussion

The aim of this study was to investigate the prevalence of three STHs in children living in northeast Texas. The study questions were: 1. Is there any indication of STH infection (*Ascaris*, hookworm, or *Trichuris*) in northeast Texas children as evidenced by the presence of microscopic identification of ova in fecal samples? Answer: There is no indication of STH in this population. 2. If there is detection, what are the relative intensities of parasitic infection in these children? Answer: This is a moot point, there was no detection of STH. 3. If there is evidence of STH infection, do prevalence rates and intensities differ among demographic groups? Answer: If strictly STH infection, again, we cannot answer this. But looking at only *Blastocystis* infection it is apparent that age is significantly related to infection (the younger the child the more likely to be infected), and number of children in the household is also a significant factor (the more children the more likely to be infected). 4. If there is evidence of STH infection, is there evidence of poly-infection (more than one parasite) in individuals? Answer: Again, there was no detection of STH.

However, we did find other organisms. We identified 21 children with parasitic protozoa (9.5%): Of those, 9 children were infected with *B. hominis* (4.1%) and 7 children with other pathogenic protozoa (*Dientamoeba fragilis*, *Giardia lamblia*, or *Enterobius vermicularis*- 3.2%). Another 5 children were identified with non-pathogenic protozoa (2.3%).

4.1 Recent epidemiologic/soil studies for comparison

Since 2017, when we accomplished our study, new research in the U.S. has emerged. Particularly interesting is research using new testing technology. *En masse* DNA detection arose over the last decade through quantitative polymerase chain reaction (qPCR) testing [32], whereby several organisms can be detected simultaneously. We summarize three studies, below, two of which were done in either disadvantaged populations or in areas considered low social-economic status (SES). The two studies test people; the third study reports on soil testing.

First, a 2017 study in Alabama tested stool from a small rural community of 66 African American individuals: 34.5% were positive for hookworm, 7.3% for *Strongyloides stercoralis* and 1.8% for *Entamoeba histolytica*. No whipworm or Ascaris. This community showed high rates of raw sewage in the home (>50%) [33]. Of interest is the high hookworm identification, but no whipworm or *Ascaris*, as these three STH often are found together. Nor was any *Blastocystis* detected, which is prevalent throughout the South U.S. The stool test utilized was qPCR.

Second, a 2020 investigation in a depressed Texas community, also used qPCR. Even though this central-Texas community was peri-urban there was no municipal service for electricity or water. There were many reports of stray dogs in this community; also, 44% of the households reported signs of septic system failure. The researchers found a 16.5% sero-prevalence of *Strongyloides stercoralis*. From stool testing they found that 62.8% of the subjects were positive for *Blastocystis* spp., and 2.3% for *Giardia lamblia* [31]. Here it is interesting to note that the STH *Strongyloides* was not detected from stool but from serum antibodies, indicating infection from possibly many years in the past. The authors of this study highlight that there was little evidence of people migrating in or out of the area. These researchers associated the high *Blastocystis* prevalence to the poor sanitation situation in the area.

And thirdly, we outline a geographically large-ranging soil study from 2024, which sampled about 500 soil samples across 37 sites, located among five communities in the U.S. South, also using qPCR. Blackburn and colleagues mentioned that *Blastocystis* spp. was revealed in 19.0% of soil samples, indicating unsanitary conditions for humans. In addition, they found evidence of two of the three major STHs in soil (*Trichuris* at 1.8%, hookworm at 0.4% of soil samples). Strangely, *Ascaris* was not detected. By community, contamination rates were very different with southwestern Alabama showing the most contamination (39.6%) and southern Texas showing the least (6.9%). The authors concluded that the DNA burden of parasites were highest in communities with the highest poverty rates [32].

Our study found no STH and a 4.1% prevalence of *Blastocystis hominis*, and 0.5% *Giardia lamblia*, in Northeast Texas children, highlighting a decline in STH, yet lingering concern due to parasitic protists.

4.2 *Blastocystis*: Profiles and challenges

During our initial epidemiological survey, the primary focus was on identifying STHs and derive a prevalence figure among an East Texas population. However, no helminths were detected. On the other hand, there was a higher prevalence of

Blastocystis than any other infectious agent. The identification of *Blastocystis* led to a shift in the study's focus, offering potential new insights into *Blastocystis*, which has a controversial interface with humans. There is a debate whether this organism a pathogenic, beneficial, or commensal agent. We offer new data, opening avenues for future investigation into *Blastocystis*'s epidemiological and clinical significance.

The next few paragraphs cite research that underlies the harmful vs. beneficial debate dealing with *Blastocystis*. Wawrzyniak and colleagues [21] mention that the *Blastocystis* protist has been implicated in irritable bowel syndrome (IBS), cutaneous lesions, and various clinical gastrointestinal symptoms. In Argentina, *Blastocystis* has been associated with poor skin conditions [26]. On the other hand, Lukes et al. [27] claim that *Blastocystis* never seems to migrate out of the gut, as do micro-pathogens which cause lesions, abscesses and inflammation along the way. Rather, it seems to colonize the gut and retain homeostasis. According to Tito et al., ST3 is the most prevalent subtype in individuals with or without IBS [28]; ST4 seems to be prevalent in only asymptomatic individuals. However, [26] and [21] cite evidence to the contrary, mentioning that there is a high prevalence of ST4 also in ill individuals. Wawrzyniak and colleagues [21] mention that the *Blastocystis* protist has been implicated in irritable bowel syndrome (IBS), cutaneous lesions, and various clinical gastrointestinal symptoms. In Argentina, *Blastocystis* has been associated with poor skin conditions [26]. On the other hand, Lukes et al. [27] claim that *Blastocystis* never seems to migrate out of the gut, as do other micro-pathogens which cause lesions, abscesses and inflammation along the way. Rather, it seems to colonize the gut and retain homeostasis. According to Tito et al., ST3 is the most prevalent subtype in individuals with or without IBS; ST4 seems to be prevalent in only asymptomatic individuals [26]. However, there is evidence to the contrary which show high rates of ST4 also in ill individuals [26].

In a recent study with Colombian children, *B. hominis* manifested in 12.6% of their stool. Of those, ST3 was the most prevalent subtype. In addition, of those infected with *B. hominis* nearly three fourths (71.9%) were asymptomatic, and the only significant co-infection with *B. hominis* was *Endolimax nana*, a benign gut protozoan [26]. A tilt in gut acidity or alkalinity may nudge the *B. hominis* microbe from a neutral state to a harmful state [26].In a recent study with Colombian children, *B. hominis* manifested in 12.6% of them. Of those, ST3 was the most prevalent subtype. In addition, of those children infected with *B. hominis* nearly three fourths (71.9%) were asymptomatic, and the only significant co-infection with *B. hominis* was *Endolimax nana*, a benign gut protozoan [26]. A tilt in gut acidity or alkalinity may nudge the *B. hominis* microbe from a neutral state to a harmful state [26].

Ciesielski et al. calls *B. hominis* a "nonpathogen (27); p. 1260)." Our study, presented in this chapter, sides with *B. hominis* being pathogenic (marginal association with caregivers reports of their child's illness). Ciesielski et al. calls *B. hominis* a "nonpathogen [24]; p. 1260)." Our study, presented in this chapter, sides with *B. hominis* being pathogenic (we show a marginal association with caregivers' reports of their child's illness).

These next three paragraphs discuss other patterns of *Blastocystis*. High risk populations include those with close contact to animals, those in SES-depressed areas (lowered hygiene), particularly among children in these areas, and immunocompromised individuals [21]. In a Texas study, 62.8% of the subjects were positive for *B. hominis* infection in a low-income community, but the same stool test failed to find any STH [31].

In a different stool survey with Texas children, Escobedo et al. [25] found *B. hominis* prevalence at 13.2%. Compared to other gut-parasites, *B. hominis* was more prevalence by a factor of 4-to-1. The high prevalence is confirmed by Amin [22] who showed that of all stool specimens tested, 23% were positive for *B. hominis*, and of those with any parasite detected, *B. hominis* was detected at a ratio of 3-to-1 over every other intestinal infection caused by an identifiable agent. Yet data from Ciesielski et al. [24] show that, in high risk adults, that relationship is inverse. Amin speculated that *B. hominis* prevalence is increasing in the U.S [22]. In a different stool survey with Texas children, Escobedo et al. [25] found *B. hominis* prevalence at 13.2%. Compared to other gut-parasites, *B. hominis* was more prevalent by a factor of 4-to-1. The high prevalence is confirmed by Amin [22] who showed that of all stool specimens tested, 23% were positive for *B. hominis*, and of those with any parasite detected, *B. hominis* was detected at a ratio of 3-to-1 over every other intestinal infection caused by an identifiable agent. Yet data from Ciesielski et al. [24] show that, in high risk adults, that relationship is inverse. Amin speculated that *B. hominis* prevalence is increasing in the U.S [22].

Ramirez et al., [26] found no demographic variable associated with *B. hominis* infection in children. We contradict this from our study that in showing that age is a significant predictor in distinguishing *B. hominis* from other pathogens, that is, the younger one is, the more likely one will contract *B. hominis* (the age gradient supports the studies described above). Furthermore, polyparasitism was rare in our study, which is consistent with other studies showing *B. hominis* seemingly "crowding out" other parasitic pathogens.

4.3 Speculation about possible determinants

In the Introduction section we listed four concerns that may significantly impact current intestinal parasite infection, or the reporting thereof. These next paragraphs summarize our outlook on 1. Migration, 2. Climate change, 3. Social and cultural influence, and 4. Testing techniques.

The next four paragraphs deal with the topic of migration. We found 9.5% overall prevalence from our children's study; 4.1% were infected with *B. hominis* alone. Compared to Mexico, however, current prevalence figures with STH in Texas seem diminutive [16]. Gutierrez-Jimenez et al. cited children's studies conducted within Mexico, showing protist prevalence [16]. One study done in Guadalajara children shows a prevalence of *Giardia lamblia* at 1.2% and *B. hominis* at 0.9%. In Merida, another study shows *B. hominis* prevalence at 10.5% and *G. lamblia* at 7.6%, again in children [16].

Concerning migrants or refugees, three decades ago Ciesielski et al. [24] reported a 1.1% prevalence for *Ascaris*, 5.7% to 7.2% for *Trichuris*, 5.7% to 8.8% for hookworm, and 0.6% to 1.1% for *B. hominis*, in North Carolina migrant farmworkers.

Two studies dealing with refugees to the U.S., one a review, return a complicated picture because of the many countries involved, and the required health screenings refugees take, both before travel and after passage to the U.S. A study with refugees in California, from 2013, found relatively small proportions of intestinal parasite infection (0.0% prevalence for *Ascaris*, 0.2% for *Trichuris*, 1.1% for hookworm, and 1.1% for *B. hominis*) [29]. Interestingly they found, also, a marginal trend for increasing STH prevalence with increasing age of the subject, and for protists to decrease in proportion with increasing age. We concur with this last observation in dealing with *B. hominis*: we found that the youngest children were more likely to be infected with *B. hominis*. Lastly, a review of refugee studies, by Smith Darr et al. [34] is more alarmist in tone as they summarize intestinal parasite prevalences from 9 to 19%

in refugees to the U.S.; unfortunately, they were not more specific than this. They did, however, mention that *Giardia lamblia* was the most frequent parasite found in refugees to the U.S.

We see no reason to believe that migrants and refugees are allowing an influx of intestinal parasites to enter the U.S. Thus, the indigenous Texas infection rate of both STHs and protists seems to be as high as anything seen in mobile populations. However, it appears that STH prevalence in Texas is decreasing over time while protist prevalence may be increasing.

The next three paragraphs are about earth's changing climate and parasites. Climate change poses a different challenge in thinking through intestinal parasite ecology, often because the consequences are complex and the ability to predict future outcomes are uncertain. Blum et al. [35] attempt to predict what would happen to STHs in the face of what we know about climate change. In general, they write, there will be an increase in parasite infectivity rates. More specifically, hookworms are mentioned as species that will benefit the most. In Africa, hookworms could very well emerge as a dominant STH, because of their tolerance for higher temperatures. In Asia, ascariasis will thrive in more arid areas. These authors were not conclusive about scenarios involving the U.S.

On the contrary, Chammartin et al. show that STH prevalence is decreasing in South America, since 2005, in spite of climate change [36].

A review paper by Weaver et al. [37] tried to draw conclusions with STH and climate change; Javanmard et al. [38] do the same with *Blastocystis*. Both of these articles argue that there definitely will be epidemiologic changes by climate change, impinging on STH and *Blastocystis* infection, because of sensitive feedback loops. Neither team, however, could conclude what these changes may be. But what is salient is that both research teams claim that the changing social conditions of humans are more important in determining intestinal parasite epidemiology than changing environment. For example, according to Weaver et al., we can expect climate change to drive low SES levels to even lower levels, which may increase STH prevalence [37]. Whether this is a pertinent conclusion for U.S. citizens remains doubtful.

The next four paragraphs mention cultural change. Rapid cultural change, accompanied by shifts in human behavior, offer another layer of complexity when discussing humans and their relationship with parasites. Cultural change in this context includes lifestyle and environmental changes. These changes include reduced exposure to soil and animals, changes in diet, and increased exposure to pollutants and antibiotics [39], disrupting the structure of ecosystems through roadways, water systems, deforestation, human settlements, and commercial development [2, 40].

As mentioned previously, cultural behaviors taking place across different geographic regions directly affect the epidemiology of parasitic infection in human populations [40, 41]. The hygiene hypothesis involves the understanding that as we exist in increasingly hygienic environments we decrease our exposure to microbes that lead to an overactive immune system [42, 43]. As expected, high-income countries with improved sanitation, food sterilization, and usage of antibiotics have lower microbiota diversity. Researchers have found that this reduced microbiota diversity correlates with a lower incidence of parasite infections and a higher prevalence of autoimmune disorders [5, 39]. Advancements in the medical field have led to efforts to eradicate parasitic infections with little understanding of how these shifts in microbiota populations will affect our gut microbiome overall. A massive 1995 deworming program in school-age children in Mexico, for example, resulted in immediate shifts in the composition of the microbiota, including an increased infection of *B. hominis* [4]. Emerging evidence suggests several non-bacterial organisms, including protozoa and helminths, may act as commensals or even provide immunologic benefit [5]. *B. hominis* has been found to cause illness in some individuals, while others remain asymptomatic. Asymptomatic individuals carrying *B. hominis* have been found to have a more diverse microbiota compared to their symptomatic counterparts [4].

Our data show that younger children are more likely to become infected with *B. hominis* than other children. Our data also show more infection in families with more children. Family-size may be influenced culturally according to social norms. In addition, the tension between family resources and family-size amplifies a feedback loop with larger families facing challenging deficits and shortages, exacerbating lack of prevention.

The mounting evidence involving the role that the microbiome places in clinical manifestation [5] underscores the importance of continued exploration into how parasites influence humans. Understanding of infection patterns and their effect on the human body may be utilized in order to correctly assess modern health problems [2].

This last paragraph closes the Discussion section in briefly mentioning testing techniques. We found in our study a 9.5% overall prevalence of intestinal parasites and a 4.1% prevalence of mere *Blastocystis* infection. These are certainly underreported figures since 1. O&P tests are less sensitive than more advanced technology testing [7, 38]. And, 2. Only one fecal sample was submitted per child for testing, whereas with O&P it is recommended to submit more than one sample. On the other hand, what we did find is within the prevalence range of several other studies we have summarized in this chapter.

4.4 Limitations, strengths, recommendations

In our Texas study, recruiting efforts reached 481 caregivers, an excess of the established goal.

We saw a positive trend in stool return rates as the study continued, from 25.3% (mid-June 2017) to 31.3% (mid-July), to the last month of the study (mid-August) of 43.9%. This indicates that it takes a few months for improved study efficiency and messaging from recruiters to caregivers. Furthermore, the response rate increased once we left behind urban clinic sites and moved into the rural areas, with individualized collection plans, devised by the CHW.

In collecting stool specimens, we achieved about half of the expected goal. There is a poor "response" rate even when the caregiver is recruited in-person, educated, and given a cash incentive. That rate appears to hover around 25–45%. This should not have surprised us considering the "ick" factor associated with handling stool, the busy lives of caregivers, and perhaps caregivers' denial of susceptibility or mistrust in services [44]. In addition, it is harder to recruit caregivers in rural settings, or caregivers of ethnic minorities. Other studies also suffer from difficulty in obtaining stool specimens [30, 33].

Our results show that, of 221 stool specimens returned to the laboratory, 41 were recorded as inappropriate or incomplete because of improper collection (18.6%). In some cases collection timing was not utilized properly, in other cases laboratory requisition forms were not filled out properly. This subset of error indicates that caregivers were either not properly educated in stool collection techniques or, if they were, caregivers did not pay sufficient attention. Furthermore, 9 laboratory results were received by this study that did not match with any questionnaire information.

The survey questions were designed to capture possible associations between transmission factors and parasitic infections. Two specific and important questions the study failed to assess, however, were sex of the child and travel history. In addition, better probing of children's symptoms could have been worked out on the questionnaire. The sample size of infected children was small enough (n = 16) to hamstring data analysis conclusions due to a lack in statistical power. Recruitment was not randomized, leading to likely bias.

Moreover, the calendar induced a natural break in activities and consequent loss of potential participants and laboratory specimens, during entire weeks surrounding a summer national holiday. On top of this, many families traveled over the summer months since children are traditionally out of school.

Lasty, like the Escobedo study [25], our limitations include a probable undercount of intestinal parasites since only one stool was collected per child, and a standard microscopy test was used without fluorescence methods or staining for acid-fast organisms. McKenna et al. [33] mention that the O&P microscopy test is only 50–85% sensitive. On the other hand, Ramirez et al. [45] agree that a test like PCR is more sensitive, but by only 3.3% (that is, O&P "...microscopy was sensitive enough... [p. 8/13]").

We recommend for future studies to include a ramp up period of two weeks, whereby training and administrative connections are secured before recruiting starts. On top of this, include a pilot period of one week of actual recruiting but with special attention to recruiting feedback. Rural areas need more attention from management and more lines of support should be built into this component of future programs. Further investigation concerning why caregivers who were recruited but did not volunteer their children's stool is merited. This could be done through focus groups. Lastly, further investigation into the children's health status should be considered. Travel history, allergy status and other symptoms could be better gleaned to uncover new information or check reliability of laboratory testing.

5. Conclusion

The aim of this study was to investigate the prevalence of three STHs in children living in northeast Texas. The study questions were mostly not answered because no evidence of STH was found. However, we did find other organisms. We identified 21 children with parasitic protozoa (9.5%): Of those, 9 children were infected with *B. hominis* (4.1%) and 7 children with other pathogenic protozoa (*Dientamoeba fragilis*, *Giardia lamblia*, or *Enterobius vermicularis*- 3.2%). Another 5 children were identified with non-pathogenic protozoa (2.3%).

Looking at only *Blastocystis* infection it is apparent that age is significantly related to infection (the younger the more likely to be infected), and number of children in the household is also a significant factor (the more children the more likely to be infected).

There seems to be a real decline in STHs in this area, over the course of several decades. We speculate that widespread and sustained sanitation piques this decline. We conjecture that *Blastocystis* is filling this gap.

Acknowledgements

We would like to thank the Texas Department of State Health Services in Austin for this opportunity, and the personnel at three wonderful clinics in our area: St.

Paul's Children's Clinic in Tyler Texas, the DSHS/Gregg Co. Immunization clinic, and Wellpoint in Longview Texas. Lastly, we thank all CHWs who worked on this study for their perceptive input.

Conflict of interest

The authors declare no conflict of interest.

Author details

William Sorensen*, Rebecca Swindall, Valerie Smith and Cheryl Cooper
University of Texas at Tyler, Tyler Texas, United States

*Address all correspondence to: wsorensen@uttyler.edu

References

[1] Perry GH. Parasites and human evolution. Evolutionary Anthropology: Issues, News, and Reviews. 2014;**23**(6):218-228

[2] Thomas F, Daoust SP, Raymond M. Can we understand modern humans without considering pathogens? Evolutionary Applications. 2012;**5**(4):368-379

[3] Bañuls A-L, Thomas F, Renaud F. Of parasites and men. Infection, Genetics and Evolution. 2013;**20**:61-70

[4] Partida-Rodríguez O, Serrano-Vázquez A, Nieves-Ramírez ME, Moran P, Rojas L, Portillo T, et al. Human intestinal microbiota: Interaction between parasites and the host immune response. Archives of Medical Research. 2017;**48**(8):690-700

[5] Ianiro G, Iorio A, Porcari S, Masucci L, Sanguinetti M, Perno CF, et al. How the gut parasitome affects human health. Therapeutic Advances in Gastroenterology. 2022;**15**:17562848221091524

[6] Buonfrate D, Tamarozzi F, Paradies P, Watts MR, Bradbury RS, Bisoffi Z. The diagnosis of human and companion animal Strongyloides stercoralis infection: Challenges and solutions. A Scoping Review. Advances in Parasitology. 2022;**118**:1-84

[7] Eberhard M, Gabrielli A, Savioli L, Heymann D. Ascariasis. Hookworm Disease. Trichuriasis. Control of Communicable Diseases Manual. 19th ed. Washington, DC: American Public Health Association; 2008

[8] Sorensen WC, Cappello M, Bell D, DiFedele LM, Brown MA. Poly-helminth infection in east Guatemalan school children. Journal of Global Infectious Diseases. 2011;**3**(1):25-31

[9] Birch CL, Anast BP. The changing distribution of helminthic diseases in the United States. Journal of the American Medical Association. 1957;**164**(2):121-126

[10] Birn A-E, Pillay Y, Holtz TH. Textbook of Global Health. 4th ed. New York, NY: Oxford University Press; 2017

[11] Lynn MK, Morrissey JA, Conserve DF. Soil-transmitted helminths in the USA: A review of five common parasites and future directions for avenues of enhanced epidemiologic inquiry. Current Tropical Medicine Reports. 2021;**8**:32-42

[12] Starr MC, Montgomery SP. Soil-transmitted helminthiasis in the United States: A systematic review—1940-2010. The American Journal of Tropical Medicine and Hygiene. 2011;**85**(4):680

[13] Hotez PJ. Neglected infections of poverty in the United States of America. PLoS Neglected Tropical Diseases. 2008;**2**(6):e256

[14] Cooper CM. Enumeration and Health-Related Characteristics of Hired Farm Workers in Cherokee County. Texas: Texas Woman's University; 2005

[15] Hotez PJ, Bottazzi ME, Dumonteil E, Valenzuela JG, Kamhawi S, Ortega J, et al. Texas and Mexico: Sharing a legacy of poverty and neglected tropical diseases. PLoS Neglected Tropical Diseases. 2012;**6**(3):e1497

[16] Gutiérrez-Jiménez J, Luna-Cazáres LM, Vidal JE. Malnutrition and

Intestinal Parasites: Mexico Perspectives. Handbook of Famine, Starvation, and Nutrient Deprivation from Biology to Policy. Cham: Springer International Publishing; 2017. pp. 1-18

[17] Upton R. Incidence and severity of hookworm infestation in East Texas. American Journal of Public Health and the Nations Health. 1936;**26**(9):924-926

[18] Health Facts Profile (2014-2015): Texas Department of State Health Services; 2019. Available from: https://healthdata.dshs.texas.gov/dashboard/archive/surveys-and-profiles/health-facts-profiles/health-facts-profile-2014-2015

[19] Garcia LS. Dientamoeba fragilis, one of the neglected intestinal protozoa. Journal of Clinical Microbiology. 2016;**54**(9):2243-2250

[20] Alfellani MA, Taner-Mulla D, Jacob AS, Imeede CA, Yoshikawa H, Stensvold CR, et al. Genetic diversity of blastocystis in livestock and zoo animals. Protist. 2013;**164**(4):497-509

[21] Wawrzyniak I, Poirier P, Viscogliosi E, Dionigia M, Texier C, Delbac F, et al. Blastocystis, an unrecognized parasite: An overview of pathogenesis and diagnosis. Therapeutic Advances in Infectious Disease. 2013;**1**(5):167-178

[22] Amin OM. Seasonal prevalence of intestinal parasites in the United States during 2000. The American Journal of Tropical Medicine and Hygiene. 2002;**66**(6):799-803

[23] Graczyk TK, Shiff CK, Tamang L, Munsaka F, Beitin AM, Moss WJ. The association of blastocystis hominis and endolimax nana with diarrheal stools in Zambian school-age children. Parasitology Research. 2005;**98**:38-43

[24] Ciesielski SD, Seed JR, Ortiz JC, Metts J. Intestinal parasites among North Carolina migrant farmworkers. American Journal of Public Health. 1992;**82**(9):1258-1262

[25] Escobedo LG, Homedes N, Von Alt K, Escobedo MA. Intestinal parasites in children from three West Texas border communities. Journal of School Health. 2004;**74**(10):411-414

[26] Ramírez JD, Flórez C, Olivera M, Bernal MC, Giraldo JC. Blastocystis subtyping and its association with intestinal parasites in children from different geographical regions of Colombia. PLoS One. 2017;**12**(2):e0172586

[27] Lukeš J, Stensvold CR, Jirků-Pomajbíková K, Wegener PL. Are human intestinal eukaryotes beneficial or commensals? PLoS Pathogens. 2015;**11**(8):e1005039

[28] Tito RY, Chaffron S, Caenepeel C, Lima-Mendez G, Wang J, Vieira-Silva S, et al. Population-level analysis of blastocystis subtype prevalence and variation in the human gut microbiota. Gut. 2019;**68**(7):1180-1189

[29] Chang AH, Perry S, Du JN, Agunbiade A, Polesky A, Parsonnet J. Decreasing intestinal parasites in recent northern California refugees. The American Journal of Tropical Medicine and Hygiene. 2013;**88**(1):191

[30] Osborne J, Wilson C, Moore V, Gregory T, Flight I, Young G. Sample preference for colorectal cancer screening tests: Blood or stool? Open Journal of Preventive Medicine. 2012;**2**(3):326-331

[31] Singer R, Xu TH, Herrera LNS, Villar MJ, Faust KM, Hotez PJ, et al.

Prevalence of intestinal parasites in a low-income Texas community. The American Journal of Tropical Medicine and Hygiene. 2020;**102**(6):1386

[32] Blackburn CC, Yan SM, McCormick D, Herrera LN, Iordanov RB, Bailey MD, et al. Parasitic contamination of soil in the southern United States. The American Journal of Tropical Medicine and Hygiene. 2024;**111**(3):506

[33] McKenna ML, McAtee S, Bryan PE, Jeun R, Ward T, Kraus J, et al. Human intestinal parasite burden and poor sanitation in rural Alabama. The American Journal of Tropical Medicine and Hygiene. 2017;**97**(5):1623

[34] Smith Darr J, Conn DB. Importation and transmission of parasitic and other infectious diseases associated with international adoptees and refugees immigrating into the United States of America. BioMed Research International. 2015;**2015**(1):763715

[35] Blum AJ, Hotez PJ. Global "Worming": Climate Change and its Projected General Impact on Human Helminth Infections. CA USA: Public Library of Science San Francisco; 2018. p. e0006370

[36] Chammartin F, Scholte RG, Guimarães LH, Tanner M, Utzinger J, Vounatsou P. Soil-transmitted helminth infection in South America: A systematic review and geostatistical meta-analysis. The Lancet Infectious Diseases. 2013;**13**(6):507-518

[37] Weaver HJ, Hawdon JM, Hoberg EP. Soil-transmitted helminthiases: Implications of climate change and human behavior. Trends in Parasitology. 2010;**26**(12):574-581

[38] Javanmard E, Niyyati M, Ghasemi E, Mirjalali H, Aghdaei HA, Zali MR. Impacts of human development index and climate conditions on prevalence of blastocystis: A systematic review and meta-analysis. Acta Tropica. 2018;**185**:193-203

[39] Ehlers S, Kaufmann SH. Infection, inflammation, and chronic diseases: Consequences of a modern lifestyle. Trends in Immunology. 2010;**31**(5):184-190

[40] Patz JA, Graczyk TK, Geller N, Vittor AY. Effects of environmental change on emerging parasitic diseases. International Journal for Parasitology. 2000;**30**(12-13):1395-1405

[41] Petney TN. Environmental, cultural and social changes and their influence on parasite infections. International Journal for Parasitology. 2001;**31**(9):919-932

[42] Guarner F, Bourdet-Sicard R, Brandtzaeg P, Gill HS, McGuirk P, Van Eden W, et al. Mechanisms of disease: The hygiene hypothesis revisited. Nature Clinical Practice Gastroenterology & Hepatology. 2006;**3**(5):275-284

[43] Yazdanbakhsh M, Matricardi PM. Parasites and the hygiene hypothesis: Regulating the immune system? Clinical Reviews in Allergy & Immunology. 2004;**26**:15-23

[44] Natale-Pereira A, Enard KR, Nevarez L, Jones LA. The role of patient navigators in eliminating health disparities. Cancer. 2011;**117**(S15):3541-3550

[45] Ramirez AG, Munoz E, Parma DL, Michalek JE, Holden AEC, Phillips TD, et al. Lifestyle and clinical correlates of hepatocellular carcinoma in South Texas: A matched case-control study. Clinical Gastroenterology and Hepatology. 2017;**15**(8):1311-1312

Chapter 8

Understanding the Diagnosing of Canine Ehrlichiosis: A Comprehensive Review

Monica E.T. Alcón-Chino and Salvatore G. De-Simone

Abstract

Canine Ehrlichiosis is a zoonotic disease transmitted by ticks, posing a global challenge to veterinary and public health. The prevalence of *Ehrlichiosis canis* varies across regions, emphasizing the need for a comprehensive approach to understanding and combating this illness. This chapter explores its complex pathogenesis, highlighting how the bacterium manipulates the host's immune response, leading to diverse clinical manifestations. Diagnostic methods, from traditional microscopy to molecular techniques and serology, are critically assessed for their strengths and limitations. By recognizing these nuances, the review equips practitioners with the knowledge for informed decision-making. A key focus is advocating for an integrated "One Health" approach, leveraging genomics, proteomics, and artificial intelligence to improve diagnostics and develop innovative treatments globally. This collaborative framework acknowledges the link between human, animal, and environmental health, offering a holistic strategy against canine Ehrlichiosis. The review synthesizes scientific literature and emphasizes methodological rigor, providing a foundation for future research and interventions. With a commitment to "One Health" principles and advanced technologies, efforts can mitigate the disease's impact and protect both animal and human well-being.

Keywords: Ehrlichiosis, Hemoparasites, *Rhipicephalus sanguineous*, *Ehrlichia canis*, tick, diagnostic, vaccine

1. Introduction

Canine Ehrlichiosis, caused by Ehrlichia's obligate intracellular pleomorphic bacterium, primarily *Ehrlichia canis,* is a significant concern within veterinary and public health [1]. This tick-borne zoonosis mainly affects dogs and poses a risk to other animals such as sheep, goats, cattle, horses [2], and humans [3]. The prevalence of *E. canis* infection is notable in areas with tropical or temperate climates [4, 5], where tick proliferation is influenced by environmental factors alongside ecological and socio-economic elements [6]. Upon infection, the disease may manifest acutely, subclinically, or chronically, displaying diverse clinical signs such as fever, anorexia, anemia, thrombocytopenia, hemorrhages, lymphadenopathy, splenomegaly, uveitis, and polyarthritis [7]. Diagnosis of canine Ehrlichiosis presents a challenge, necessitating a combination of direct and indirect methods, each with limitations in sensitivity, specificity, availability, and cost [8].

Treatment of the disease typically relies on antibiotics, primarily doxycycline, albeit effectiveness and affordability vary [9–11]. Despite treatment efforts, prevention of canine Ehrlichiosis hinges on tick control and immunoprophylaxis, yet a commercially available vaccine remains elusive [12, 13]. Consequently, canine Ehrlichiosis stands as a zoonotic threat to public and animal health, demanding an integrated "One Health" approach for mitigation. This article aims to review the scientific literature on canine Ehrlichiosis, exploring future perspectives and recent advances in genomics, proteomics, and artificial intelligence technologies to enhance diagnostic accuracy, identify therapeutic targets and biomarkers, and develop preventive strategies on a global scale.

2. Methodology

This research was conducted based on an exploratory bibliographic study using the literature review method [14]. For this purpose, literature was obtained from three databases: PubMed, Web of Science, and EBSCO.

In the review, inclusion criteria were established considering the relevance of the content to the addressed topic, the quality of the study, and a temporal cutoff of the last twenty decades. Duplicate studies focusing on species other than dogs and studies not directly addressing canine Ehrlichiosis were excluded.

For the search strategy, a combination of the following descriptors and Boolean operators has been applied: "treatment" AND "canine ehrlichiosis" or "*Ehrlichia canis*" AND "diagnosis" AND "epidemiology." RayyanTM Web (https://www.rayyan.ai) helped organize the bibliographic data and eliminate duplicates. Subsequently, the titles and abstracts were evaluated, followed by a full-text examination using the eligibility criteria. After a thorough reading, ten articles from PubMed, seven from Web of Science, and three from EBSCO were selected, totaling 20 articles that guided the research.

The collected data were analyzed and synthesized to provide a comprehensive overview of canine Ehrlichiosis, including aspects related to epidemiology, diagnosis, treatment, and disease prevention. Additionally, future perspectives and technological advances that may contribute to effectively managing this zoonosis were explored.

3. Ehrlichia and its morphology

Ehrlichia species are Gram-negative bacteria that infect phagocytic bone marrow-derived cells in mammalian hosts [15–17]. These bacteria measure from 0.5 to 2 mm in diameter and lead an obligate intracellular existence inside cytoplasmic vacuoles, where they divide by binary fission to form clusters of bacteria called morulae. Many *Ehrlichia* species spend part of their normal life cycle in an arthropod host, most commonly a hardshell tick [15, 17–19]. Transovarial transmission of *Ehrlichia* species appears inefficient in ticks, and mammalian hosts are presumed to play an important role in maintaining and propagating *Ehrlichia* species in nature.

Ehrlichia genus encompasses six species: *E. canis*, *E. chaffeensis*, *E. ewingii*, *E. muris*, *E. ruminantium*, and *E. mineirensis* [19, 20]. While E. *chaffeensis, E. muris*, and *E. ewingii* have been linked to Ehrlichiosis in humans [21], reports indicate that *E. ewingii* and *E. chaffeensis* can infect dogs [4, 22]. Thus, Ehrlichiosis presents in two manifestations in both species: Canine monocytic Ehrlichiosis (CME), primarily caused by *E. canis*, and Canine Granulocytic ehrlichiosis (CGE), induced by *E. ewingii* [4]. Human monocytic Ehrlichiosis (HME) involves *E. chaffeensis*, while *E. ewingii* contributes to human granulocytic Ehrlichiosis (HGE) alongside agents like *Anaplasma phagocytophilum* and *Neorickettsia sennetsu* [23–25].

Given the diversity of *Ehrlichia* species, understanding their structural and morphological characteristics is crucial for elucidating their pathogenic mechanisms. Ehrlichia exhibits two distinct morphological forms throughout its life cycle: reticulate and dense-core cells. As a Gram-negative bacterium, it undergoes morphological variations and is surrounded by a thin, undulated outer membrane. This membrane shares structural characteristics with other Gram-negative bacteria, notably featuring a more complex cell wall with a higher content of amino acids and lipids. These structural attributes play a key role in the bacterium's ability to persist within host cells, evade immune responses, and establish infection, thereby contributing to the pathogenesis of both human and canine Ehrlichiosis [26, 27]. However, unlike most Gram-negative bacteria, Ehrlichia avoids the expression of lipopolysaccharide (LPS) and peptidoglycan on its surface, evading recognition by human leukocyte receptors and vector hemocytes, thereby thwarting elimination [2, 28].

4. Tick biological cycle

The *Rhipicephalus sanguineus* tick is the primary biological vector for *transmitting E. canis* to dogs, although other tick species also possess this capability [5, 29, 30]. Consequently, dogs function as the principal host for *R. sanguineus,* concurrently acting as reservoirs due to prolonged bacteremia [31, 32]. However, *R. sanguineus* infests other hosts, including small mammals and large animals, such as humans [5].

The transmission of canine Ehrlichiosis initiates when a tick feeds on a previously infected host, thereby acquiring *E. canis* [33, 34]. Throughout its biological cycle, the tick progresses through four life stages: egg, larva, nymph, and adult. While larvae, nymphs, and adults partake in blood meals and can acquire *E. canis*, only nymphs and adults can transmit the pathogen. Larvae, having not been previously exposed to the pathogen, cannot transmit it. Consequently, transstadial transmission, where the pathogen persists across the various life stages of the tick, is feasible, but transovarian transmission does not occur [33, 34]. Subsequently, during the nymph and adult life cycle, the tick may transmit the bacteria to other hosts during subsequent blood meals.

The prevalence of *E. canis* typically peaks during warmer periods of the year in tropical and subtropical regions, correlating with the tick's life cycle (**Figure 1**).

5. Epidemiology of canine Ehrlichiosis

Canine Ehrlichiosis exhibits a widespread global distribution, particularly prevalent in regions with tropical and subtropical climates [35]. Noteworthy studies shed light on the disease's prevalence across various continents.

Judy and colleagues conducted a comprehensive assessment spanning 2016 to 2021 in Africa, analyzing 400 samples from Kenya and Tanzania using the IDEXX SNAP 4Dx™ Plus test. Results unveiled a seropositivity of 31% (29/245) in Kenya and

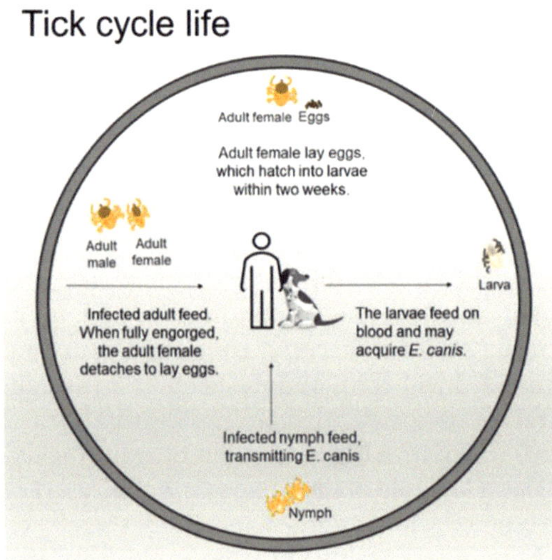

Figure 1.
The cycle of canine Ehrlichiosis. When a previously infected host feeds the tick, the biological cycle of E. canis *in the tick goes through four life stages: egg, larva, nymph, and adult.*

a surprising 69% (63/155) in Tanzania, underscoring the significant dissemination of Ehrlichiosis in the region [36]. In contrast, a study in Europe by Miró et al. over 5 years (2016–2020), covering samples from 35 countries, revealed an intriguing trend. Despite an increase in the number of tests conducted, there was a decline in Ehrlichia spp. positivity, with seropositivity dropping from 4.3 to 3.4% [12].

Reference	Year	Location	Diagnostic method	Prevalence
[41]	2019	Belém, Pará	PCR	109/276 (39.4%)
[42]	2019	Cuiabá, Mato Grosso	IFA and PCR	9/20 (45.0%)
[38]	2020	Caatinga, Northeast	Serology and PCR	61–75% 13/147 (8.8%)
[31]	2020	49 municipalities across North, Northeast, Midwest, South, and Southeast	ELISA	456/814 (56.0%)
[43]	2021	Belém, Pará	PCR	6/50 (12%)
[39]	2022	Goiás, Midwest	IFA	156/264 (59.1%)
[33]	2022	Ceará, Northeast	PCR and serology	21/153 (13.7%)
[40]	2022	São Paulo, SP	IFA and real-time PCR	32/54 (59.3%)
[44]	2023	Barão de Melgaço, Pantanal	PCR	157/369 (42.5%)
[45]	2023	Amazon, Indigenous Communities	PCR and sequencing	40/327 (12.2%)
[46]	2024	Rio Grande do Norte	PCR	16/120 (13.3%)
[47]	2024	Ceará, Northeast	RT-PCR and IFA	Sobral: 9.9%, Alcântara: 5.6%
[48]	2024	Porto Seguro, Bahia	PCR	110/730 (15.1%)

Table 1.
Prevalence of E. canis *in dogs in Brazil.*

In Latin America, evidence from Argentina indicates *an E. canis* infection prevalence ranging between 13.5% and 37.5% in symptomatic dogs. In Paraguay, a study in domestic dogs reported a seroprevalence of 23.5%, accompanied by a molecular prevalence of 11.8%. Similarly, in Peru, a seroprevalence of 16.5% was recorded in a cohort of 140 dogs [37].

Previous studies in Brazil have highlighted variability in the seroprevalence of canine Ehrlichiosis, which is influenced by regional differences across the country. Studies conducted between 2019 and 2024 provide insights into the distribution of Ehrlichiosis within Brazilian territory. **Table 1** summarizes the diagnostic methods, prevalence rates, and respective study locations. The states of Goiás and São Paulo reported the highest prevalence rates, approximately 59%, whereas the lowest incidence was observed in the Northeastern region, specifically in the Caatinga biome, with 8.8% [38–40]. These variations may reflect regional differences in canine exposure to the pathogen and differences in the sensitivity and specificity of the diagnostic methods used. Despite the availability of epidemiological data on the disease in Brazil, underreporting remains a significant challenge.

6. Pathogenesis and systemic pathophysiology

6.1 Pathogenesis in canine Ehrlichiosis

Upon tick infection, *E. canis* dissemination begins within the epithelial cells of the intestine, progressing to the tick's hemocytes and salivary gland cells [42]. Transmission to dogs occurs when infected ticks feed on blood, transferring the infective form of *E. canis* and their salivary secretions, which contain molecules facilitating pathogen acquisition and transmission, alongside exhibiting anticoagulant and anti-inflammatory properties [49].

Within the vertebrate host, the bacteria infiltrate monocytes, forming intracellular aggregates known as "morulas." Multiplication transpires within the phagolysosome and vacuoles of the host cell, affording isolation and protection from the immune system [50]. After 7–12 days post-infection, morulae are released into the bloodstream, infecting other cells. This interaction between infected and uninfected cells within blood vessels can incite vasculitis and perivascular migration of macrophages and lymphocytes. Predominant multiplication within macrophages and lymphocytes can lead to splenomegaly, hepatomegaly, and lymphadenopathy [11, 25, 51].

During host-pathogen interaction, various glycoproteins (GP) like GP19, gp36, gp140, and O-glycan, alongside outer membrane proteins such as P28/OMP and TRP 120, are pivotal for growth, accentuating the significance of these immunogenic outer membrane-associated proteins for pathogen replication within macrophages both in vitro and in vivo [20, 52–54]. Studies conducted by McBride and colleagues underscore the importance of the TRP 120 protein in mediating *E. canis* and host-cell interaction, influencing adhesion and internalization by phagosomes [20, 54–56]. This capability enables bacteria to modulate the host's immune response, diminishing reactive oxygen species production and impeding host cell apoptosis. Additionally, the gp200 gene plays a critical role in immune response modulation, facilitating immune system evasion and the potential to differentiate distinct pathogen strains [57, 58].

The onset of the immune response, from initial exposure to symptom manifestation in canine Ehrlichiosis, encompasses an incubation period spanning 8–20 days [59]. Subsequently, the disease progresses through acute, chronic, and subclinical phases, with the latter potentially persisting for several years without evident symptoms, underscoring the complexity and variability of *E. canis* infection within the host [60].

6.2 Multisystemic pathophysiological alterations in canine Ehrlichiosis

The clinical manifestations of *Ehrlichia canis* infection are diverse; however, the most frequently observed signs include depression, lethargy, weight loss, anorexia, pyrexia, lymphadenomegaly, and splenomegaly. A defining feature of *E. canis* infection is the presence of hematologic abnormalities, particularly anemia, thrombocytopenia, and leukopenia, which are critical indicators of disease progression [11].

6.2.1 Hematopoietic and immune system dysfunction

The hallmark of *E. canis* infection is hematologic abnormalities, notably anemia, thrombocytopenia, and leukopenia. These alterations are attributed to direct effects on hematopoietic progenitor cells and immune-mediated destruction. Dogs in both acute and chronic phases may show normocytic normochromic anemia and varying degrees of pancytopenia, which are more characteristic of the chronic phase [61]. The disease also triggers a dysregulated immune response, with increased proinflammatory cytokines such as TNF-α, IFN-γ, and IL-6, leading to systemic inflammatory effects. In addition to its anti-inflammatory properties, IL-10 plays a key immunoregulatory role. An imbalance in cytokines is likely a key mechanism contributing to the pathogenesis and tissue damage seen in dogs with canine monocytic Ehrlichiosis (CME) [62, 63].

6.2.2 Renal dysfunction

Renal involvement in Ehrlichiosis is increasingly reported, especially in chronic and subclinical stages. Alterations include elevated blood urea nitrogen (BUN), serum creatinine, and persistent proteinuria. Hyposthenuria and increased urinary protein-creatinine ratios suggest early glomerular damage. These findings are consistent with early or progressing chronic kidney disease (CKD). Studies have shown associations between hypocalcemia, low urine specific gravity, and elevated protein-creatinine ratio (UPC) in seropositive animals, reinforcing the hypothesis of renal impairment induced by *E. canis* infection. The deposition of immune complexes and tissue hypoxia resulting from anemia are also relevant pathogenic factors for renal dysfunction [64–66].

6.2.3 Hepatic alterations

Liver involvement can be assessed using ultrasonographic techniques and biochemical markers, elastography, and histopathological analysis. However, Liver enzyme elevations, including alanine aminotransferase (ALT), aspartate aminotransferase (AST), and alkaline phosphatase (ALP), may be observed, particularly in the acute phase. These reflect hepatocellular injury and possible hepatic inflammation. Increased serum butyrylcholinesterase (BChE) activity has also been documented, which correlates with inflammatory activity and can serve as an additional biomarker for hepatic pathophysiological alterations and systemic response during the acute phase [59, 61, 63, 67].

7. Immune response

Both cellular and humoral immune responses are pivotal in defense against *E. canis*. CD4+ and CD8+ T cells play significant roles in the cellular immune response, crucial for resisting infections caused by this bacterium [68]. During E. *canis* infection, CD4 T lymphocytes secrete cytokines like IFN-γ and TNF-α, which can modulate the inflammatory response or confer protection to the host [3, 69]. The protective immune response involves IFN-γ and Th1 secretion. However, components of tick saliva act as host immunomodulators during blood meals, reducing the production of IL-9, IL-2, and IL-4 in Th1 cells stimulated by IFN-γ.

Additionally, Castro and colleagues observed differences in MHCII molecule expression between lymphoid tissues and inflammatory infiltrates in organs of dogs with CME, along with an increase in the IgG2 subclass and a decrease in IgG1 and IgE [70, 71]. Following E. *canis* infection, immunoglobulin release occurs in the blood circulation. IgA appears approximately 4–7 days later and IgM 15 days later, while initial IgG levels are relatively low. IgG titers (**Figure 2**) notably increase as the infection progresses, predominantly comprising the IgG2 subclass during both acute and convalescent phases [10, 55, 70, 72].

However, the pathogen also exhibits immune system evasion mechanisms during infection. Two studies noted a decrease in MHC II expression, suggesting an evasion mechanism by *E. canis* [49, 54]. Another observed evasion mechanism is the absence of LPS in *E. canis*, which, upon infecting leukocytes, aids their circulation through the vascular system, facilitating bacterial spread throughout the host's body and potentially enhancing survival in cellular vacuoles [15].

In immunocompetent mice, the spectrum of models for Ehrlichiosis ranges from incomplete infection to uniform lethal outcomes, depending on the *Ehrlichia* species, the dosage of inoculum, and the inoculation method. CD4+ T lymphocytes and

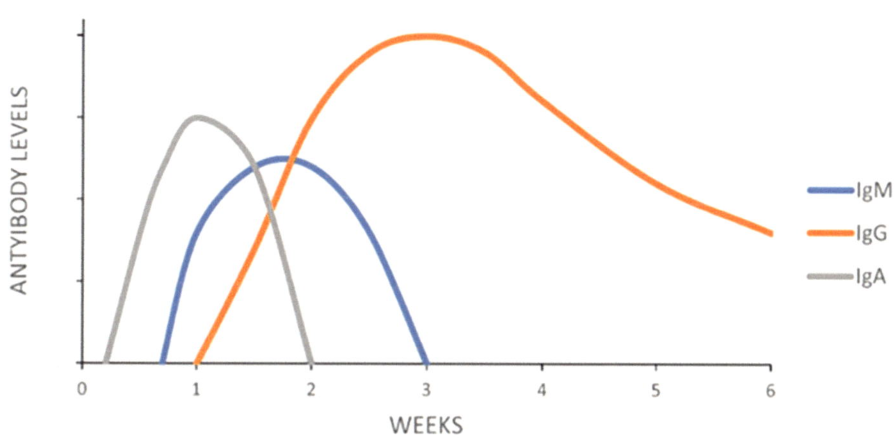

Figure 2.
Antibody response about E. canis *infection and time.*

gamma interferon orchestrate effective immunity. Lethal infections result from an early surge in proinflammatory cytokines and the excessive TNF alpha and IL-10 production by CD8+ T lymphocytes [62, 63]. Fatal Ehrlichiosis is also linked to TLR 9/ MyD88 signaling, leading to the upregulation of multiple inflammasome complexes and the hepatic mononuclear cells' secretion of IL-1 beta, IL-1 alpha, and IL-18 [73]. The involvement of both canonical and noncanonical inflammasome pathways, with IL-18 playing a harmful role and caspase 1 providing protection, can be suggested. Autophagy facilitates Ehrlichia infection, while MyD88 signaling impedes it by suppressing autophagy induction and flux [51].

Activation of caspase 11 during infection of hepatocytes by lethal *Ehrlichia* species, following interferon alpha receptor signaling, triggers inflammasome-dependent IL-1 beta production, extracellular secretion of HMGB1, and pyroptosis, indicating a pathway to toxic shock [73]. Elevated HMGB1 levels in lethal Ehrlichiosis imply its involvement in this shock. Studies on primary bone marrow-derived macrophages infected by highly or mildly avirulent Ehrlichia reveal distinct M1 and M2 macrophage polarization patterns. These patterns correlate with the generation of pathogenic CD8 T cells and neutrophils and excessive inflammation in one scenario and with the robust expansion of protective Th1 and NKT cells, inflammation resolution, and infection clearance in the other [50].

8. Clinical signs

Canine monocytic Ehrlichiosis (CME) presents a polysystemic disease with clinical or subclinical manifestation (**Table 2**). The clinical course of infection begins in the acute phase. This initial stage, lasting 15–30 days, typically exhibits more pronounced symptoms. Bacteria multiply in mononuclear cells during this phase, spreading within the host. Clinical signs include fever, loss of appetite and weight, petechiae, and other symptoms [70, 74]. Afterward, the infection may lead to complete recovery or transition to the subclinical phase. It is characterized by asymptomatic presentation for 6–9 weeks or persistent absence of clear clinical signs over several years.

Nevertheless, it may cause non-regenerative anemia, leukopenia, and thrombocytopenia [70, 75]. The infection can sometimes progress to the chronic phase, which resembles an autoimmune condition impacting the host's immune system. Symptoms mirror those of the acute phase but are more severe. It represents a prolonged and persistent stage of

Stage of infection	Common symptoms	Frequency of symptoms
Acute phase	Fever, lethargy, anorexia, lymphadenopathy, splenomegaly, thrombocytopenia, normochromic normocytic anemia, leukopenia.	High frequency
Subclinical phase	Asymptomatic or mild and nonspecific symptoms include anemia, thrombocytopenia, and hyperproteinemia.	Low frequency
Chronic phase	Variable symptoms include severe anemia, thrombocytopenia, severe bone marrow aplasia, pancytopenia, sepsis, severe bleeding, and myelosuppression.	Variable frequency

Table 2.
Frequency of presenting signs and symptoms observed during the different phases of Ehrlichia canis *infection in dogs.*

the infection, with intensified symptoms such as glomerulonephritis, nephrotic syndrome, bone marrow suppression leading to pancytopenia, and susceptibility to secondary infections [59, 76]. The complexity of *E. canis* infection is evident through this broad range of clinical manifestations. Additionally, proteins related to evasion, adherence, DNA repair, and efflux pumps play a role in pathogenesis and bacterial virulence [77]. The varying virulence of *E. canis* strains contributes to differing disease severities.

9. Diagnosis

Diagnosing canine Ehrlichiosis entails amalgamating clinical and epidemiological data with direct or indirect methods to confirm the suspicion, guiding appropriate treatment, and epidemiological control, which is crucial for both veterinary and public health, given the zoonotic nature of Ehrlichiosis [70].

9.1 Microscopy

Microscopic analysis enables the identification of *E. canis* bacteria in various clinical samples, including peripheral blood, bone marrow, and biological fluids. Confirmation of canine Ehrlichiosis relies on detecting microcolonies or morulae in the cytoplasm of specific cells, like monocytes or leukocytes [34, 78]. This method is most effective during the acute phase, although its sensitivity diminishes in chronic and subclinical phases. Expertise is required to differentiate between morulae and other tissue structures [11, 74, 79].

9.2 Molecular

Polymerase chain reaction (PCR) assays are increasingly utilized because they can detect minute amounts of genetic material with high precision, providing evidence of active infection and superior sensitivity to conventional microscopy [13, 34, 80]. Despite the wide use of PCR, discrepancies between PCR and microscopic results underscore the need for cautious interpretation [81]. Quantitative real-time PCR (qPCR) and multiplex PCR assays enhance sensitivity and enable simultaneous detection of multiple *Ehrlichia* species [82]. However, some studies report lower sensitivity than conventional PCR [83, 84].

9.3 Serology

Serological tests, including indirect immunofluorescence reaction test (IFAT) and enzyme-linked immunosorbent assay (ELISA), detect antibodies against *E. canis* immunoreactive proteins [60, 85]. Commercial tests for both methods are available, with varying sensitivities and specificities compared to the "gold standard" IFAT [86]. Limitations exist in serological tests, particularly in distinguishing acute from chronic infection and defining previous exposure, prompting research into new protein targets for improved diagnosis [87–89].

9.4 Imaging techniques

Imaging is crucial in assessing systemic complications of canine Ehrlichiosis, in addition to laboratory-based methods. Thoracic radiography may help identify

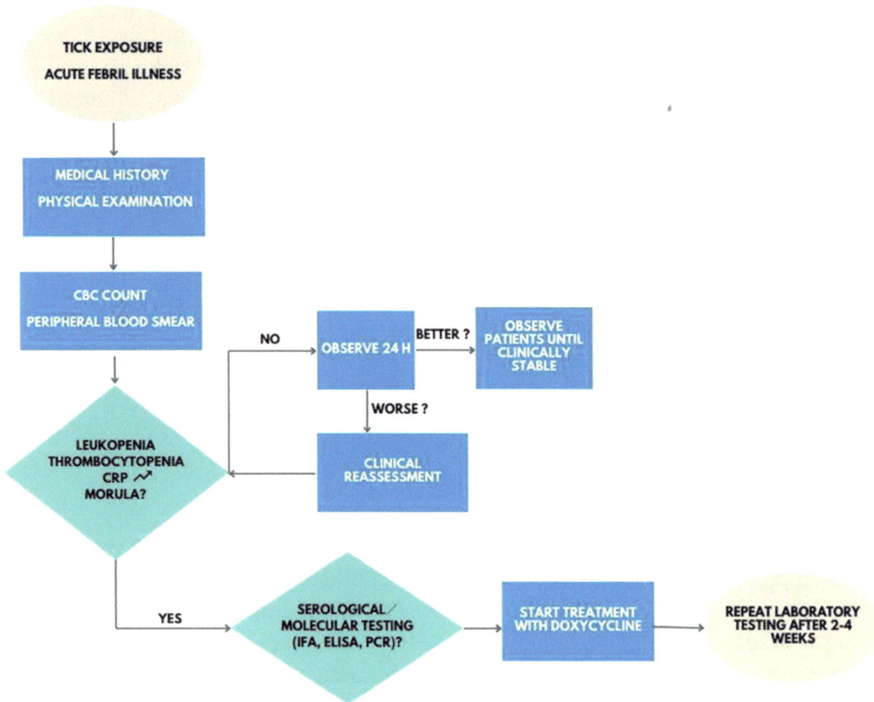

Figure 3.
Suggested clinical, laboratory, and treatment approaches for patients with a history of recent exposure to ticks or a confirmed tick bite who present with a nonspecific febrile illness. CBC, complete blood cell; CRP, C-reactive protein; IFA, indirect fluorescent antibody.

lymphadenopathy and pulmonary hemorrhage, while abdominal ultrasound detects splenomegaly and hepatic/renal alterations. In severe cases, magnetic resonance imaging (MRI) provides valuable insights into neurological and meningeal involvement, which can be associated with advanced stages of the disease. While imaging does not replace direct pathogen detection, it enhances diagnostic accuracy and helps guide clinical management by identifying disease severity and potential complications [67, 90, 91].

Recently, an innovative study combined statistics artificial intelligence (AI) and machine learning (ML) techniques to identify biomarkers by analyzing the transcriptome of patients with cardiovascular diseases (CVD). Eighteen transcriptomic biomarkers were identified with 96% accuracy [92]. This approach may contribute to the early diagnosis of tick-borne diseases.

In summary, a multifaceted approach combining different diagnostic methods is essential for accurate diagnosis, treatment, and control of canine Ehrlichiosis (**Figure 3**).

10. Treatment

Some factors can influence the underdiagnosis of the disease, such as the physiopathogenesis of Ehrlichiosis in each phase. Thus, adequate treatment may not occur [11]. When diagnosed, treatment involves using antibiotics such as doxycycline, tetracycline, or rifampicin. Currently, the treatment presented as standard therapy still uses doxycycline antibiotics. Doxycycline may be administered orally at 10 mg/kg of dog body weight, divided into two daily doses, for 28 days. This drug is effective in the treatment of canine Ehrlichiosis. Although effective in the treatment of canine Ehrlichiosis, prolonged administration of the drug may be associated with adverse effects, such as anorexia, vomiting, diarrhea, and hepatic toxicity [60].

On the other hand, Cardoso and colleagues observed an increase in IL-1β and monocytes, aggravating the inflammatory process [93]. Additionally, reports of bacterial resistance to doxycycline have been described [11, 94]. In addition to the challenges associated with the use of doxycycline, the treatment of canine Ehrlichiosis is also complicated by the difficulty in early diagnosis since symptoms can be nonspecific and, like other clinical conditions, leading to the chronic form of the disease [11, 74].

Given the need for new therapeutic strategies for canine Ehrlichiosis, research is being conducted to evaluate the effectiveness of alternative treatments, including the use of plant extracts and combinations of drugs. A study demonstrated the in vitro efficacy of the plant *Ageratum conyzoides*. They evaluated the viability of DH82 cells against the aqueous fraction of the *Ageratum conyzoides* extract associated with doxycycline, which demonstrated the ability to eliminate or suppress *E. canis* [95].

Protocol	Drug(s)	Dose/duration	Indication	Advantages	Limitations
Standard monotherapy [93]	Doxycycline	10 mg/kg PO, once or twice daily, for 28 days	All CME stages	Highly effective intracellular penetration reduces cytokine imbalance	Side effects, hepatotoxicity, emerging resistance
Alternative [97]	Minocycline	10–12 mg/kg PO, twice daily for 14–28 days	Non-acute infections or doxycycline intolerance	Similar efficacy to doxycycline, oral use	Limited clinical data, potential effects
Alternative [98]	oxytetracycline	22 mg/kg for 3 days, PO for 14 days	Moderate to severe CME	Rapid clinical response	Requires hospitalization, venous access potential, renal toxicity
Alternative [98]	Imidocarb dipropionate	6.6 mg/kg SC; repeat after 14 days	Chronic or refractory cases	Effective against rickettsial pathogens	Painful injection, hepatic/renal toxicity risk
Non-standard antibiotic [99]	Rifampicin	10–15 mg/kg PO, once daily, for 21 days	Drug-resistant infections	Alternative mechanism of action, reduced bacterial load	Hepatotoxicity, limited veterinary data, slow efficacy
Experimental combination [95]	Doxycycline + *Ageratum conyzoides* extract	Dose variable, tested in vitro	Alternative with synergistic potential	Reduced MIC of doxycycline by 5.83× in vitro	Not yet validated in vivo

Table 3.
Overview of therapeutic protocols for Canine Monocytic Ehrlichiosis (CME).

Intervention	Indication	Rationale	Limitations
Fluid therapy [99, 100]	Dehydration, hypoperfusion	Restores hydration, supports perfusion	Requires inpatient care
Blood transfusion [101]	Severe anemia or hemorrhage	Restores oxygen-carrying capacity and coagulation	Risk of transfusion reaction; costly
Hepatoprotective agents (e.g., silymarin, SAMe) [102]	Elevated liver enzymes	Protects liver from drug toxicity	Limited veterinary evidence
Filgrastim [96]	Non-regenerative pancytopenia	Stimulates bone marrow activity; experimental improvement	High-cost, experimental use

Table 4.
Supportive care strategies for Canine Monocytic Ehrlichiosis (CME).

Furthermore, an in vitro study [82] administered filgrastim in dogs with canine monocytic Ehrlichiosis and non-regenerative pancytopenia showed significant improvement in clinical outcomes [96].

Minocycline, a drug belonging to the tetracycline family, has been successfully used to treat canine Ehrlichiosis and can be an effective alternative to doxycycline for clearing *E. canis* from the blood in non-acute infections [97]. In this context, alternative or adjunctive therapies may be considered in cases of drug intolerance, suspected resistance, or treatment failure. A summary of protocols is presented below in **Table 3**.

In some cases, blood transfusions in animals with severe anemia or hemorrhage are used as a complement to treatment with doxycycline, helping to correct blood abnormalities and improve tissue oxygenation [100]. Supportive measures are essential to improve treatment outcomes, especially in moderate or chronic CME (**Table 4**). They help stabilize systemic functions, reduce inflammation, and manage complications.

11. Future outlook and recent advances

The management of canine anaplasmosis hinges on identifying vectors/reservoirs, managing tick vectors, and preventing iatrogenic/mechanical transmission. Strategies for controlling human disease involve minimizing activities with high-risk tick exposure (like gardening and hiking), ensuring safe blood transfusions, avoiding immunosuppression when possible, and identifying and managing reservoirs/vectors [103].

Advancements in genomics and proteomics have facilitated the identification of *E. canis* proteins. In addition, reducing virulence-associated genes has enhanced our understanding of host-pathogen interactions [104]. These advancements also allow us to observe alterations in the composition of proteins present in the blood serum during infection [105]. The pathogen's ability to disrupt the host's immune response poses diagnostic challenges, but screening antigenic protein epitopes with automated systems has improved research outcomes [106, 107].

Genetic variability in bacteria, a consequence of mutation and genetic recombination, presents challenges for diagnosis and vaccination [108]. Studies combining genomics, bioinformatics, and immunological screening have identified novel immunoreactive proteins from *E. chaffeensis* and *E. canis*, potentially serving as therapeutic targets and predictive biomarkers [109].

Comparative genomics has elucidated intraspecific variability in Ehrlichia bacteria, aiding in understanding the genetic basis of different clinical manifestations. Markers like the "TEDSVSAPA" repeat motif found in Australian trp36 sequences offer insights for phylogenetic and epidemiological studies of *E. canis* [110, 111].

Immune response molecules are increasingly utilized as biomarkers for tick-borne diseases [112]. These biomarkers play a pivotal role not only in monitoring infection but also in identifying potential vaccine targets. In this context, Biomarkers of Infection (BMI) and Biomarkers of Protection (BMP) stand out [113]. CXCL13, for instance, shows promise in diagnosing Lyme neuroborreliosis, with studies comparing assay methods to enhance sensitivity and specificity [114]. Additionally, innovative approaches combining statistics, artificial intelligence (AI), and machine learning (ML) techniques have identified transcriptomic biomarkers for cardiovascular diseases (CVD), potentially enabling early diagnosis of tick-borne diseases [92].

These advancements underscore the multidisciplinary efforts to improve diagnostics, understand disease mechanisms, and develop targeted interventions for canine Ehrlichiosis and related conditions.

12. Conclusions

Canine Ehrlichiosis presents a significant challenge due to its extensive dissemination and the difficulties associated with diagnosis and treatment. The wide-ranging clinical manifestations and the presence of various species highlight these difficulties. Despite the widespread use of the antibiotic doxycycline for treatment, some studies have reported resistance to this medication. Consequently, continuous research on novel therapeutic approaches may help reduce the morbidity and mortality of canine Ehrlichiosis. The ongoing investigation of new therapeutic approaches could contribute to reducing the morbidity and mortality associated with canine Ehrlichiosis.

On the other hand, the pathogenesis of the disease has demonstrated the complexity of interactions between *E. canis* and the host immune system, with evasion mechanisms contributing to pathogen persistence. The acute, chronic, and subclinical phases demonstrate variability in clinical presentation, while the immune response, both cellular and humoral, plays a crucial role in defense against infection.

However, integrated approaches considering clinical, epidemiological, and laboratory methods are essential for diagnosis. Furthermore, comparative genomics has been instrumental in understanding the intraspecific variability and evolution of *E. canis*. Proteomics provides a more comprehensive view of changes in protein expression associated with infection. Techniques, including protein microarrays, have made high-throughput analysis possible, contributing to the identification of new therapeutic targets and biomarkers for tick-borne diseases like Lyme neuroborreliosis. Automated systems for screening antigenic protein epitopes have demonstrated the value of increasing diagnostic sensitivity and specificity. Furthermore, integrating artificial intelligence and machine learning holds promise for revolutionizing early disease diagnosis, such as canine Ehrlichiosis. This development offers new perspectives for adopting a "One Health" approach considering the interconnectedness of human, animal, and environmental health.

The ongoing advancements in understanding and diagnosing canine Ehrlichiosis are transforming disease management strategies. With continued research and technological innovation, veterinarians can expect improved diagnostic accuracy, early detection, and better treatment outcomes, ultimately enhancing canine health and welfare.

Acknowledgements

M.E.T.A.C. is a doctoral fellow from the Post-Graduation Program in Science and Biotechnology from the Federal Fluminense University.

Parts of this chapter were previously published in the following preprint: Alcón-Chino, M. E. and De-Simone, S. G. 2024 "Advancements in Understanding and Diagnosing Canine Ehrlichiosis: A Comprehensive Review" Preprints. https://doi.org/10.20944/preprints202404.0490.v1

Conflict of interest

The authors declare no conflicts of interest.

Author details

Monica E.T. Alcón-Chino[1,3] and Salvatore G. De-Simone[1,2,3]*

1 Center for Technological Development in Health (CDTS)/National Institute of Science and Technology for Innovation in Neglected Population Diseases (INCT-IDPN), Oswaldo Cruz Foundation (FIOCRUZ), Rio de Janeiro, RJ, Brazil

2 Laboratory of Epidemiology and Molecular Systematics (LESM), Oswaldo Cruz Institut, FIOCRUZ, Rio de Janeiro, RJ, Brazil

3 Post-Graduation Program in Science and Biotechnology, Department of Molecular and Cellular Biology, Biology Institute, Federal Fluminense University, Niteroi, RJ, Brazil

*Address all correspondence to: salvatore.simone@fiocruz.br

References

[1] Dumler JS, Barbet AF, Bekker CP, Dasch GA, Palmer GH, Ray SC, et al. Reorganization of genera in the families Rickettsiaceae and Anaplasmataceae in the order Rickettsiales: Unification of some species of Ehrlichia with Anaplasma, Cowdria with Ehrlichia and Ehrlichia with Neorickettsia, descriptions of six new species combinations and designation of *Ehrlichia equi* and 'HGE agent' as subjective synonyms of *Ehrlichia phagocytophila*. International Journal of Systematic and Evolutionary Microbiology. 2001;**51**:2145-2165. DOI: 10.1099/00207713-51-6-2145

[2] Rikihisa Y. Molecular events involved in cellular invasion by *Ehrlichia chaffeensis* and *Anaplasma phagocytophilum*. Veterinary Parasitology. 2010;**167**:155-166. DOI: 10.1016/j.vetpar.2009.9.017

[3] Saito TB, Walker DH. Ehrlichioses: An important one health opportunity. Veterinary Science. 2016;**3**(3):20. DOI: 10.3390/vetsci3030020

[4] Beall MJ, Alleman AR, Breitschwerdt EB, Cohn LA, Couto CG, Dryden MW, et al. Seroprevalence of *Ehrlichia canis*, *Ehrlichia chaffeensis,* and *Ehrlichia ewingii* in dogs in North America. Parasites & Vectors. 2012;**5**:29. DOI: 10.1186/1756-3305-5-29

[5] Sanches GS, Villar M, Couto J, Ferrolho J, Fernández de Mera IG, André MR, et al. Comparative proteomic analysis of *Rhipicephalus sanguineus* sensu lato (Acari: Ixodidae) tropical and temperate lineages: Uncovering differences during *Ehrlichia canis* infection. Frontiers in Cellular and Infection Microbiology. 2020;**10**:611113. DOI: 10.3389/fcimb.2020.611113

[6] Dantas-Torres F. Canine vector-borne diseases in Brazil. Parasites & Vectors. 2008;**1**:25. DOI: 10.1186/1756-3305-1-25

[7] De Castro MB, Machado RZ, de Aquino LP, Alessi AC, Costa MT. Experimental acute canine monocytic ehrlichiosis: Clinicopathological and immunopathological findings. Veterinary Parasitology. 2004;**119**:73-86. DOI: 10.1016/j.vetpar.2003.10.012

[8] René-Martellet M, Lebert I, Chêne J, Massot R, Leon M, Leal A, et al. Diagnosis and incidence risk of clinical canine monocytic Ehrlichiosis under field conditions in Southern Europe. Parasites & Vectors. 2015;**8**:3. DOI: 10.1186/s13071-014-0613-4

[9] Harris S, Waner T, Strauss-Ayali D, Bark H, Jongejan F, Hecht G, et al. Dynamics of IgG1 and IgG2 subclass response in dogs naturally and experimentally infected with *Ehrlichia canis*. Veterinary Parasitology. 2001;**99**:63-71. DOI: 10.1016/s0304-4017(01) 00450-2

[10] Waner T, Harrus S, Jongejan F, Bark H, Keysary A, Cornelissen AW. Significance of serological testing for ehrlichial diseases in dogs with special emphasis on the diagnosis of canine monocytic Ehrlichiosis caused by *Ehrlichia canis*. Veterinary Parasitology. 2001;**95**:1-15. DOI: 10.1016/s0304-4017(00)00407-6

[11] Mylonakis ME, Harrus S, Breitschwerdt EB. An update on the treatment of canine monocytic Ehrlichiosis (*Ehrlichia canis*). Veterinary Journal. 2019;**246**:45-53. DOI: 10.1016/j.tvjl.2019.01.015

[12] Maggi RG, Krämer F. A review on the occurrence of companion vector-borne

diseases in pet animals in Latin America. Parasites & Vectors. 2019;**12**:145. DOI: 10.1186/s 13071-019-3407-x

[13] Sainz Á, Roura X, Miró G, Estrada-Peña A, Kohn B, Harrus S, et al. Guideline for veterinary practitioners on canine Ehrlichiosis and anaplasmosis in Europe. Parasites & Vectors. 2015;**8**:75. DOI: 10.1186/s13071-015-0649-0

[14] Sukhera J. Narrative reviews in medical education: Key steps for researchers. Journal of Graduate Medical Education. 2022;**14**:418-419. DOI: 10.4300/jgme-d-22-00481.1

[15] Rikihisa Y. The tribe Ehrlichia and Ehrlichial diseases. Clinical Microbiology Reviews. 1991;**4**:286-308. DOI: 10.1128/cmr.4.3.286

[16] Walker DH, Dumler JS. Emergence of ehrlichioses as human health problems. Emerging Infectious Diseases. 1996;**2**(1):18-29. DOI: 10.3201/eid0201.960102

[17] Dumler JS, Bakken JSH, ehrlichioses. Newly recognized infections transmitted by ticks. Annual Review of Medicine. 1998;**49**:201-213. DOI: 10.1146/annurev.med.49.1.201

[18] Guccione C, Colomba C, Iaria C, Cascio A. Rickettsiales in the WHO European region: An update from a one health perspective. Parasites & Vectors. 2023;**16**(1):41. DOI: 10.1186/s13071-022-05646-4

[19] Dumler JS, Bakken JS. Ehrlichial diseases of humans: Emerging tick-borne infections. Clinical Infectious Diseases. 1995;**20**:1102-1110. DOI: 10.1093/clinids/20.5.110

[20] Cruz AC, Zweygarth E, Ribeiro MF, da Silveira JA, de la Fuente J, Grubhoffer L, et al. New species of Ehrlichia isolated from *Rhipicephalus* (Boophilus) *microplus* shows an ortholog of the *E. canis* major immunogenic glycoprotein gp36 with a new sequence of tandem repeats. Parasites & Vectors. 2012;**5**:291. DOI: 10.1186/1756-3305-5-291

[21] Poolsawat N, Sangchuai S, Jaroensak T, Watthanadirek-Wijidwong A, Srionrod N, Minsakorn S, et al. Molecular occurrence and genetic diversity of *Ehrlichia canis* in naturally infected dogs from Thailand. Scientific Reports. 2023;**13**(1):20394. DOI: 10.1038/s41598-023-47784-4

[22] Goodman RA, Hawkins EC, Olby NJ, Grinder CB, Hegarty B, Breitschwerdt EB. Molecular identification of *Ehrlichia ewingii* infection in dogs: 15 cases (1997-2001). Journal of the American Veterinary Medical Association. 2003;**222**:1102-1107. DOI: 10.2460/javma.2003.222.1102

[23] Olano JP, Walker DH. Human ehrlichioses. The Medical Clinics of North America. 2002;**86**:375-392. DOI: 10.1016/s0025-7125(03)00093-2

[24] Oteo JA, Brouqui P. Ehrlichiosis and human anaplasmosis. Enfermedades Infecciosas y Microbiología Clínica. 2005;**23**:375-380. DOI: 10.1157/13076178

[25] Popov VL, Yu X, Walker DH. The 120 kDa outer membrane protein of *Ehrlichia chaffeensis*: Preferential expression on dense-core cells and gene expression in *Escherichia coli* associated with attachment and entry. Microbial Pathogenesis. 2000;**28**:71-80. DOI: 10.1006/mpat.1999.0327

[26] Ge Y, Rikihisa Y. Surface-exposed proteins of *Ehrlichia chaffeensis*. Infection and Immunity. 2007;**75**:3833-3841. DOI: 10. 1128/iai.00188-07

[27] Dunning Hotopp JC, Lin M, Madupu R, Crabtree J, Angiuoli SV, Eisen JA, et al. Comparative genomics of emerging human ehrlichiosis agents. PLoS Genetics. 2006;**2**:e21. DOI: 10.1371/journal. pgen.0020021

[28] Dantas-Torres F. The brown dog tick, *Rhipicephalus sanguineus* (Latreille, 1806) (Acari: Ixodidae): From taxonomy to control. Veterinary Parasitology. 2008;**152**:173-185. DOI: 10.1016/j.vetpar.2007.12.030

[29] Diakou A, Sofroniou D, Paoletti B, Tamvakis A, Kolencik S, Dimzas D, et al. Ticks, fleas, and harbored pathogens from dogs and cats in Cyprus. Pathogens. 2022;**11**(12):1403. DOI: 10.3390/pathogens11121403

[30] Movilla R, García C, Siebert S, Roura X. Country-wide serological evaluation of canine prevalence for *Anaplasma spp*., *Borrelia burgdorferi* (sensu lato), *Dirofilaria immitis* and *Ehrlichia canis* in Mexico. Parasites & Vectors. 2016;**9**:421. DOI: 10.1186/s13071-016-1686-z

[31] Taques I, Campos ANS, Kavasaki ML, de Almeida SLH, de Aguiar DM. Geographic distribution of *Ehrlichia canis* TRP genotypes in Brazil. Veterinary Sciences. 2020;7:165. DOI: 10.3390/vetsci7040165

[32] Bremer WG, Schaefer JJ, Wagner ER, Ewing SA, Rikihisa Y, Needham GR, et al. Transstadial and intrastadial experimental transmission of *Ehrlichia canis* by male *Rhipicephalus sanguineus*. Veterinary Parasitology. 2005;**131**:95-105. DOI: 10.1016/j.vetpar.2005.04.030

[33] Fonsêca ADV, Oliveira LMB, Jorge FR, Cavalcante RO, Bevilaqua CML, Pinto FJM, et al. Occurrence of tick-borne pathogens in dogs in a coastal region of the state of Ceará, Northeastern Brazil. Revista Brasileira de Parasitologia Veterinária. 2022;**31**:e021321. DOI: 10.1590/s1984-29612022010

[34] Diniz P, Moura de Aguiar D. Ehrlichiosis and Anaplasmosis: An update. The Veterinary Clinics of North America. Small Animal Practice. 2022;**52**:1225-1266. DOI: 10.1016/j.cvsm.2022.07.002

[35] Judy L, David K, Peter K, Dhaval S. Canine ehrlichiosis seropositivity and associated factors in Kenya and Tanzania: A retrospective study. BMC Veterinary Research. 2023;**19**:175. DOI: 10.1186/s12917-023-03746-6

[36] Miró G, Wright I, Michael H, Burton W, Hegarty E, Rodón J, et al. Seropositivity of main vector-borne pathogens in dogs across Europe. Parasites & Vectors. 2022;**15**:189. DOI: 10.1186/s13071-022-05316-5

[37] Aguiar DM, Cavalcante GT, Pinter A, Gennari SM, Camargo LM, Labruna MB. Prevalence of *Ehrlichia canis* (Rickettsiales: Anaplasmataceae) in dogs and *Rhipicephalus sanguineus* (Acari: Ixodidae) ticks from Brazil. Journal of Medical Entomology. 2007;**44**:126-132. DOI: 10.1603/0022-2585(2007)44[126:poecra]2.0.co;2

[38] de Oliveira GMB, da Silva IWG, da Cruz Ferreira EAM, de Azevedo Serpa MC, Silva CAN, Dutra V, et al. Tick-borne pathogens in dogs, wild small mammals and their ectoparasites in the semiarid Caatinga biome, northeastern Brazil. Ticks and Tick-borne Diseases. 2020;**11**:101409. DOI: 10.1016/j.ttbdis.2020.101409

[39] Paula WVDF, Taques ÍIGG, Miranda VC, Barreto ALG, Paula LGFD, Martins DB, et al.

Seroprevalence and hematological abnormalities associated with *Ehrlichia canis* in dogs referred to a veterinary teaching hospital in central-western Brazil. Ciência Rural. 2022;**52**:e20201131. DOI: 10.1590/0103-8478cr20201131

[40] Queiroz S, Aguiar D, Silva Junior E, Reggiani D, Carvalho T, Agopian R, et al. Detection and laboratory findings due to *Ehrlichia canis* in dogs from the south area of São Paulo – SP, Brazil. Brazilian Journal of Global Health. 2022;**2**(7):1-5

[41] Brandão VMD, Barrozo PHM, Sousa LO, Santos RCD, Schwanke K, Sampaio Junior FD, et al. Molecular detection of *Ehrlichia canis* and *Anaplasma platys* in dogs from the municipality of Belém, State of Pará, Brazil. Ciência Rural. 2019;**49**:e20190414. DOI: 10.1590/0103-8478cr20190414

[42] Costa JS, Melo ALT, Witter R, Pacheco TA, Chitarra CS, Carvalho ITS, et al. Molecular detection of *Ehrlichia canis* in *Rhipicephalus sanguineus* (s.l.) ticks in dogs and their domestic environment in Cuiaba, MT, Brazil. Brazilian Journal of Veterinary Research and Animal Science. 2019;**56**(2):e153661

[43] Guimarães MDCN, de Aguiar PT, Monteiro TRM, dos Santos CDC, Costa JC, Valente KF, et al. Occurrence of tick-borne diseases in domestic dogs in Belém, Pará, Brazil. Acta Veterinaria Brasilica. 2021;**15**:323-329. DOI: 10.21708/avb.2021.15.4.10133

[44] Pereira ME, Canei DH, Carvalho MR, Dias ÁFLR, de Almeida A, Nakazato L, et al. Molecular prevalence and factors associated with *Ehrlichia canis* infection in dogs from the North Pantanal wetland, Brazil. Veterinary World. 2023;**16**:1209-1213. DOI: 10.14202/vetworld.2023.1209-1213

[45] Minervino AHH, Marcili A, Moraes-Filho J, Lima JTR, Soares HS, Malheiros AF, et al. Molecular detection of tick-borne pathogens in dogs from indigenous communities, Amazon, Brazil. Vector-Borne and Zoonotic Diseases. 2023;**23**:458-464. DOI: 10.1089/vbz.2023.0014

[46] Nogueira LLC, Braga JFV, Sousa RLP, Araújo BVS, Guimarães ALCG, Carmo LDAO, et al. Occurrence of pathogens transmitted by Rhipicephalus sanguineus sensu lato ticks in dogs in the semiarid region of Rio Grande do Norte state, Brazil. Pesquisa Veterinaria Brasileira. 2024;**44**:e07366. DOI: 10.1590/1678-5150-PVB-7366

[47] Fernandes NNU, Jorge FR, Costa VMD, Rodrigues A, Magalhães MML, Junior RSL, et al. Evaluating the circulation of *Ehrlichia canis* and Rickettsia spp. in domestic dogs from a semiarid region in Brazil. Veterinary Parasitology, Regional Studies and Reports. 2024;**52**:101041. DOI: 10.1016/j.vprsr.2024.101041

[48] Carvalho JPDS, Calazans APF, Oliveira GMSD, Alves LF, Santos LDM, Silva FB, et al. Epidemiologia de Ehrlichia canis: aspectos hematológicos, bioquímicos, fatores associados e moleculares em cães hígidos no município de Porto Seguro, Bahia, Brasil. Semina: Ciencias Agrarias. 2024;**45**:659-676. DOI: 10.5433/1679-0359.2024v45n3p659

[49] Harrus S, Waner T, Friedmann-Morvinski D, Fishman Z, Bark H, Harmelin A. Down-regulation of MHC class II receptors of DH82 cells, following infection with *Ehrlichia canis*. Veterinary Immunology and Immunopathology. 2003;**96**:239-243. DOI: 10.1016/j.vetimm.2003.08.005

[50] Ismail N, Sharma A, Soong L, Walker DH. Review: Protective

immunity and immunopathology of Ehrlichiosis. Zoonoses (Burlington). 2022;**2**:10.15212/zoonoses-2022-0009. DOI: 10.15212/zoonoses-2022-0009

[51] Sharma AK, Ismail N. Noncanonical inflammasome pathway: The role of cell death and inflammation in Ehrlichiosis. Cells. 2023;**12**:2597. DOI: 10.3390/cells12222597

[52] Cárdenas AM, Doyle CK, Zhang X, Nethery K, Corstvet RE, Walker DH, et al. Enzyme-linked immunosorbent assay with conserved immunoreactive glycoproteins gp36 and gp19 has enhanced sensitivity and provides species-specific immunodiagnosis of *Ehrlichia canis* infection. Clinical and Vaccine Immunology. 2007;**14**:123-128. DOI: 10.1128/cvi.00361-06

[53] McBride JW, Walker DH. Molecular and cellular pathobiology of Ehrlichia infection: Targets for new therapeutics and immunomodulation strategies. Expert Reviews in Molecular Medicine. 2011;**13**:e3. DOI: 10.1017/s1462399410 001730

[54] Zhang X, Luo T, Keysary A, Baneth G, Miyashiro S, Strenger C, et al. Genetic and antigenic diversities of major immunoreactive proteins in globally distributed *Ehrlichia canis* strains. Clinical and Vaccine Immunology. 2008;**15**:1080-1088. DOI: 10.1128/cvi.00482-07

[55] McBride JW, Corstvet RE, Gaunt SD, Boudreaux C, Guedry T, Walker DH. Kinetics of antibody response to Ehrlichia canis immunoreactive proteins. Infection and Immunity. 2003;**71**:2516-2524. DOI: 10.1128/iai.71.5.2516-2524.2003

[56] Byerly CD, Patterson LL, McBride JW. Ehrlichia TRP effectors: Moonlighting, mimicry and infection. Pathogens and Disease. 2021;**79**:ftab026. DOI: 10.1093/femspd/ftab026

[57] Nethery KA, Doyle CK, Zhang X, McBride JW. *Ehrlichia canis* gp200 contains dominant species-specific antibody epitopes in terminal acidic domains. Infection and Immunity. 2007;**75**:4900-4908. DOI: 10.1128/iai.00041-07

[58] Parthiban ABR, Palavesam A, Srinivasan S, Mohanan A, Ghosh S, Krishnaswamy Gopalan T. Molecular characterization of *Ehrlichia canis* from naturally infected dogs reveals a novel Asiatic-lineage and co-circulation of multiple lineages in India. Research in Veterinary Science. 2024;**175**:105311. DOI: 10.1016/j.rvsc.2024.105311

[59] Mylonakis ME, Theodorou KN. Canine monocytic Ehrlichiosis: An update on diagnosis and treatment. Acta Veterinaria. 2017;**67**:299-317. DOI: 10.1515/acve-2017-0025

[60] Aziz MU, Hussain S, Song B, Ghauri HN, Zeb J, Sparagano OA. Ehrlichiosis in dogs: A comprehensive review about the pathogen and its vectors with emphasis on south and east Asian countries. Veterinary Sciences. 2022;**10**(1):21. DOI: 10.3390/vetsci10010021

[61] Verma S, Srivastava MK, Tiwari J, Srivastava A, Sachan R, Bhatt S, et al. Study of haematological and biochemical alterations in clinical cases of canine Ehrlichiosis to understand the clinical picture of the disease. Journal of Advances in Microbiology. 2024;**24**:48-56. DOI: 10.9734/jamb/2024/v24i6832

[62] Stanilov I, Gospodinova K, Petrov V, Miteva L, Tsachev I, Stanilova S. Enhanced production of IL-10 in PCR-positive dogs infected with *E. canis* and *A. phagocytophilum* facilitate specific

immune responses. Microorganisms. 2024;**12**:12. DOI: 10.3390/microorganisms12122516

[63] do Carmo GM, Crivellenti LZ, Bottari NB, Machado G, Borin-Crivellenti S, Moresco RN, et al. Butyrylcholinesterase as a marker of inflammation and liver injury in the acute and subclinical phases of canine Ehrlichiosis. Comparative Immunology, Microbiology and Infectious Diseases. 2015;**43**:16-21. DOI: 10.1016/j.cimid.2015.09.005

[64] de Almeida VGF, Xavier M d S, da Cunha NC, Teixeira R d S, Bax JC, Almosny NRP. Clinical and laboratory profile of dogs seroreactive to Ehrlichiosis treated at the Veterinary Medical Teaching Hospital in Niterói, State of Rio de Janeiro, Brazil. Acta Scientiae Veterinariae. 2021;**49**:1824. DOI: 10.22456/1679-9216.116039

[65] Pereira ME, Canei DH, Trevisan YPA, Maruyama FH, de Assis PN, Pavan E, et al. Urinary NGAL and KIM-1 in canine monocytic Ehrlichiosis. Veterinary Sciences. 2025;**12**:105. DOI: 10.3390/vetsci12020105

[66] Moraes LF, Takahira RK, Golim MA. Hematological and renal function evaluation in dogs with IMHA. Acta Scientiae Veterinariae. 2017;**45**:12. DOI: 10.22456/1679-9216.80789

[67] Singh A, Srivastava MK, Gupta KK. Ultrasonographic assessment of important abdominal organs in a dog naturally infected with *Ehrlichia canis*. Veterinary Practitioner. 2021;**22**:64-66

[68] Feng HM, Walker DH. Mechanisms of immunity to *Ehrlichia muris*: A model of monocytotropic Ehrlichiosis. Infection and Immunity. 2004;**72**:966-971. DOI: 10.1128/IAI.72. 2.966-971.2004

[69] Winslow GM, Bitsaktsis C. Immunity to the Ehrlichiae: New tools and recent developments. Current Opinion in Infectious Diseases. 2005;**18**:217-221. DOI: 10.1097/01.qco.00001683 81.86024.cf

[70] Harrus S, Waner T. Diagnosis of canine monocytotropic Ehrlichiosis (*Ehrlichia canis*): An overview. Veterinary Journal. 2011;**187**:292-296. DOI: 10.1016/j.tvjl.2010.02.001

[71] Castro MB, Szabó MPJ, Aquino L, Dagnoni AS, Alessi AC, Costa MT, et al. Immunophenotypical and pathological changes in dogs experimentally infected with *Ehrlichia canis*. Revista Brasileira de Parasitologia Veterinária. 2022;**31**:e021621. DOI: 10.1590/s1984-29612022020

[72] Davis SK, Selva KJ, Kent SJ, Chung AW. Serum IgA Fc effector functions in infectious disease and cancer. Immunology and Cell Biology. 2020;**98**:276-286. DOI: 10.1111/imcb.12306

[73] Tominello TR, Oliveira ERA, Hussain SS, Elfert A, Wells J, Golden B, et al. Emerging roles of autophagy and inflammasome in Ehrlichiosis. Frontiers in Immunology. 2019;**10**:1011. DOI: 10.3389/fimmu.2019.01011

[74] Mylonakis ME, Ceron JJ, Leontides L, Siarkou VI, Martinez S, Tvarijonaviciute A, et al. Serum acute phase proteins as clinical phase indicators and outcome predictors in naturally occurring canine monocytic Ehrlichiosis. Journal of Veterinary Internal Medicine. 2011;**25**:811-817. DOI: 10.1111/j.1939-1676.2011.0728.x

[75] Shipov A, Klement E, Reuveni-Tager L, Waner T, Harrus S. Prognostic indicators for canine monocytic Ehrlichiosis. Veterinary Parasitology.

2008;**153**:131-138. DOI: 10.1016/j.vetpar.2008.01.009

[76] Rodríguez-Alarcón CA, Beristain-Ruiz DM, Olivares-Muñoz A, Quezada-Casasola A, Pérez-Casio F, Álvarez-Martínez JA, et al. Demonstrating the presence of *Ehrlichia canis* DNA from different tissues of dogs with suspected subclinical Ehrlichiosis. Parasites & Vectors. 2020;**13**:518. DOI: 10.1186/s13071-020-04363-0

[77] Wang Y, Nair ADS, Alhassan A, Jaworski DC, Liu H, Trinkl K, et al. Multiple *Ehrlichia chaffeensis* genes critical for its persistent infection in a vertebrate host are identified by random mutagenesis coupled with in vivo infection assessment. Infection and Immunity. 2020;**88**(10):e00316-e00320. DOI: 10.1128/iai.00316-20

[78] Franco-Zetina M, Adame-Gallegos J, Dzul-Rosado K. Effectivity of diagnostic methods for the detection of human and canine monocytic Ehrlichiosis. Revista Chilena de Infectología. 2019;**36**:650-655. DOI: 10.4067/s0716-10182019000500650

[79] Wichianchot S, Hongsrichan N, Maneeruttanarungroj C, Pinlaor S, Iamrod K, Purisarn A, et al. A newly developed droplet digital PCR for *Ehrlichia canis* detection: Comparisons to conventional PCR and blood smear techniques. The Journal of Veterinary Medical Science. 2022;**84**:831-840. DOI: 10.1292/jvms.22-0086

[80] Nakaghi AC, Machado RZ, Ferro JA, Labruna MB, Chryssafidis AL, André MR, et al. Sensitivity evaluation of a single-step PCR assay using *Ehrlichia can*is p28 gene as a target and its application in diagnosis of canine Ehrlichiosis. Revista Brasileira de Parasitologia Veterinária. 2010;**19**(2):75-79

[81] Silva L, Oliveira P, Campos A, Silva V, Saturnino K, Braga Î, et al. Misdiagnosis of canine monocytic Ehrlichiosis: Why do we still risk animal lives? Brazilian Journal of Veterinary Research and Animal Science. 2023;**60**:e213508. DOI: 10.11606/issn.1678-4456. bjvras.2023.213508

[82] Kledmanee K, Suwanpakdee S, Krajangwong S, Chatsiriwech J, Suksai P, Suwannachat P, et al. Development of multiplex polymerase chain reaction for detection of *Ehrlichia canis, Babesia spp* and *Hepatozoon canis* in canine blood. The Southeast Asian Journal of Tropical Medicine and Public Health. 2009;**40**:35-39

[83] Bilgiç HB, Karagenç T, Simuunza M, Shiels B, Tait A, Eren H, et al. Development of a multiplex PCR assay for simultaneous detection of *Theileria annulata*, *Babesia bovis* and *Anaplasma marginale* in cattle. Experimental Parasitology. 2013;**133**:222-229. DOI: 10.1016/j.exppara.2012.11.005

[84] Azhahianambi P, Jyothimol G, Baranidharan G, Aravind M, Ram Narendran R, Latha BR, et al. Evaluation of multiplex PCR assay for detection of Babesia spp, *Ehrlichia canis* and *Trypanosoma evansi* in dogs. Acta Tropica. 2018;**188**:58-67. DOI: 10.1016/j.actatropica.2018.08.028

[85] Stillman BA, Monn M, Liu J, Thatcher B, Foster P, Andrews B, et al. Performance of a commercially available in-clinic ELISA for detection of antibodies against *Anaplasma phagocytophilum*, *Anaplasma platys*, *Borrelia burgdorferi*, *Ehrlichia canis*, and *Ehrlichia ewingii* and *Dirofilaria immitis* antigen in dogs. Journal of the American Veterinary Medical Association. 2014;**245**:80-86. DOI: 10.2460/javma. 245.1.8

[86] Liu J, Drexel J, Andrews B, Eberts M, Breitschwerdt E, Chandrashekar R.

Comparative evaluation of 2 In-clinic assays for vector-borne disease testing in dogs. Topics in Companion Animal Medicine. 2018;**33**:114-118. DOI: 10.1053/j.tcam.2018.09.003

[87] Bélanger M, Sorenson HL, France MK, Bowie MV, Barbet AF, Breitschwerdt EB, et al. Comparison of serological detection methods for diagnosis of *Ehrlichia canis* infections in dogs. Journal of Clinical Microbiology. 2002;**40**:3506-3508. DOI: 10.1128/jcm.40.9.3506-3508.2002

[88] Harris S, Alleman AR, Bark H, Mahan SM, Waner T. Comparison of three enzyme-linked immunosorbent assays with the indirect immunofluorescent antibody test for the diagnosis of canine infection with *Ehrlichia canis*. Veterinary Microbiology. 2002;**86**:361-368. DOI: 10.1016/s0378-1135(02)00022-6.4

[89] Kaewmongkol S, Suwan E, Sirinarumitr T, Jittapalapong S, Fenwick SG, Kaewmongkol G. Detection of specific IgM and IgG antibodies in acute canine monocytic Ehrlichiosis that recognize recombinant gp36 antigens. Heliyon. 2020;**6**:e04409. DOI: 10.1016/j.heliyon. 2020.e04409

[90] Dona FD, Gomes SA, Andriuc RA, Garosi L, Tauro A. Magnetic resonance findings of meningoencephalitis in a dog seroreactive to *Ehrlichia canis* in United Kingdom. Veterinary Record Case Reports. 2021;**9**:e50. DOI: 10.1002/vrc2.50

[91] Garcia RM, da Silva CPC, Pchevuzinske LM, Portilho FVR, Siqueira AK, Takahira RK, et al. Pleural effusion-related *Nocardia otitidiscaviarum*, *Anaplasma platys* and *Ehrlichia canis* coinfection in a dog. Brazilian Journal of Microbiology. 2023;**54**:2497-2504. DOI: 10.1007/s42770-023-01029-8

[92] DeGroat W, Abdelhalim H, Patel K, Mendhe D, Zeeshan S, Ahmed Z. Discovering biomarkers associated and predicting cardiovascular disease with high accuracy using a novel nexus of machine learning techniques for precision medicine. Scientific Reports. 2024;**14**:1. DOI: 10.1038/s41598-023-50600-8

[93] Cardoso SP, Honorio-França AC, França DCH, Silva LPS, Fagundes-Triches DLG, Neves MCB, et al. Effects of doxycycline treatment on hematological parameters, viscosity, and cytokines in canine monocytic Ehrlichiosis. Biology (Basel). 2023;**12**(8):1137. DOI: 10.3390/biology 12081137

[94] Del Fiol Fde S, Lopes LC, Toledo MI, Barberato-Filho S. Prescription patterns and antibiotic use in community-based infections. Revista da Sociedade Brasileira de Medicina Tropical. 2010;**43**:68-72. DOI: 10.1590/s0037-86822010000100015

[95] Marques do Rosário CJR, de Aguiar DM, Lima CAA, Coutinho DF, Pereira JG, Melo FA, et al. Association of polar fraction of *Ageratum conyzoides* from the Brazilian Amazon with doxycycline against infection of macrophages with *Ehrlichia canis*. South African Journal of Botany. 2023;**155**:90-97. DOI: 10.1016/j.sajb.2023.02.017

[96] Palacios M, Arteaga R, Calvo G. High-dose filgrastim treatment of non-regenerative pancytopenia associated with chronic canine Ehrlichiosis. Topics in Companion Animal Medicine. 2017;**32**:28-30. DOI: 10.1053/j.tcam.2017.05.005

[97] Jenkins S, Ketzis JK, Dundas J, Scorpio D. Efficacy of minocycline in naturally occurring nonacute *Ehrlichia canis* infection in dogs. Journal

of Veterinary Internal Medicine. 2018;**32**:217-221. DOI: 10.1111/jvim.14842

[98] Gamit PG, Patel AR, Mehta SA, Mavadiya SV, Patel MD, Parmar SM, et al. Clinico-diagnostic and therapeutic management of Ehrlichiosis in dog. Indian Journal of Animal Research. 2024;**58**:1529-1535. DOI: 10.18805/IJAR.B-5243

[99] Zhang J, Wang J, Kelly PJ, Zhang Y, Li M, Li J, et al. Experimental infection and coinfection with Chinese strains of *Ehrlichia canis* and Babesia vogeli in intact and splenectomized dogs: Insights on clinical, hematologic and treatment responses. Veterinary Parasitology. 2023;**323**:110032. DOI: 10.1016/j.vetpar.2023.110032

[100] Kasondra A, Gupta S, Bhai G, Saini VK. Therapeutic management of canine Ehrlichiosis with aid of blood transfusion: A case report. Journal of Parasitic Diseases. 2017;**41**:395-397. DOI: 10.1007/s12639-016-0813-2

[101] Bothrel JPM, Maciel LA, Oliveira LAT, Costa LF, Araújo I. Hematological findings of canine Ehrlichiosis: A case study. Research, Society and Development. 2024;**13**:e3513646021. DOI: 10.33448/rsd-v13i6.46021

[102] Sá IDSS, Sá R d S, Almeida LF d A, Araujo MSA, Lisboa Neto AF d LN, Silva JCFS, et al. Erliquiose canina: Relato de caso. Pubvet. 2018;**12**:1-6. DOI: 10.22256/pubvet.v12n6a118.1-6

[103] Atif FA, Mehnaz S, Qamar MF, Roheen T, Sajid MS, Ehtisham-Ul-Haque S, et al. Epidemiology, diagnosis, and control of canine infectious cyclic thrombocytopenia and granulocytic anaplasmosis: Emerging diseases of veterinary and public health significance. Veterinary Sciences. 2021;**8**:312. DOI: 10.3390/vetsci 8120312

[104] Zhang J, Wang J, Wang C. Whole genome sequencing and comparative analysis of the first *Ehrlichia canis* isolate in China. Microorganisms. 2024;**12**. DOI: 10.3390/microorganisms12010125

[105] Escribano D, Cihan H, Martínez-Subiela S, Levent P, Kocaturk M, Aytug N, et al. Changes in serum proteins in dogs with *Ehrlichia canis* infection. Microbial Pathogenesis. 2017;**113**:34-39. DOI: 10.1016/j.micpath.2017. 10.024

[106] Luo T, Zhang X, McBride JW. Major species-specific antibody epitopes of the *Ehrlichia chaffeensis* p120 and *E. canis* p140 orthologs in surface-exposed tandem repeat regions. Clinical and Vaccine Immunology. 2009;**16**:982-990. DOI: 10.1128/CVI.00048-09

[107] Luo T, Patel JG, Zhang X, McBride JW. Antibody reactive immunomes of *Ehrlichia chaffeensis* and *E. canis* are diverse and defined by conformational antigenic determinants. Frontiers in Cellular and Infection Microbiology. 2024;**13**:1321291. DOI: 10.3389/fcimb. 2023. 1321291

[108] van Schaik EJ, Fratzke AP, Gregory AE, Dumaine JE, Samuel JE. Vaccine development: Obligate intracellular bacteria new tools, old pathogens: The current state of vaccines against obligate intracellular bacteria. Frontiers in Cellular and Infection Microbiology. 2024;**14**:1282183. DOI: 10.3389/fcimb.2024.1282183

[109] Luo T, Patel JG, Zhang X, Walker DH, McBride JW. Immunoreactive protein repertoires of *Ehrlichia chaffeensis* and *E. canis* reveal the dominance of hypothetical proteins and conformation-dependent antibody epitopes. Infection and Immunity. 2021;**89**:e0022421. DOI: 10.1128/iai.00224-21

[110] Setubal JC, Almeida NF, Wattam AR. Comparative genomics for prokaryotes. Methods in Molecular Biology. 2018;**1704**:55-78. DOI: 10.1007/978-1-4939-7463-4_3

[111] Neave MJ, Mileto P, Joseph A, Reid TJ, Scott A, Williams DT, et al. Comparative genomic analysis of the first *Ehrlichia canis* detections in Australia. Ticks and Tick-borne Diseases. 2022;**13**:101909. DOI: 10.1016/j.ttbdis.2022.101909

[112] Magni R, Luchini A, Liotta L, Molestina RE. Proteomic analysis reveals pathogen-derived biomarkers of acute babesiosis in erythrocytes, plasma, and urine of infected hamsters. Parasitology Research. 2020;**119**:2227-2235. DOI: 10.1007/s00436-020-06712-5

[113] Pretorius A, Nefefe T, Thema N, Liebenberg J, Steyn H, van Kleef M. Screening for immune biomarkers associated with infection or protection against *Ehrlichia ruminantium* by RNA-sequencing analysis. Microbial Pathogenesis. 2024;**189**:106588. DOI: 10.1016/j.micpath.2024.106588

[114] Haglund S, Lager M, Gyllemark P, Andersson G, Ekelund O, Sundqvist M, et al. CXCL13 in laboratory diagnosis of Lyme neuroborreliosis-the performance of the recomBead and ReaScan CXCL13 assays in human cerebrospinal fluid samples. European Journal of Clinical Microbiology & Infectious Diseases. 2022;**41**:175-179. DOI: 10.1007/s10096-021-04350-y

Chapter 9

Aqueous Affairs of Red Blood Cell: Variations That Alter Parasite Growth

Priya Agrohi, Raja Babu Kushwah and Prashant K. Mallick

Abstract

Volume regulation is an important aspect of red blood cell (RBC) physiology that facilitates efficient transport of oxygen throughout the body. Ion channels are the key player in volume regulation allowing the movement of water and ions across the cell membrane. Dysfunction in ion channel activity can disturb the precise balance of ion transport and volume regulation, leading to the development of various disorders. Hereditary defects in RBC are well-known to provide protection against severe malaria. However, RBC's volume disorders may also impact on malaria protection which needs thorough investigation. In recent years, PIEZO1 and ATP2B4 genes were discovered to be involved in RBC volume homeostasis. These genes through calcium-activated potassium channel (Gardos channels) regulate RBC volume and may be involved in protection against severe malaria in humans. This chapter is an attempt to cover the dynamic interplay of RBC's volume regulation and its role in protection against severe malaria. This chapter also aims to provide insight on the complexity of genetic variants of human RBC that may affect malaria pathogenesis.

Keywords: *Plasmodium falciparum*, red blood cell, ion-channels, calcium homeostasis, ATP2B4, PIEZO1

1. Introduction

Red blood cell (RBC) act as an abode of malaria parasite during infection. Erythrocytic phase of malaria parasite is important for its asexual multiplication and survival [1]. Merozoites are completely developed within RBC and then released into the blood circulation. These are small, polarized, pear-shaped cells committed to invade uninfected RBC [2]. Merozoite consists of rhoptries and microneme having proteases, phospholipases, and lipids that aid in the invasion by inducing structural change on the RBC membrane [3]. A tight junction between the merozoite and RBC membrane facilitates its invasion [4]. Various parasite ligands are involved in the merozoite invasion with associated receptors on the surface of RBC. Erythrocyte binding antigen (EBA) family of proteins are the most important parasite ligands that are associated with glycophorins on RBC as receptor [5]. Another important

IntechOpen

category of parasite ligand is the reticulocyte binding proteins which interact with the complement receptor 1 (CR1) and basigin (CD147) as receptors [6]. Along with these ligands, merozoite surface proteins (MSP) are also strong candidates for invasion that mediate primary interaction with RBC [7]. Both ligands and receptors remain under natural selection, and polymorphisms on RBC membrane protein may reduce the invasion efficiency of parasite to ultimately show protection against severity of malaria [8].

After successful invasion, it alters RBC membrane, attains growth, replicates, and bursts to initiate another cycle of invasion which causes malaria pathogenesis [9]. On the other hand, various polymorphisms in RBC proteins have been reported to reduce malaria pathogenesis [10, 11]. These reported polymorphisms are either associated with ineffective invasion of merozoites or reduced growth and development within RBC, which in turn are associated with protection against the severity of malaria. Polymorphism in transporters of RBC ion channels can affect the RBC shape and volume [8, 12–15]. The mechanistic explanation of how RBC volume affects the severity of malaria is an ongoing area of research. The dysregulation of membrane ion transport results into dehydration of RBC with increased fraction of dense RBC, which further reduces parasite invasion and growth [16–19]. Dehydration of RBC is also a feature of different hemoglobinopathies that lowers parasitemia and severity of disease [18]. These hemoglobinopathy disorders are highly prevalent in malaria-endemic populations [20, 21]. RBC-related monogenic inherited diseases are most common due to selective pressure of malaria [17, 22]. This selective force is particularly high in malaria-endemic areas since these regions experienced high malaria transmission for a long period provide plenty of opportunity for natural selection to shape the human genome [23]. This chapter will provide an insight to RBC's volume homeostasis that has importance in its own life cycle and how any alteration may affect the life cycle of human malaria parasites. It will focus on the variations in the channels involved in RBC volume homeostasis and their role in malaria protection. Additionally, it will explore other genetic variations present in proteins of the RBC membrane and cytoplasm and their potential role against malaria that may provide us valuable insights to improvised therapeutic strategies against malaria.

2. Coexistence of RBC and malaria parasite

2.1 Malaria parasite life cycle within RBC

Red blood cells are prime target for the malaria parasite because of their abundance, lack of a nucleus, and availability of hemoglobin as a nutrition source [17]. RBC plays a key role in life cycle of malaria parasite as it is involved in survival and proliferation of parasite [1]. Human malaria begins with sporozoites being inoculated into the skin of a human by a female Anopheles mosquito. The sporozoites enter the liver by blood vessels and subsequently invade liver cells by passing through Kupffer cells [24]. In hepatocytes a parasite goes through schizogony where it divides into thousands of merozoites [25]. After the maturation of merozoites, infected hepatocytes rupture and released into bloodstream, where these enter into the RBC and initiate a new cycle of schizogony, where the haploid genome of parasite replicates asexually [26, 27]. During development inside RBC, parasites go through the ring, trophozoite, and schizont stage [17]. The adult schizont may comprise multiple (16–32) daughter merozoites and are released to invade fresh RBC once infected RBC (iRBC) gets ruptured [28]. This erythrocytic cycle in *Plasmodium malariae* takes around 72 hours, 48 hours for *Plasmodium vivax*, *Plasmodium falciparum,* and *Plasmodium ovale* and 24 hours for *Plasmodium knowlesi* [29, 30]. Apart from merozoites, ruptured RBC also produces numerous metabolic by-products, such as hemozoin, which is formed during digestion of hemoglobin. These by-product triggers immune system and causes various clinical symptoms such as fever, headache, and chills in human. Some patients may progress into severe form of malaria (cerebral malaria), acidosis, severe anemia, and death [31].

2.2 Malaria evolutionary force on RBC

Mutual evolution at both host and parasite has been observed due to long-term cellular interaction during infection [32]. In parasite the diversification is observed among proteins involved in invasion of RBC, and host showed the signature of selection on proteins interacting during parasite invasion, its growth, and host immunological genes [33]. As malaria parasite and human host co-evolved, genetic disorders are well-known to alter aspects of RBC biology and influence the malaria susceptibility or pathogenicity. In the erythrocytic phase of *P. falciparum*, first step of RBC and merozoite interaction is very important, and various parasite ligands are involved in its invasion with cognate receptor on the surface of RBC [5, 6, 34, 35]. Throughout the extensive evolutionary history of malaria parasites and humans, RBC has undergone various adaptive changes which include modifications in the receptors present on its surface which contribute to protection against parasite invasion in diverse geographic populations across the globe. Notable examples of such adaptations include mutations in glycophorin, complement receptor 1 (CR1), and band 3 protein. After the invasion, parasite grow and replicate inside RBC. This intracellular development is accompanied by several structural, biochemical, and functional alterations in RBC [9]. RBC proteins such as hemoglobin, intracellular enzymes, RBC ion channels, RBC surface proteins, and proteins associated with RBC shape and volume have been observed to reduce malaria pathogenesis [8, 11–15].

2.3 Relationship between RBC volume, calcium channels, and malaria protection

RBC volume dysregulation and malaria protection is an active area of research. The mechanisms behind the impact of RBC dehydration on malaria protection are still not fully decoded *in vivo*. However, *in vitro* studies showed that hydration of RBC plays a key role in parasite invasion and may result in the reduction of invasion efficiency or it becomes resistant to invasion of parasite [18]. Calcium channels play a key role in regulation of ion concentration and cell volume. These are indirectly involved in volume regulation by controlling the activity of other ion channels that directly affect RBC volume [36, 37]. RBC calcium homeostasis is maintained primarily by the calcium channels PMCA1 (plasma membrane calcium ATPase 1), PMCA4 (plasma membrane calcium ATPase 4), PIEZO1 (piezo type mechanosensitive ion channel component 1), eNMDARs (erythroid N-methyl D-aspartate receptor), and Gardos channels. Gardos channel is important in volume regulation of RBC and activated by increased intracellular calcium concentration. This channel plays a role during RVD by decreasing the ionic concentration inside RBC which causes efflux of potassium (K^+) ion followed by loss of water [38]. Out of all these channels, ATPase plasma membrane calcium transporting 4 (ATP2B4) and PIEZO1 emerge as strong candidates in malaria protection at various parts of the world. Both genes are involved in calcium homeostasis and dehydration of RBC. In human RBC, ATP2B4 gene encodes plasma membrane calcium ATPase (PMCA4). PMCA4 is an active calcium pump in RBC membrane and is involved in regulation of cellular calcium level [36]. Recently PIEZO1 channel is also identified in RBC membrane as a mechanosensitive, non-selective cation channel, and it is also permeable for calcium [39]. It also involved in RBC volume regulation by robust calcium influx [40, 41]. Clinical severity in sickle cell disease was observed due to RBC dehydration [42], and in contrast same phenomenon is involved in protection from malaria parasite [18]. This finding is supported in different malaria endemic population by GWAS and population-based studies, where genetic variation present in calcium channels of RBC has been linked with protection to severe *P. falciparum* malaria [11, 43–46].

3. RBC volume regulation mechanisms

3.1 Passive mechanisms

Natural function of red blood cell and its volume are maintained by the complex interaction between semi-permeable cell membrane and osmotic gradient. Understanding interaction permeability and osmotic gradient is essential to study the role of RBC in oxygen transport and in different diseases related to RBC physiology [47]. RBC membrane is selectively permeable, allows the free movement of water molecules (100 μm/s), and impermeable to most of the solutes inside the cell. Aquaporin water channels are essential for water exchange and osmotic water exchange, which supports in osmoregulation depending on the external environment [48]. Electrical neutrality persists on both sides of the plasma membrane at a steady state of cell, and diffusible ion concentrations remain equivalent on both sides of semi-permeable membrane as per Gibbs-Donnan equilibrium [49]. However, overall concentration of intracellular molecules is significantly higher than the concentration of extracellular molecules due to the existence of non-diffusible intracellular protein. Because of this concentration gradient, obligatory water movement occurs and creates osmotic gradient, so at steady state, this osmosis can cause cell swelling and eventually cell death [50]. In active transport of ions, Na^+/K^+ ATPase is the main player, where three sodium (Na^+) ions pump out of the cell in exchange for two potassium (K^+) ions to prevent cellular osmoexplosion [51].

3.1.1 Aquaporins

Aquaporins (AQP) are one of the major contributors in osmoregulation of a cell. These are integral membrane proteins which facilitate bidirectional water flow driven by osmotic pressure [52]. Along with water it also transports gases, glycerol, ammonia, and ions in a selective manner. In mammals, 13 aquaporins from AQP0 to AQP12 have been identified which are different in their water permeability and size [53, 54]. All AQPs possess a conserved structure consisting of six transmembrane alpha-helices which form a barrel-like configuration and two short alpha-helix domains on periplasmic and cytoplasmic side of the barrel. These domains contain asparagine-proline-alanine (NPA) motif which is AQP family's signature, also viewed as the "hourglass model" [55]. RBC has AQP1, formerly known as CHIP28 (channel-forming integral protein 28) is the most studied in water channels [56], and it is also expressed on central nervous system (CNS), kidneys, inner ears, lungs, eyes, and skeletal muscles [57]. One of the rare blood group systems, i.e., Colton blood group (CO) has been associated with AQP1 [58].

3.2 Active mechanisms

RBC volume regulation involves both passive and active mechanism, together these mechanisms ensure that the volume of RBC remains within the range for overall physiological balance. The primary means to regulate RBC volume is by means of control on the cell's solute concentration across plasma membrane results in modulation of intracellular water content [59]. Different ion channels present in RBC membrane are responsible for achieving electrochemical concentration gradient and hence regulate the cell volume. At steady-state, osmoexplosion is prevented, and RBC volume is maintained by Na^+/K^+ ATPase. It actively transports K^+ ions into the cell and Na^+ ions out of the cell, against their electrochemical gradients [51]. The K^+ ions further recycled through K^+ channels, and ATP is rapidly resynthesized from ADP and inorganic phosphate. This mechanism is called double Donnan mechanism or pump-leak balance, as shown in **Figure 1** [48].

RBC can readjust their volume rapidly in response to various environment changes like in transient anisotonic conditions. This readjustment is mediated by number of channels and transporters which results in the net flow of osmolytes and osmotically obligated water, as described in **Table 1**. However, cell experience hypertonic and hypotonic stress after that [48]. There are two ways of regulating cell volume in anisotonic conditions; regulatory volume increase (RVI) and regulatory volume decrease (RVD) in hypertonic and hypotonic conditions, respectively [60].

In hypertonic environment when osmotic cell shrinkage occurs, RVI is achieved by net influx of sodium chloride (NaCl) and water. There are three different cotransporter-mediated mechanisms responsible for RVI; (1) operation of Cl^- – HCO^{3-} antiporters (anion exchanger AE or band 3) and Na^+-H^+ antiporter (NHE)

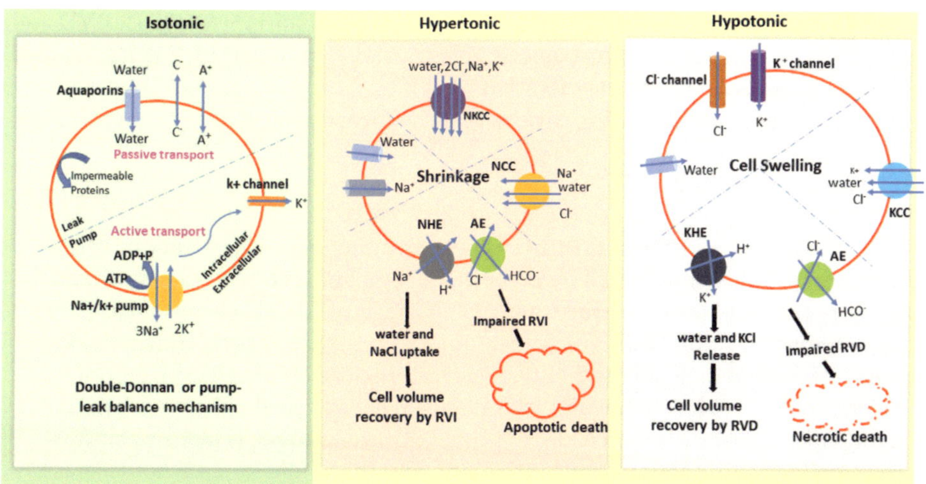

Figure 1.
Schematic illustration of the mechanisms for regulatory volume increase (RVI) and regulatory volume decrease (RVD) under different physiological conditions. In steady state under isotonic conditions, cell volume regulation occurred by the "double-Donnan" or "pump-leak balance" mechanism via the Na⁺, K⁺ pump in RBC. In hypertonic and hypotonic conditions, RVI and RVD occurred by different ion channels (see in text for details).

RBC transporter/ channels	Gene	Disorders
Na^+/K^+ ATPase	ATP1A1, ATP1B1 (ATPase Na^+/K^+ Transporting Subunit Alpha 1)	
NHE	SLC9A1 (Solute Carrier Family 9 Member A1)	
AE band 3	SLC4A1 (Solute Carrier Family 4 Member 1 or Diego Blood Group)	Southeast Asian Ovalocytosis
Na^+-Cl^- symporter (NCC)	SLC12A3 (Solute Carrier Family 12 Member 3)	
Na^+-K^+-$2Cl^-$ symporter (NKCC)	SLC12A1 (Solute Carrier Family 12 Member 1)	
K^+ and Cl^- symporter (KCC)	SLC12A4 (Solute Carrier Family 12 Member 4)	
Gardos channels	KCNN4 (Potassium Calcium-Activated Channel Subfamily N Member 4)	Hereditary Xerocytosis, Dehydrated Hereditary Stomatocytosis
PMCA	ATP2B4 (ATPase Plasma Membrane Ca2+ Transporting 4)	RBC dehydration in malaria resistance in humans
PIEZO1	PIEZO1 (Piezo Type Mechanosensitive Ion Channel Component 1)	Dehydrated Hereditary Stomatocytosis Hereditary Xerocytosis

Table 1.
Ion channels involved in RBC volume regulation and its associated disorders.

parallelly, (2) operation of Na^+-Cl^- symporter (NCC), (3) operation of Na^+-K^+-$2Cl^-$ symporter (NKCC) in different cell type [61–63]. In hypotonic condition when osmotic cell swelling occurs, RVD is achieved by net potassium chloride (KCl) efflux. RBC transporters involved in this are K^+ and Cl^- symporter (KCC) or Cl^- channels like K^+-Cl^- symporter, Cl^--$HCO3^-$ (AE or band 3 protein) antiporters [64]. RVD and RVI are essential in maintaining osmotic balance and ensure that RBC neither swells or shrinks excessively to preserve its structural integrity. It also allows RBC to adapt as per external environment during diverse physiological conditions.

3.3 Calcium channels in RBC

Calcium ions (Ca^{2+}) are indirectly involved in either osmotic balance or hydration activity of RBC; however, it involves in the regulation of different ion channels which play prominent role during water homeostasis of RBC [37]. Apart from this, calcium homeostasis of a cell is important for various reasons as calcium acts as a universal signaling molecule and also involves in regulation of cell cycle, motility, and structural integrity [65]. RBC differentiation is also relied on Ca^{2+}-dependent signaling [65]. After differentiation, mature RBC lacks intracellular calcium storage organelles such as endoplasmic reticulum, and the whole calcium homeostasis depends on the calcium channels of plasma membrane. A balance between active calcium extrusion and passive calcium influx supports in the maintenance of low cytoplasmic calcium concentration Ca^{2+} (30–60 nM) as compared to high blood calcium concentration (1.8 mM) [36]. Low intracellular calcium concentration is important for RBC physiology as it can become dehydrated, if not able to maintain the low intracellular calcium concentration, as in the case of sickle cell disease and RBC aging. During increased intracellular calcium, a calcium-activated potassium channel, i.e., Gardos channels become activated which causes potassium efflux, water loss, and consequently, RBC volume loss called as Gardos effect [66, 67].

4. Genetic evolutions in RBC towards tolerance to malaria

Malaria has been a strong evolutionary force that can be evidenced at different populations which have developed independent genetic variations for protection against severe malaria [68]. Most of the genetic variation developed is related to the RBC structure and function [9]. Major of the protective variations lie among surface proteins of RBC involved in parasite invasion and proteins involved in RBC's physiology affecting parasite growth and replication. Below is the detailed description of variation in proteins of RBC cell membrane and changes induced by malaria parasite selection pressure affecting its physiology.

4.1 Variations on RBC cell membrane affecting parasite invasion

4.1.1 Glycophorins and MNS blood group

Glycophorins are the most abundant sialo-glycoproteins on human erythrocyte membranes which act as receptors for various pathogens, including *Plasmodium spp.* Genetic variations in the glycophorin region (GYPA, GYPB, and GYPE genes) on chromosome-4 are of interest, particularly the Dantu hybrid glycophorin variant associated with a 40% reduction in severe malaria incidence in East African communities [69]. Glycophorins play a key role in malaria parasite invasion of erythrocytes, with GPA and GPB served as receptors for *P. falciparum* ligands like EBA-175 [70]. The GYPA and GYPB genes also contribute to the MNS blood group system [71], and their fusion produced the rare blood group Dantu [72]. Absence of glycophorins on RBC surfaces is linked with protection against malaria. An En(a-) mutation lacking Glycophorin A is associated with *P. falciparum* malaria protection [73–75] and a haplotype, including GYPA, GYPB, and Dantu, provided 33% protection from severe falciparum malaria [8, 76]. Dantu's effect on *P. falciparum* merozoite invasion of RBC is linked to changes in the RBC surface protein repertoire. Video microscopy revealed a significant correlation between RBC tension and merozoite invasion, with Dantu cells exhibited higher average surface tension, providing an explanation for the protection from malaria [77].

4.1.2 SLC4A (hereditary elliptocytosis)

Band 3, encoded by the SLC4A gene, is an important glycoprotein in the RBC membrane. It facilitates chloride and bicarbonate exchange and also vital for carbon dioxide respiration [78]. Band 3 also plays a key role in *P. falciparum* invasion as a host receptor for merozoite surface protein 1 (MSP1) [7]. Heterozygous deletion of codons in band 3 causes the ovalocytotic phenotype in a RBC membrane disorder called as Southeast Asian ovalocytosis (SAO) [79]. Individuals with heterozygous SAO show reduced RBC anion transport and altered RBC membrane protein structures [80]. Interestingly, SAO mutations confer resistance to both *P. vivax* and *P. falciparum* malaria [81, 82]. Homozygotes for the ovalocytosis allele may face mortality risks, but heterozygotes have an advantage against malaria [83]. The protective mechanism involves an aberrant band 3 protein binding tightly to ankyrin in cytoskeleton, increasing RBC stiffness and resisting invasion of malaria parasite [84].

4.1.3 DARC

DARC (Duffy antigen receptor for chemokines), is a glycosylated membrane protein with seven transmembrane domains encoded by FY gene. It acts as a non-specific receptor for various chemokines and serves as the entry receptor for *P. vivax* [85] and *P. knowlesi* [86, 87]. The FY*ES allele is associated with the absence of the Duffy antigen, and prevalent in Sub-Saharan Africa, indicates strong positive natural selection due to its role in malaria resistance [88, 89]. Polymorphism in DARC is one of the key examples of malaria exerting selective pressure on the human genome [86, 88, 90, 91].

4.1.4 ADGRE1 (EMR1)

EGF-Like Module Receptor 1 (EMR1) encodes a transmembrane glycoprotein resembling G protein-coupled receptors, having cell-adhesion and cell-cell interaction properties [92]. EMR1 is associated with malaria susceptibility as polymorphisms (e.g., rs373533) showed associations with malaria-associated seizures and hyperpyrexia among African populations [93, 94]. A genome-wide study on *P. chabaudi* observed significant changes in DNA methylation, affecting the expression of seven genes, including EMR1. These alterations were associated with differentially methylated promoters, suggesting a potential epigenetic influence on the host's response to malaria. Its exact role in malaria protection remains unclear, however, highlighted the complex relationship between epigenetic modifications and malaria protection [95].

4.1.5 ABCB6

ATP binding cassette subfamily B member 6 (ABCB6), a member of the ATP-binding cassette transporter family, acts as a porphyrin transporter in nucleated cells for heme biosynthesis. ABCB6 is responsible for the Lan blood group antigen on RBC. Individuals lacking Lan (Lan null) are asymptomatic, and ABCB6's role in adult human erythrocytes is unclear [96, 97]. Erythrocytes lacking the Lan protein demonstrate protection to invasion by *P. falciparum* parasites. Interestingly porphyrin accumulation or porphyrin-induced toxicity is not the reason behind this protection, which implies that in Lan null RBC, protective role operates independently of LAN's porphyrin transport function.

4.2 Variations in RBC physiology affecting parasite growth

RBC physiological variation includes gene responsible for altered growth of parasite inside RBC; it includes oxidative stressed genes, hemoglobinopathies, enzymopathies, and RBC volume alteration [68]. The role of oxidative stress in the early clearance of iRBC is closely linked to the activity of key genes, such as G6PD and NOS2. G6PD plays a key role in maintaining cellular redox balance, while NOS2 contributes to the generation of reactive nitrogen species, collectively influencing the dynamics of iRBC clearance during the course of infection [98].

4.2.1 G6PD

Glucose-6-phosphate dehydrogenase (G6PD) gene on the X-chromosome encodes key enzyme protecting erythrocytes from oxidative stress caused by reactive oxygen species. G6PD deficiency, an X-linked recessive condition affecting around 400 million people globally, is associated with a reduced risk of malaria [99]. G6PD-deficient RBC showed a reduction in growth of *P. falciparum* parasite in in vitro study [100]. Studies in African children demonstrated a 46–58% lower risk of severe malaria in G6PD-deficient individuals supporting a selective advantage in malaria-prone regions [101]. The most common G6PD variant named Mahidol is associated with reduced *P. vivax* density in Southeast Asia and showed strong positive selection over the past 1500 years driven by malaria [102].

4.2.2 NOS2

Inducible nitric oxide synthase (iNOS) encoded by the nitric oxide synthase 2 (NOS2) gene generates nitric oxide (NO), a free radical with antiparasitic effects. However, NO's immunosuppressive impact and its potential role in malaria protection is unclear. In a Gabonese study, the A954C allele of NOS2 was associated with elevated NO synthase activity, providing protection from severe malaria and reinfection [103]. Another study conducted among Tanzanian and Kenyan children suggested that polymorphisms in the NOS2 gene promoter region enhance NO production, which has a potential antimalarial effect [104].

4.2.3 Hemoglobinopathies

Hemoglobinopathies are the genetic abnormalities in hemoglobin's structure and function. It encompasses variations like structural hemoglobin anomalies and thalassemia, affecting the production of hemoglobin. The Hemoglobin Subunit Alpha (HBA) genes (HBA1 and HBA2) and Hemoglobin Subunit Beta (HBB) gene, encoding α- and β-globins, respectively, are located on chromosomes 11 and 16 [105]. One variable HBB gene is HbAS allele causes sickle cell trait, a polymorphism observed at 10% frequency in many malaria-endemic regions [106]. HbAS leads to sickle-shaped erythrocytes under low oxygen conditions, offering protection against severe malaria. This protection is linked to mechanisms like enhanced phagocytosis of infected HbAS erythrocytes and reduced parasite growth and invasion [107–110] and shows 10-fold lower risk of severe malaria [111, 112].

Hemoglobin C carriers also demonstrate protection against malaria [113]. Hemoglobin C alters the surface characteristics of *P. falciparum*-infected erythrocytes, reduces its adhesion to endothelial cells, and minimizes sequestration in the microvasculature. Various association studies, including one in the Luo tribe of Kenya, provide evidence of the HBB gene's role in malaria resistance. Overall, these genetic variations showcase the intricate interplay between hemoglobinopathies and malaria susceptibility, highlighting the complex evolutionary adaptations in diverse populations [114].

4.3 Variations among RBC calcium channels affecting parasite growth

Recent studies have expanded our understanding about the evolutionary adaptations in humans and suggested that calcium channels also play a key role in malaria protection. Understanding how variations in calcium channels affect the RBC's response to parasite infection may add a new layer to the whole phenomenon. Here are some of the recently discovered genetic variation related to calcium channels.

4.3.1 PIEZO1 (FAM38A)

PIEZO1 is a mechanosensitive, non-selective cation channel. It aids in sensing mechanical stimuli in various multicellular organisms [115]. In vertebrates, PIEZO1 and PIEZO2 are present with homologs in invertebrates regulating blood pressure and RBC volume [116, 117]. Gain-of-function mutations in PIEZO1 gene have been associated with dehydrated hereditary stomatocytosis (DHS) [118, 119]. A new gain-of-function mutation observed in PIEZO1 gene, prevalent in one-third of people of African decedent has been shown inhibited Plasmodium infection [45]. This mutation (E756Ddel) characterized by TCC deletion specifically removes one glutamic acid from a stretch of seven in wild type. This deletion leads to increased calcium influx in RBC and activates the Gardos channel to cause RBC dehydration. Mouse model for hereditary xerocytosis (HX) has demonstrated that Plasmodium infection does not generate experimental cerebral malaria in these mice due to PIEZO1 activation among RBC and T cells [45]. The heterozygosity for E756del did not provide additive protection in sickle cell trait (HbAS) patients, whereas homozygosity was linked to an increased risk of severe illness, implying an epistatic interaction between HbAS and PIEZO1 E756del. Surface protein analysis in heterozygotes revealed low expression of the *P. falciparum* virulence protein named *Plasmodium falciparum* erythrocyte membrane protein-1 (PfEMP-1) [120]. Despite this, a study conducted in Ghana observed no significant association between them [121]. The actual mechanism of protection is not known but compound Yoda-1, a PIEZO1 activator, prevents *P. falciparum* invasion into RBC without affecting intraerythrocytic growth, and suggests a mechanism unrelated to RBC dehydration or ion imbalance [122].

4.3.2 ATP2B4

The ATP2B4 gene encodes a P-type primary ion transport ATPase that removes bivalent Ca^{2+} ion from the eukaryotic cell against high concentration gradient and play important role in calcium homeostasis. PMCA4 serves as a key exporter of Ca^{2+} ion in case of human RBC and expression analysis showed a lower PMCA4 expression caused an impaired calcium efflux from the RBC. About 1.58 to 1.67-fold higher overall Ca^{2+} ion levels were observed in RBC with low PMCA4 when compared to RBC with average level of PMCA4. This study observed mutations in the promoter region that was highly correlated with this lower PMCA4 protein levels [123]. Till date, Gardos-mediated dehydration of RBC due to the mutant ATP2B4 gene is only possible mechanism explained for the malaria protection, and mechanistic link is yet to be established [44]. Population-based and in vitro studies showed variation in ATP2B4 gene is associated with increased MCHC [11] that protect from mild and severe malaria [10, 124]. In addition, low PMCA expression [44, 123] reduced parasite density [125] and slow growth of falciparum [126], which may attribute to protection against severity in malaria [18]. Recent study showed inhibition of PMCA4 by aurintricarboxylic acid (ATA), and Resveratrol can cease the growth of *P. falciparum* inside RBC [127].

4.3.3 KCNN4

KCNN4 (Potassium Calcium-Activated Channel Subfamily N Member 4) gene encodes for Gardos channels which are calcium-activated potassium channels and regulated by intracellular calcium. Its activation is followed by membrane hyperpolarization and loss of KCl and water from the RBC. Its role in malaria protection in sickle cell disease is uncertain, and the Gardos channels inhibitor Senicapoc effectively reduced RBC dehydration. The compound Senicapoc demonstrated inhibition of Plasmodium development inside RBC in in vitro studies. While, administration of Senicapoc led to a reduction in *Plasmodium yoelii* parasitemia in mice, indicating its potential as an antimalarial agent through its influence on RBC hydration dynamics [46].

Interestingly, various ion channels within red blood cells, including those discussed here, have been associated with disorders related to cell volume regulation, such as stomatocytosis, dehydrated hereditary xerocytosis, and ovalocytosis (as illustrated in **Table 1**). These volume-related disorders have been intriguingly linked with protection against malaria in diverse human populations residing in malaria-endemic regions [17]. These volume-related variations underscore the interactions among malaria protection and RBC volume regulation. It presents different prospects for the development of novel therapeutic approaches and for the improvement of our knowledge of the complex interaction between human hosts and malaria parasites.

4.4 Disorders in RBC volume regulation in response to malaria pressure

Erythrocyte dehydration is classified into primary and secondary categories. Primary disorders, such as hereditary xerocytosis syndromes, are intrinsic volume regulation disorders that directly lead to erythrocyte dehydration. On the other hand, secondary dehydration is linked to various diseases which influence the RBC hydration. In both classes, understanding the role of ion channels is important not just for understanding problems associated with RBC dehydration but also for investigating possible links to disease like malaria, where changes in RBC hydration state affect its defenses against the malaria parasite. Disorders like hemoglobinopathies, thalassemia, sickle cell disease, hereditary spherocytosis, and Southeast Asian ovalocytosis showed a significant role of erythrocyte dehydration in associated pathophysiology [128]. One more RBC condition known as hereditary xerocytosis (HX) is also marked by increased cellular dehydration. Dehydration of red blood cells has been linked with mutations in genes including PIEZO1, KCNN4, and ATP2B4. It is interesting to note that these genes have been linked to both providing protection against malaria and the pathophysiology of HX. Prior research has linked PIEZO1 and KNCC4 to RBC dehydration but no direct association has been found between ATP2B4 and any dehydration disorder. However, increased calcium levels in RBC, which are facilitated by these genes, activate the Gardos channels, resulting in cellular dehydration, which is the hallmark of HX. The resultant alterations in RBC hydration contribute to a protective effect against malaria [18], highlighting the intricate interplay between genetic factors, ion homeostasis, and the RBC's response to malaria.

5. Conclusions

The role of membrane proteins, enzymopathies, and RBC hemoglobinopathies in malaria protection has been thoroughly investigated. However, limited knowledge of altered volume in RBC due to defects in calcium channels need more investigations to add new perspective toward the context of malaria susceptibility. The Gardos effect, activated by calcium influx, influences RBC dehydration and also linked to the

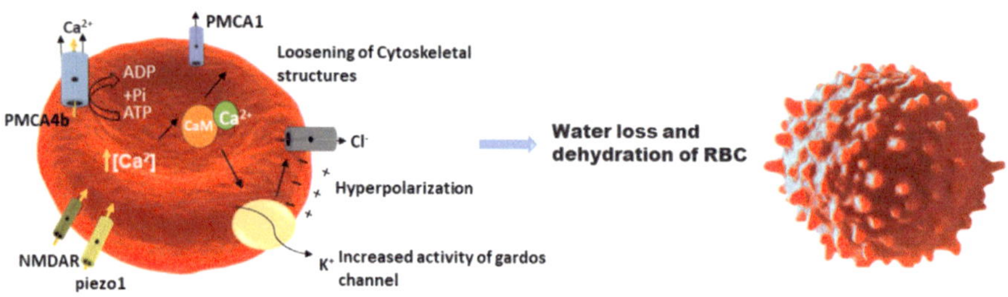

Figure 2.
Calcium ion channels of red blood cell (RBC). Mutation in these channels leads to increased intracellular Ca^{2+} ion concentration (depicted by yellow arrow). This increased intracellular calcium concentration triggers the hyperpolarization, loosening of cytoskeleton, and Gardos effect, leading to excessive potassium efflux through Gardos channels and subsequent loss of water from the RBC. Consequently, the RBC undergoes dehydration.

severity in malaria outcomes. In conclusion, studies of RBC volume-regulating ion channels—specifically, calcium channels, and their role on malaria protection provide a unique perspective in the context of malaria susceptibility.

Pharmaceutical research on inhibitors to Gardos channels and PMCA and activators of PIEZO1 highlight the potential of targeted treatment strategies in case of malaria. The compound Senicapoc, a Gardos channels inhibitor, inhibits growth of *P. falciparum* as well as treats RBC's dehydration in sickle cell disease. The compound Yoda-1 showed collective inhibition of PMCA and activation of PIEZO1 that indicates complex relationship between calcium homeostasis and malaria as it prevents invasion of Plasmodium. Despite the previous research, a complete understanding of links between alterations of RBC volume, calcium channels, and malaria protection remains a growing narrative. This chapter is an attempt to navigate the unexplored areas of research in calcium homeostasis of RBC, and it is anticipated to serve as a foundation for avenues toward new approaches in the fight against malaria (**Figure 2**).

Conflict of interest

The authors declare no conflict of interest.

Author details

Priya Agrohi[1,2], Raja Babu Kushwah[3] and Prashant K. Mallick[1,2]*

1 National Institute of Malaria Research, New Delhi, India

2 Academy of Scientific and Innovative Research (AcSIR), Ghaziabad, Uttar Pradesh, India

3 Texas A&M University, USA

*Address all correspondence to: pkmmrc01@gmail.com

References

[1] Burns AL et al. Targeting malaria parasite invasion of red blood cells as an antimalarial strategy. FEMS Microbiology Reviews. 2019;**43**(3):223-238. DOI: 10.1093/femsre/fuz005

[2] White NJ, Pukrittayakamee S, Hien TT, Faiz MA, Mokuolu OA, Dondorp AM. Malaria. The Lancet. 2014;**383**(9918):723-735. DOI: 10.1016/S0140-6736(13)60024-0

[3] Bannister L, Mitchell G. The ins, outs and roundabouts of malaria. Trends in Parasitology. 2003;**19**(5):209-213. DOI: 10.1016/S1471-4922(03)00086-2

[4] Keeley A, Soldati D. The glideosome: A molecular machine powering motility and host-cell invasion by apicomplexa. Trends in Cell Biology. 2004;**14**(10):528-532. DOI: 10.1016/j.tcb.2004.08.002

[5] Tham W-H, Healer J, Cowman AF. Erythrocyte and reticulocyte binding-like proteins of *Plasmodium falciparum*. Trends in Parasitology. 2012;**28**(1):23-30. DOI: 10.1016/j.pt.2011.10.002

[6] Crosnier C et al. Basigin is a receptor essential for erythrocyte invasion by *Plasmodium falciparum*. Nature. 2011;**480**(7378):534-537. DOI: 10.1038/nature10606

[7] Baldwin M et al. Human erythrocyte band 3 functions as a receptor for the sialic acid-independent invasion of *Plasmodium falciparum*. Role of the RhopH3-MSP1 complex. Biochimica et Biophysica Acta. 2014;**1843**(12):2855-2870. DOI: 10.1016/j.bbamcr.2014.08.008

[8] Leffler EM et al. Resistance to malaria through structural variation of red blood cell invasion receptors. Science. 2017;**356**(6343):eaam6393. DOI: 10.1126/science.aam6393

[9] Cooke B, Mohandas N, Coppel R. The malaria-infected red blood cell: Structural and functional changes. In: Advances in Parasitology. Vol. 50. Academic Press; 2001. pp. 1-86. DOI: 10.1016/S0065-308X(01)50029-9

[10] Band G et al. Insights into malaria susceptibility using genome-wide data on 17,000 individuals from Africa, Asia and Oceania. Nature Communications. 2019;**10**:5732. DOI: 10.1038/s41467-019-13480-z

[11] Malaria Genomic Epidemiology Network and Malaria Genomic Epidemiology Network. Reappraisal of known malaria resistance loci in a large multicenter study. Nature Genetics. 2014;**46**(11):1197-1204. DOI: 10.1038/ng.3107

[12] Weatherall DJ. Common genetic disorders of the red cell and the malaria hypothesis. Annals of Tropical Medicine and Parasitology. 1987;**81**(5):539-548. DOI: 10.1080/00034983.1987.11812155

[13] Weatherall DJ. Single gene disorders or complex traits: Lessons from the thalassaemias and other monogenic diseases. BMJ. 2000;**321**(7269):1117-1120. DOI: 10.1136/bmj.321.7269.1117

[14] Weatherall DJ. Thalassaemia and malaria, revisited. Annals of Tropical Medicine and Parasitology. 1997;**91**(7):885-890. DOI: 10.1080/00034983.1997.11813215

[15] Weatherall DJ. Genetic variation and susceptibility to infection: The red cell and malaria. British Journal of

Haematology. 2008;**141**(3):276-286. DOI: 10.1111/j.1365-2141.2008.07085.x

[16] Ilboudo Y et al. Genome-wide association study of erythrocyte density in sickle cell disease patients. Blood Cells, Molecules & Diseases. 2017;**65**:60-65. DOI: 10.1016/j.bcmd.2017.05.005

[17] Mohandas N, An X. Malaria and human red blood cells. Medical Microbiology & Immunology (Berl.). 2012;**201**(4):593-598. DOI: 10.1007/s00430-012-0272-z

[18] Tiffert T, Lew VL, Ginsburg H, Krugliak M, Croisille L, Mohandas N. The hydration state of human red blood cells and their susceptibility to invasion by *Plasmodium falciparum*. Blood. 2005;**105**(12):4853-4860. DOI: 10.1182/blood-2004-12-4948

[19] Lew VL, Bookchin RM. Ion transport pathology in the mechanism of sickle cell dehydration. Physiological Reviews. 2005;**85**(1):179-200. DOI: 10.1152/physrev.00052.2003

[20] Bunyaratvej A, Fucharoen S, Greenbaum A, Mohandas N. Hydration of red cells in alpha and beta thalassemias differs. A useful approach to distinguish between these red cell phenotypes. American Journal of Clinical Pathology. 1994;**102**(2):217-222. DOI: 10.1093/ajcp/102.2.217

[21] Tripette J et al. Effects of hydration and dehydration on blood rheology in sickle cell trait carriers during exercise. American Journal of Physiology-Heart and Circulatory Physiology. 2010;**299**(3):H908-H914. DOI: 10.1152/ajpheart.00298.2010

[22] Evans AG, Wellems TE. Coevolutionary genetics of plasmodium malaria parasites and their human Hosts1. Integrative and Comparative Biology. 2002;**42**(2):401-407. DOI: 10.1093/icb/42.2.401

[23] Trape J-F et al. The Dielmo project: A longitudinal study of natural malaria infection and the mechanisms of protective immunity in a community living in a holoendemic area of senegal. The American Journal of Tropical Medicine and Hygiene. 1994;**51**(2):123-137. DOI: 10.4269/ajtmh.1994.51.123

[24] Meis JF, Verhave JP, Jap PH, Meuwissen JH. An ultrastructural study on the role of Kupffer cells in the process of infection by *Plasmodium berghei* sporozoites in rats. Parasitology. 1983;**86**(Pt 2):231-242. DOI: 10.1017/s003118200005040x

[25] Prudêncio M, Rodriguez A, Mota MM. The silent path to thousands of merozoites: The Plasmodium liver stage. Nature Reviews. Microbiology. 2006;**4**(11):849-856. DOI: 10.1038/nrmicro1529

[26] Gerald N, Mahajan B, Kumar S. Mitosis in the human malaria parasite *Plasmodium falciparum*. Eukaryotic Cell. 2011;**10**(4):474-482. DOI: 10.1128/EC.00314-10

[27] Simon CS, Stürmer VS, Guizetti J. How many is enough?—Challenges of multinucleated cell division in malaria parasites. Frontiers in Cellular and Infection Microbiology. 2021;**11**:658616. Available from: https://www.frontiersin.org/articles/10.3389/fcimb.2021.658616 [Accessed: January 31, 2024]

[28] Bannister LH, Hopkins JM, Fowler RE, Krishna S, Mitchell GH. A brief illustrated guide to the ultrastructure of *Plasmodium falciparum* asexual blood stages. Parasitology Today (Personal Ed.). 2000;**16**(10):427-433. DOI: 10.1016/s0169-4758(00)01755-5

[29] Singh B, Daneshvar C. Human infections and detection of plasmodium knowlesi. Clinical Microbiology Reviews. 2013;**26**(2):165-184. DOI: 10.1128/CMR.00079-12

[30] Garnham PCC. Malaria Parasites and Other Haemosporidia. [Online]. 1966. Available from: https://www.cabdirect.org/cabdirect/abstract/19672901312. [Accessed: January 31, 2024]

[31] Dalapati T, Moore JM. Hemozoin: A complex molecule with complex activities. Current Clinical Microbiology Reports. 2021;**8**(2):87-102. DOI: 10.1007/s40588-021-00166-8

[32] Su X, Zhang C, Joy DA. Host-malaria parasite interactions and impacts on mutual evolution. Frontiers in Cellular and Infection Microbiology. 2020;**10**:587933. DOI: 10.3389/fcimb.2020.587933

[33] Kariuki SN, Williams TN. Human genetics and malaria resistance. Human Genetics. 2020;**139**(6-7):801-811. DOI: 10.1007/s00439-020-02142-6

[34] Cowman AF, Crabb BS. Invasion of red blood cells by malaria parasites. Cell. 2006;**124**(4):755-766. DOI: 10.1016/j.cell.2006.02.006

[35] Goel VK, Li X, Chen H, Liu S-C, Chishti AH, Oh SS. Band 3 is a host receptor binding merozoite surface protein 1 during the *Plasmodium falciparum* invasion of erythrocytes. Proceedings of the National Academy of Sciences of the United States of America. 2003;**100**(9):5164-5169. DOI: 10.1073/pnas.0834959100

[36] Kaestner L, Bogdanova A, Egee S. Calcium channels and calcium-regulated channels in human red blood cells. Advances in Experimental Medicine and Biology. 2020;**1131**:625-648. DOI: 10.1007/978-3-030-12457-1_25

[37] Jansen J et al. Mechanistic ion channel interactions in red cells of patients with Gárdos channelopathy. Blood Advances. 2021;**5**(17):3303-3308. DOI: 10.1182/bloodadvances.2020003823

[38] Rapetti-Mauss R et al. A mutation in the Gardos channel is associated with hereditary xerocytosis. Blood. 2015;**126**(11):1273-1280. DOI: 10.1182/blood-2015-04-642496

[39] Volkers L, Mechioukhi Y, Coste B. Piezo channels: From structure to function. Pflügers Archiv. 2015;**467**(1):95-99. DOI: 10.1007/s00424-014-1578-z

[40] Gottlieb PA, Sachs F. Piezo1: Properties of a cation selective mechanical channel. Channels Austin Tex. 2012;**6**(4):214-219. DOI: 10.4161/chan.21050

[41] Cahalan SM, Lukacs V, Ranade SS, Chien S, Bandell M, Patapoutian A. Piezo1 links mechanical forces to red blood cell volume. eLife. 2015;**4**:e07370. DOI: 10.7554/eLife.07370

[42] Bartolucci P et al. Erythrocyte density in sickle cell syndromes is associated with specific clinical manifestations and hemolysis. Blood. 2012;**120**(15):3136-3141. DOI: 10.1182/blood-2012-04-424184

[43] Bedu-Addo G, Meese S, Mockenhaupt FP. An ATP2B4 polymorphism protects against malaria in pregnancy. The Journal of Infectious Diseases. 2013;**207**(10):1600-1603. DOI: 10.1093/infdis/jit070

[44] Lessard S et al. An erythroid-specific ATP2B4 enhancer mediates red blood cell hydration and malaria susceptibility. The Journal of Clinical Investigation. 2017;**127**(8):3065-3074. DOI: 10.1172/JCI94378

[45] Ma S et al. Common PIEZO1 allele in African populations causes RBC dehydration and attenuates plasmodium infection. Cell. 2018;**173**(2):443-455.e12. DOI: 10.1016/j.cell.2018.02.047

[46] Tubman VN et al. The clinically tested Gardos channel inhibitor senicapoc exhibits antimalarial activity. Antimicrobial Agents and Chemotherapy. 2016;**60**(1):613-616. DOI: 10.1128/AAC.01668-15

[47] Cossins AR, Gibson JS. Volume-sensitive transport systems and volume homeostasis in vertebrate red blood cells. The Journal of Experimental Biology. 1997;**200**(2):343-352. DOI: 10.1242/jeb.200.2.343

[48] Okada Y. Ion channels and transporters involved in cell volume regulation and sensor mechanisms. Cell Biochemistry and Biophysics. 2004;**41**(2):233-258. DOI: 10.1385/CBB:41:2:233

[49] Leaf A. On the mechanism of fluid exchange of tissues in vitro. The Biochemical Journal. 1956;**62**(2):241-248. DOI: 10.1042/bj0620241

[50] Lang F et al. Functional significance of cell volume regulatory mechanisms. Physiological Reviews. 1998;**78**(1):247-306. DOI: 10.1152/physrev.1998.78.1.247

[51] Donnan FG. Theory of membrane equilibria and membrane potentials in the presence of non-dialysing electrolytes. A contribution to physical-chemical physiology. Journal of Membrane Science. 1995;**100**(1):45-55. DOI: 10.1016/0376-7388(94)00297-C

[52] Agre P. The aquaporin water channels. Proceedings of the American Thoracic Society. 2006;**3**(1):5. DOI: 10.1513/pats.200510-109JH

[53] Kong W, Yang S, Wang Y, Bendahmane M, Fu X. Genome-wide identification and characterization of aquaporin gene family in beta vulgaris. PeerJ. 2017;**5**:e3747. DOI: 10.7717/peerj.3747

[54] Nesverova V, Törnroth-Horsefield S. Phosphorylation-dependent regulation of mammalian aquaporins. Cells. 2019;**8**(2):82. DOI: 10.3390/cells8020082

[55] Scheuring S et al. High resolution AFM topographs of the Escherichia coli water channel aquaporin Z. The EMBO Journal. 1999;**18**(18):4981-4987. DOI: 10.1093/emboj/18.18.4981

[56] Preston GM, Carroll TP, Guggino WB, Agre P. Appearance of water channels in xenopus oocytes expressing red cell CHIP28 protein. Science. 1992;**256**(5055):385-387. DOI: 10.1126/science.256.5055.385

[57] Wagner K, Unger L, Salman MM, Kitchen P, Bill RM, Yool AJ. Signaling mechanisms and pharmacological modulators governing diverse aquaporin functions in human health and disease. International Journal of Molecular Sciences. 2022;**23**(3):1388. DOI: 10.3390/ijms23031388

[58] Smith BL, Preston GM, Spring FA, Anstee DJ, Agre P. Human red cell aquaporin CHIP. I. Molecular characterization of ABH and colton blood group antigens. The Journal of Clinical Investigation. 1994;**94**(3):1043-1049

[59] Svetina S. Theoretical bases for the role of red blood cell shape in the regulation of its volume. Frontiers in Physiology. 2020;**11**:544. DOI: 10.3389/fphys.2020.00544

[60] Hoffmann EK, Lambert IH, Pedersen SF. Physiology of cell volume regulation in vertebrates. Physiological Reviews. 2009;**89**(1):193-277. DOI: 10.1152/physrev.00037.2007

[61] Hoffmann EK, Simonsen LO. Membrane mechanisms in volume and pH regulation in vertebrate cells. Physiological Reviews. 1989;**69**(2):315-382. DOI: 10.1152/physrev.1989.69.2.315

[62] Okada Y. Volume expansion-sensing outward-rectifier Cl- channel: Fresh start to the molecular identity and volume sensor. The American Journal of Physiology. 1997;**273**(3 Pt 1):C755-C789. DOI: 10.1152/ajpcell.1997.273.3.C755

[63] Baumgarten CM, Feher JJ. 21—Osmosis and regulation of cell volume. In: Sperelakis N, editor. Cell Physiology Source Book. 13th ed. San Diego: Academic Press; 2001. pp. 319-355. DOI: 10.1016/B978-012656976-6/50113-X

[64] MacLeod RJ, Hamilton JR. Separate K+ and Cl- transport pathways are activated for regulatory volume decrease in jejunal villus cells. The American Journal of Physiology. 1991;**260**(3 Pt 1):G405-G415. DOI: 10.1152/ajpgi.1991.260.3.G405

[65] Brini M, Calì T, Ottolini D, Carafoli E. Intracellular calcium homeostasis and signaling. Metal Ions in Life Sciences. 2013;**12**:119-168. DOI: 10.1007/978-94-007-5561-1_5

[66] Maher AD, Kuchel PW. The Gárdos channel: A review of the Ca2+–activated K+ channel in human erythrocytes. The International Journal of Biochemistry & Cell Biology. 2003;**35**(8):1182-1197. DOI: 10.1016/s1357-2725(02)00310-2

[67] Lew VL, Tiffert T. On the mechanism of human red blood cell longevity: Roles of calcium, the sodium pump, PIEZO1, and Gardos channels. Frontiers in Physiology. 2017;**8**:977. DOI: 10.3389/fphys.2017.00977

[68] Kwiatkowski DP. How malaria has affected the human genome and what human genetics can teach us about malaria. American Journal of Human Genetics. 2005;**77**(2):171-192. DOI: 10.1086/432519

[69] Amuzu DS et al. High-throughput genotyping assays for identification of glycophorin B deletion variants in population studies. Experimental Biology and Medicine. 2021;**246**(8):916-928. DOI: 10.1177/1535370220968545

[70] Jaskiewicz E, Jodłowska M, Kaczmarek R, Zerka A. Erythrocyte glycophorins as receptors for Plasmodium merozoites. Parasites & Vectors. 2019;**12**(1):317. DOI: 10.1186/s13071-019-3575-8

[71] Cooling L. Blood groups in infection and host susceptibility. Clinical Microbiology Reviews. 2015;**28**(3):801-870. DOI: 10.1128/CMR.00109-14

[72] Anstee DJ. The nature and abundance of human red cell surface glycoproteins. Journal of Immunogenetics. 1990;**17**(4-5):219-225. DOI: 10.1111/j.1744-313x.1990.tb00875.x

[73] Pasvol G, Wainscoat JS, Weatherall DJ. Erythrocytes deficiency in glycophorin resist invasion by the malarial parasite *Plasmodium falciparum*. Nature. 1982;**297**(5861):64-66. DOI: 10.1038/297064a0

[74] Siebert PD, Fukuda M. Isolation and characterization of human glycophorin A cDNA clones by a synthetic oligonucleotide approach: Nucleotide sequence and mRNA structure. Proceedings of the National Academy of Sciences of the United States of America. 1986;**83**(6):1665-1669. DOI: 10.1073/pnas.83.6.1665

[75] Pasvol G, Wilson RJ. The interaction of malaria parasites with red blood cells. British Medical Bulletin.

1982;**38**(2):133-140. DOI: 10.1093/oxfordjournals.bmb.a071749

[76] Malaria Genomic Epidemiology Network, Band G, Rockett KA, Spencer CCA, Kwiatkowski DP. A novel locus of resistance to severe malaria in a region of ancient balancing selection. Nature. 2015;**526**(7572):253-257. DOI: 10.1038/nature15390

[77] Kariuki SN et al. Red blood cell tension protects against severe malaria in the Dantu blood group. Nature. 2020;**585**(7826):579-583. DOI: 10.1038/s41586-020-2726-6

[78] Reithmeier RAF, Casey JR, Kalli AC, Sansom MSP, Alguel Y, Iwata S. Band 3, the human red cell chloride/bicarbonate anion exchanger (AE1, SLC4A1), in a structural context. Biochimica et Biophysica Acta BBA - Biomembranes. 2016;**1858**(7, Part A):1507-1532. DOI: 10.1016/j.bbamem.2016.03.030

[79] Jarolim P et al. Deletion in erythrocyte band 3 gene in malaria-resistant Southeast Asian ovalocytosis. Proceedings of the National Academy of Sciences of the United States of America. 1991;**88**(24):11022-11026. DOI: 10.1073/pnas.88.24.11022

[80] Bruce LJ et al. A band 3-based macrocomplex of integral and peripheral proteins in the RBC membrane. Blood. 2003;**101**(10):4180-4188. DOI: 10.1182/blood-2002-09-2824

[81] Allen SJ et al. Prevention of cerebral malaria in children in Papua New Guinea by southeast Asian ovalocytosis band 3. The American Journal of Tropical Medicine and Hygiene. 1999;**60**(6):1056-1060. DOI: 10.4269/ajtmh.1999.60.1056

[82] Rosanas-Urgell A et al. Reduced risk of *Plasmodium vivax* malaria in Papua New Guinean children with Southeast Asian ovalocytosis in two cohorts and a case-control study. PLoS Medicine. 2012;**9**(9):e1001305. DOI: 10.1371/journal.pmed.1001305

[83] Kidson C, Lamont G, Saul A, Nurse GT. Ovalocytic erythrocytes from Melanesians are resistant to invasion by malaria parasites in culture. Proceedings of the National Academy of Sciences of the United States of America. 1981;**78**(9):5829-5832. DOI: 10.1073/pnas.78.9.5829

[84] Liu SC et al. Molecular defect of the band 3 protein in southeast Asian ovalocytosis. The New England Journal of Medicine. 1990;**323**(22):1530-1538. DOI: 10.1056/NEJM199011293232205

[85] Grimberg BT et al. *Plasmodium vivax* invasion of human erythrocytes inhibited by antibodies directed against the duffy binding protein. PLoS Medicine. 2007;**4**(12):e337. DOI: 10.1371/journal.pmed.0040337

[86] Hadley TJ, Peiper SC. From malaria to chemokine receptor: The emerging physiologic role of the duffy blood group antigen. Blood. 1997;**89**(9):3077-3091

[87] Lim KL, et al. The duffy binding protein (PkDBPαII) of plasmodium knowlesi from peninsular malaysia and malaysian borneo show different binding activity level to human erythrocytes. Malaria Journal. 11 Aug 2017;**16**(1):331. DOI: 10.1186/s12936-017-1984-8

[88] Hamblin MT, Di Rienzo A. Detection of the signature of natural selection in humans: Evidence from the duffy blood group locus. American Journal of Human Genetics. 2000;**66**(5):1669-1679. DOI: 10.1086/302879

[89] Howes RE et al. The global distribution of the duffy blood group.

Nature Communications. 2011;**2**:266. DOI: 10.1038/ncomms1265

[90] Horuk R, Chitnis CE, Darbonne WC, Colby TJ, Rybicki A, Hadley TJ, et al. A receptor for the malarial parasite *Plasmodium vivax*: The erythrocyte chemokine receptor. Science. 1993;**261**(5125). DOI: 10.1126/science.7689250

[91] Pogo AO, Chaudhuri A. Duffy and receptors for *P. vivax* and chemotactic peptides. Transfusion Clinique et Biologique, Journal Officiel de la Société Française de Transfusion Sanguine. 1995;**2**(4):269-276. DOI: 10.1016/s1246-7820(05)80093-x

[92] Araç D et al. A novel evolutionarily conserved domain of cell-adhesion GPCRs mediates autoproteolysis. The EMBO Journal. 2012;**31**(6):1364-1378. DOI: 10.1038/emboj.2012.26

[93] Kariuki SM et al. The genetic risk of acute seizures in African children with falciparum malaria. Epilepsia. 2013;**54**(6):990-1001. DOI: 10.1111/epi.12173

[94] Apinjoh TO et al. Association of candidate gene polymorphisms and TGF-beta/IL-10 levels with malaria in three regions of Cameroon: A case-control study. Malaria Journal. 2014;**13**:236. DOI: 10.1186/1475-2875-13-236

[95] Al-Quraishy S, Dkhil MA, Abdel-Baki AAS, Delic D, Santourlidis S, Wunderlich F. Genome-wide screening identifies plasmodium chabaudi-induced modifications of DNA methylation status of Tlr1 and Tlr6 gene promoters in liver, but not spleen, of female C57BL/6 mice. Parasitology Research. 2013;**112**(11):3757-3770. DOI: 10.1007/s00436-013-3565-2

[96] Krishnamurthy PC et al. Identification of a mammalian mitochondrial porphyrin transporter. Nature. 2006;**443**(7111):586-589. DOI: 10.1038/nature05125

[97] Helias V et al. ABCB6 is dispensable for erythropoiesis and specifies the new blood group system Langereis. Nature Genetics. 2012;**44**(2):170-173. DOI: 10.1038/ng.1069

[98] López C, Saravia C, Gomez A, Hoebeke J, Patarroyo MA. Mechanisms of genetically-based resistance to malaria. Gene. 2010;**467**(1-2):1-12. DOI: 10.1016/j.gene.2010.07.008

[99] PVIVAX | knowledge sharing for relapsing malaria. PVIVAX:. Available from [Online]. https://www.vivaxmalaria.org/. [Accessed: January 27, 2024]

[100] Roth EF, Raventos Suarez C, Rinaldi A, Nagel RL. The effect of X chromosome inactivation on the inhibition of *Plasmodium falciparum* malaria growth by glucose-6-phosphate-dehydrogenase-deficient red cells. Blood. 1983;**62**(4):866-868

[101] Ruwende C et al. Natural selection of hemi- and heterozygotes for G6PD deficiency in Africa by resistance to severe malaria. Nature. 1995;**376**(6537):246-249. DOI: 10.1038/376246a0

[102] Louicharoen C et al. Positively selected G6PD-Mahidol mutation reduces *Plasmodium vivax* density in Southeast Asians. Science. 2009;**326**(5959):1546-1549. DOI: 10.1126/science.1178849

[103] Kun JF, Mordmüller B, Lell B, Lehman LG, Luckner D, Kremsner PG. Polymorphism in promoter region of inducible nitric oxide synthase gene and protection against malaria. Lancet. 1998;**351**(9098):265-266. DOI: 10.1016/S0140-6736(05)78273-8

[104] Hobbs MR et al. A new NOS2 promoter polymorphism associated with increased nitric oxide production and protection from severe malaria in Tanzanian and Kenyan children. Lancet. 2002;**360**(9344):1468-1475. DOI: 10.1016/S0140-6736(02)11474-7

[105] Wierenga KJ, Hambleton IR, Lewis NA. Survival estimates for patients with homozygous sickle-cell disease in Jamaica: A clinic-based population study. Lancet. 2001;**357**(9257):680-683. DOI: 10.1016/s0140-6736(00)04132-5

[106] Flint J, Harding RM, Boyce AJ, Clegg JB. The population genetics of the haemoglobinopathies. Baillière's Clinical Haematology. 1998;**11**(1):1-51. DOI: 10.1016/s0950-3536(98)80069-3

[107] Ayi K, Turrini F, Piga A, Arese P. Enhanced phagocytosis of ring-parasitized mutant erythrocytes: A common mechanism that may explain protection against falciparum malaria in sickle trait and beta-thalassemia trait. Blood. 2004;**104**(10):3364-3371. DOI: 10.1182/blood-2003-11-3820

[108] Akide-Ndunge OB, Ayi K, Arese P. The Haldane malaria hypothesis: Facts, artifacts, and a prophecy. Redox Report Communications in Free Radical Research. 2003;**8**(5):311-316. DOI: 10.1179/135100003225002952

[109] Roberts DJ, Williams TN. Haemoglobinopathies and resistance to malaria. Redox Report Communications in Free Radical Research. 2003;**8**(5):304-310. DOI: 10.1179/135100003225002998

[110] Cabrera G, Cot M, Migot-Nabias F, Kremsner PG, Deloron P, Luty AJF. The sickle cell trait is associated with enhanced immunoglobulin G antibody responses to *Plasmodium falciparum* variant surface antigens. The Journal of Infectious Diseases. 2005;**191**(10):1631-1638. DOI: 10.1086/429832

[111] Agarwal A et al. Hemoglobin C associated with protection from severe malaria in the Dogon of Mali, a West African population with a low prevalence of hemoglobin S. Blood. 2000;**96**(7):2358-2363

[112] Ackerman H, Usen S, Jallow M, Sisay-Joof F, Pinder M, Kwiatkowski DP. A comparison of case-control and family-based association methods: The example of sickle-cell and malaria. Annals of Human Genetics. 2005;**69**(Pt 5):559-565. DOI: 10.1111/j.1529-8817.2005.00180.x

[113] Rihet P, Flori L, Tall F, Traore AS, Fumoux F. Hemoglobin C is associated with reduced *Plasmodium falciparum* parasitemia and low risk of mild malaria attack. Human Molecular Genetics. 2004;**13**(1):1-6. DOI: 10.1093/hmg/ddh002

[114] Fairhurst RM et al. Abnormal display of PfEMP-1 on erythrocytes carrying haemoglobin C may protect against malaria. Nature. 2005;**435**(7045):1117-1121. DOI: 10.1038/nature03631

[115] Coste B et al. Piezo1 and Piezo2 are essential components of distinct mechanically activated cation channels. Science. 2010;**330**(6000):55-60. DOI: 10.1126/science.1193270

[116] Zeng W-Z et al. PIEZOs mediate neuronal sensing of blood pressure and the baroreceptor reflex. Science. 2018;**362**(6413):464-467. DOI: 10.1126/science.aau6324

[117] Kim SE, Coste B, Chadha A, Cook B, Patapoutian A. The role of drosophila piezo in mechanical nociception. Nature. 2012;**483**(7388):209-212. DOI: 10.1038/nature10801

[118] Zarychanski R et al. Mutations in the mechanotransduction protein PIEZO1 are associated with hereditary xerocytosis. Blood. 2012;**120**(9):1908-1915. DOI: 10.1182/blood-2012-04-422253

[119] Albuisson J et al. Dehydrated hereditary stomatocytosis linked to gain-of-function mutations in mechanically activated PIEZO1 ion channels. Nature Communications. 2013;**4**:1884. DOI: 10.1038/ncomms2899

[120] Nguetse CN et al. A common polymorphism in the mechanosensitive ion channel PIEZO1 is associated with protection from severe malaria in humans. Proceedings of the National Academy of Sciences of the United States of America. 2020;**117**(16):9074-9081. DOI: 10.1073/pnas.1919843117

[121] Thye T et al. Human genetic variant E756del in the ion channel PIEZO1 not associated with protection from severe malaria in a large Ghanaian study. Journal of Human Genetics. 2022;**67**(1):65-67. DOI: 10.1038/s10038-021-00958-2

[122] Lohia R et al. Pharmacological activation of PIEZO1 in human red blood cells prevents *Plasmodium falciparum* invasion. Cellular and Molecular Life Science. 2023;**80**(5):124. DOI: 10.1007/s00018-023-04773-0

[123] Zámbó B et al. Decreased calcium pump expression in human erythrocytes is connected to a minor haplotype in the ATP2B4 gene. Cell Calcium. 2017;**65**:73-79. DOI: 10.1016/j.ceca.2017.02.001

[124] Ndila CM et al. Human candidate gene polymorphisms and risk of severe malaria in children in Kilifi, Kenya: A case-control association study. Lancet Haematology. 2018;**5**(8):e333-e345. DOI: 10.1016/S2352-3026(18)30107-8

[125] Uyoga S et al. The impact of malaria-protective red blood cell polymorphisms on parasite biomass in children with severe *Plasmodium falciparum* malaria. Nature Communications. 2022;**13**(1):3307. DOI: 10.1038/s41467-022-30990-5

[126] Joof F et al. Genetic variations in human ATP2B4 gene alter *Plasmodium falciparum* in vitro growth in RBCs from Gambian adults. Malaria Journal. 2023;**22**(1):5. DOI: 10.1186/s12936-022-04359-4

[127] Adjemout M et al. Concurrent PIEZO1 activation and ATP2B4 blockade effectively reduce the risk of cerebral malaria and inhibit in vitro *Plasmodium falciparum* multiplication in red blood cells. Genes & Diseases. 2023;**10**(6):2210-2214. DOI: 10.1016/j.gendis.2023.02.029

[128] Gallagher PG. Disorders of red cell volume regulation. Current Opinion in Hematology. 2013;**20**(3):201-207. DOI: 10.1097/MOH.0b013e32835f6870